AF249144

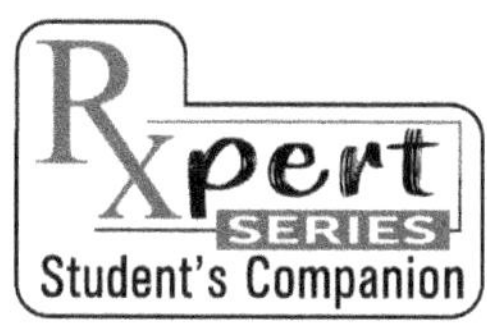

Pharmaceutical Chemistry
Theory and Practical

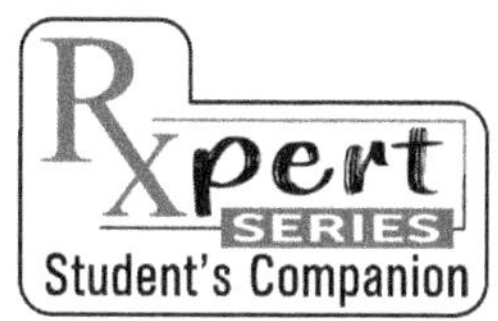

Pharmaceutical Chemistry
Theory and Practical

Prof. (Dr.) G. D. Gupta

Director-cum-Principal
ISF College of Pharmacy (An Autonomous College)
MOGA - 142 001 (Punjab)

Dr. Vivek Asati

Associate Professor
Department of Pharmaceutical Chemistry
ISF College of Pharmacy (An Autonomous College)
MOGA - 142 001 (Punjab)

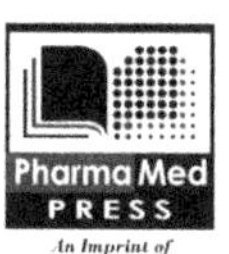

PharmaMed Press

An imprint of BSP Books Pvt. Ltd.
4-4-309/316, Giriraj Lane,
Sultan Bazar, Hyderabad - 500 095.

Pharmaceutical Chemistry: Theory and Practical
by G.D. Gupta and Vivek Asati

Published by

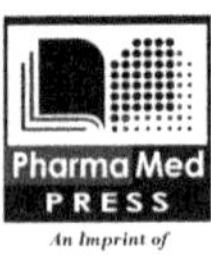

PharmaMed Press

An imprint of BSP Books Pvt. Ltd.
4-4-309/316, Giriraj Lane, Sultan Bazar, Hyderabad - 500 095.
Phone: 040-23445688; Fax: 91+40-23445611
E-mail: info@pharmamedpress.net
www.bspbooks.net/www.pharmamedpress.net

ISBN: 978-93-95039-11-6 (Hardback)

Preface

Pharmaceutical education and research have been growing quickly over the last decade. This book is a culmination of very honest and sincere efforts, keeping in view the level and aspirations of pharmacy students at the undergraduate level, in accordance with the new syllabus of the Pharmacy Council of India.

The concepts of this book include simple language with suitable descriptive figures, flow charts, the students will also discover the real pleasure of extra information through the questions in the last of each chapter. All efforts have been made to make the book student friendly.

This book is designed to impart basic knowledge on the chemical structure, storage conditions and medicinal uses of organic and inorganic chemical substances used in drugs and pharmaceuticals. Also, this book includes a description of impurities, quality control aspects of chemical substances used in pharmaceuticals.

Many observations out of our own long years of classroom experience regarding the difficulties of students have been kept in mind while presenting the subject matter. The following aspects of the chemical substances are considered such as chemical classification, chemical name, chemical structure, pharmacological uses, doses, stability and storage conditions of different types of formulations/dosage form available and their brand names.

We have tried to make things simpler and easily understandable to students, for whom this book has been written. We hope that this book will be helpful to teachers and students and help resolve both aspects as well as practical.

During this project, we have received full support and kind cooperation from the publishers of the book, who had set certain minimum standards for everyone involved. We are really thankful to them as well as their efficient staff, including the computer team, for putting in a lot of hard work with commitment and purpose.

We are also grateful to the learned authors whose works we have studied or consulted often. Despite efforts and care, there might still be a few mistakes or errors, which are understandable in a work of this magnitude. Esteemed teachers are requested to bear with us for the time being and send your valuable suggestions for strengthening this book.

Prof. (Dr.) G. D. Gupta
Dr. Vivek Asati

Contents

CHAPTER 1

Introduction to Pharmaceutical Chemistry

Introduction to Pharmaceutical Chemistry

Pharmaceutical chemistry is concerned with the drug design and synthesis of biologically active molecules/compound. The aim is to gain new chemical molecules that could enable the discovery of new pharmaceuticals or optimize already known drug structures, thereby to expand the portfolio of chemical drugs. It includes design and production of compounds that can be used for the prevention, treatment or cure of human and animal diseases. Medicinal chemistry includes the study of already existing drugs, of their biological properties and their structure-activity relationships. Pharmaceutical chemistry also includes other branches of study such as pharmacokinetics, pharmacodynamics, and drug metabolism.

Scope of Pharmaceutical Chemistry

Pharmaceutical Chemistry includes about the processes of drug development and distribution. The pharmaceutical industry is expanding day by day with the growth of medical fields worldwide. The pharmaceutical industry encompasses a wide and varied range of specialties, but one consistent element is the role of chemistry in each part of the pharmaceutical sciences. In the following areas, opportunities pertaining to pharmaceutical chemistry prevail:

(i) **Organic Chemistry:** Organic chemistry plays an important role in the pharmaceutical industry whereby knowledge of organic compounds is used to the discovery and development of new medicines.

(ii) **Computational Chemistry:** Computational chemistry is a specialty that contributes to the design of drugs as well as the drug discovery process by helping to design and study molecular structures and chemical compounds that are used as the foundation of new medicines.

(iii) Analytical Chemistry: Analytical chemistry includes pharmaceutical quality assurance and quality control ensuring the safety, stability, and efficacy of drugs and medicines. There is also a strong connection between analytic chemistry and high-performance liquid chromatography (HPLC), one of the most important analytical procedures in the drug development process. Their ability to perform complex analytical processes coupled with the skill set of managing hands-on testing.

(iv) Miscellaneous: The demand for drugs and medicines is increasing with advancements in discoveries, treatments and increasing illnesses. With the latest technologies and trends, the opportunities are also increasing with each passing year in the following areas related to pharmaceutical chemistry:

- Pharmaceutical Industry or factories
- Research Centers
- Laboratories for testing and analytical techniques
- Manufacturing industries
- Food industries
- Product marketing agencies
- Health Centers
- Clinics
- Drug Control Administration
- Medical Stores
- Colleges and Universities

Objective of Pharmaceutical Chemistry

(i) In pharmaceutical chemistry, the chemist attempts to design and synthesize a medicine or a pharmaceutical agent which will benefit humanity. Such a compound could also be called a 'drug'.

(ii) Pharmaceutical chemistry is concerned with the design (drug design) and synthesis of biologically active molecules.

(iii) The aim is to gain new chemical molecules that could enable the discovery of new pharmaceuticals or optimize already known drug structures. Although organic chemistry plays a crucial role and interact with other disciplines, such as molecular biology, structural biology, pharmacology, physical chemistry, biochemistry, pharmacokinetics, pharmaceutical technology, toxicology or with experts from the field of translational medicine, etc.

(iv) To study the relationship between the chemical structure and biological activity of a molecule (structure-activity relationships, SAR) in a quantitative sense (quantitative SAR, QSAR).

(v) Apart from the small synthetic ligands and natural products, pharmaceutical chemistry also focus on the development of modified peptides and proteins, biological agents (e.g. monoclonal antibodies), multifunctional molecular complexes and synthetic vaccines.

Sources and Types of Errors

Error refers to the difference in the standard values and the true value. Errors may be broadly divided into two categories, namely:

1. **Determinate (Systematic) Errors** - These are errors that possess a definite value with a reasonable cause and these avoidable errors may be measured and accounted for rectification. The most important errors belonging to this particular class are:

   (a) **Personal Errors:** They are exclusively caused due to 'personal equation' of an analyst and do not due to either on the prescribed procedure or methodology involved.

   (b) **Instrumental Errors:** These are invariably caused due to faulty and uncalibrated instruments, such as: pH meters, UV-spectrophotometers, potentiometers etc.

   (c) **Reagent Errors:** The errors that are solely introduced by virtue of the individual reagents, for instance, impurities inherently present in reagents; high temperature volatilization of platinum (Pt); unwanted introduction of 'foreign substances' caused by the action of reagents on either porcelain or glass apparatus.

   (d) **Constant Errors:** They are observed to be rather independent of the magnitude of the measured amount; and turn out to be relatively less significant as the magnitude enhances. Example: error of 0.10 ml is introduced in a series of titrations, hence for a specific titration needing only 10.0 ml of titrant shall represent a relative error of 1% and only 0.2% for a corresponding 50 ml of titrant consumed.

   (e) **Proportional Errors:** The absolute value of this kind of error changes with the size of the sample in such a fashion that the relative error remains constant. It is usually incorporated by a material that directly interferes in an analytical procedure.

   (f) **Errors due to Methodology:** Both improper (incorrect) sampling and incompleteness of a reaction often lead to serious errors. A few typical examples invariably encountered in titrimetric and gravimetric analysis.

(g) Additive Errors: It has been observed that the additive errors are independent of the quantum of the substances actually present in the assay.

2. **Indeterminate (Random) Errors** - As the name suggests, indeterminate errors cannot be pin-pointed to any specific well-defined reasons. These errors are mostly random in nature and ultimately give rise to high as well as low results with equal probability. They can neither be corrected nor eliminated, and therefore, form the 'ultimate limitation' on the specific measurements.

1. Repeated measurement of the same variable several times and subsequent refinement to the extent where it is simply a coincidence if the corresponding replicates eventually agree to the last digit.
2. Both unpredictable and imperceptible factors are unavoidably incorporated in the results what generally appear to be 'random fluctuations' in the measured quantity.
3. Recognition of specific definite variables which are beyond anyone's control lying very close to the performance limit of an instrument, such as: temperature variations, noise as well as drift from an electronic circuit, and vibrations caused to a building by heavy vehicular-traffic.

Sources of Error

Common sources of error include instrumental, environmental, procedural, handling of equipment and human. All of these errors can be either random or systematic depending on how they affect the results.

Errors are mainly two types random and systematic.

- **Random error** occurs due to chance. There is always some variability when a measurement is made. Random error may be caused by slight fluctuations in an instrument, the environment, or the way a measurement is read, that do not cause the same error every time.
- **Systematic error** gives measurements that are consistently different from the true value in nature, often due to limitations of either the instruments or the procedure. Systematic error is one form of bias. Bias is often caused by instruments that consistently offset the measured value from the true value.
- **Instrumental error** happens when the instruments being used are inaccurate, such as a balance that does not work. A pH meter that reads 0.5 off or a calculator that rounds incorrectly would be sources of instrument error.
- **Environmental error** happens when some factor in the environment, such as an uncommon event, leads to error. For example, if you are trying to measure

the mass of an apple on a scale, and your classroom is windy, the wind may cause the scale to read incorrectly.

- **Procedural error** occurs when different procedures are used to answer the same question and provide slightly different answers. If two people are rounding, and one rounds down and the other rounds up, this is procedural error.
- **Human error** is due to carelessness or to the limitations of human ability. Two types of human error are transcriptional error and estimation error.

Steps to Reduce the Errors

Systematic errors may be reduced substantially and significantly by adopting one of the following procedures rigidly, such as:

(i) **Calibration of Instruments, Apparatus and Applying Necessary Corrections:** Most of the instruments, commonly used in an analytical laboratory, such as: UV-Spectrophotometer, IR-Spectrophotometer, single pan electric balance, pH-meter, turbidimeter and nephelometer, polarimeter, refractometer and the like must be calibrated duly, before use so as to eliminate any possible errors. In the same manner all apparatus, namely: pipettes, burettes, volumetric flasks, thermometers, weights etc., must be calibrated duly, and the necessary corrections incorporated to the original measurements.

(ii) **Performing a Parallel Control Determination:** It essentially comprises of performing an altogether separate estimation under almost identical experimental parameters that consists of exactly the same weight of the component as is present in the unknown sample.

(iii) **Blank Determination:** It may be accomplished by performing a separate parallel estimation, without using the sample at all, and under identical experimental parameters as employed in the actual analysis of the given sample

(iv) **Cross-checking Results by Different Methods of Analysis:** In certain specific cases the accuracy of a result may be cross-checked by performing another analysis of the same substance by an altogether radically different method.

Accuracy

The accuracy represents the proximity between the standard reference and the observed value during analysis. The ability of the instrument to measure the accurate value is known as accuracy. In other words, the closeness of the measured value to a standard or true value. Accuracy is obtained by taking small readings. The small reading reduces the error of the calculation. The accuracy of the system is classified into three types as follows:

- **Point Accuracy:** The accuracy of the instrument only at a particular point on its scale is known as point accuracy.
- **Accuracy as Percentage of Scale Range:** The uniform scale range determines the accuracy of a measurement. This can be better understood with the help of the following example: Consider a thermometer having the scale range up to 500°C. The thermometer has an accuracy of ±0.5, i.e. ±0.5 percent of increase or decrease in the value of the instrument is negligible. But if the reading is more or less than 0.5°C, it is considered a high-value error.
- **Accuracy as Percentage of True Value:** Such type of accuracy of the instruments is determined by identifying the measured value regarding their true value. The accuracy of the instruments is neglected up to ± 0.5 percent from the true value.

Precision

The precision is the closeness of results obtained from analysis of the same sample repetitively.

The closeness of two or more measurements to each other is known as the precision of a substance. If you weigh a given substance five times and get 3.2 kg each time, then your measurement is very precise but not necessarily accurate. Precision is independent of accuracy. The below example will tell you about how you can be precise but not accurate and vice versa. Precision is sometimes separated into:

- **Repeatability:** The variation arising when the conditions are kept identical and repeated measurements are taken during a short time period.
- **Reproducibility:** The variation arises using the same measurement process among different instruments and operators, and over longer time periods.

Significant Figures

Significant figures (also known as the significant digits, precision or resolution) of a number in positional notation are digits in the number that are reliable and absolutely necessary to indicate the quantity of something.

If a number expressing the result of measurement of something (e.g., length, pressure, volume, or mass) has more digits than the digits allowed by the measurement resolution, only the digits allowed by the measurement resolution are reliable so only these can be significant figures.

Of the significant figures in a number, the most significant is the digit with the highest exponent value (simply the left-most significant figure), and the least significant is the digit with the lowest exponent value (simply the right-most significant figure).

Impurities in Pharmaceuticals

Impurity is a substance which is not part of the drug or medicinal substance. It is foreign substance present in the formulation other than the drug. Chemical purity means freedom from foreign matter (Impurity). The substance used in pharmaceutical field should be almost pure so that they can be used safely. It is rather difficult to obtain an almost pure substance. We find substances and chemicals with varying degree of purity because the purity of substance depends upon several factors such as their method of manufacture, type of recrystallisation or purification process.

In the pharmaceutical field, one deals with a large number of drugs, chemicals or other substance which are used in formulations. All such materials need to be pure. However, it is almost impossible to get an absolutely pure material as impurities gets incorporated into them either during manufacture, purification or storage.

Test for purity: The pharmacopoeias prescribe test for purity for substance in order to ensure their reasonable freedom from the undesirable impurities. Test for purity is in fact tests for detecting the presence of impurities and they fix the limits of tolerance for these impurities. The test for purity does not have the aim of ensuring freedom of substance from every possible impurity.

The following certain tests are carried out on the substances.

(i) **Odour and Colour:** These test are employed only when other test for purity are not applicable. Therefore, these tests have limited importance. These tests are valuable to know whether the substance is reasonably aesthetic and hygienic or not.

(ii) **Physical Constants:** Melting point, boiling point, refractive index. Optical rotation is the reliable physical constants. The determination of physical constants ensure whether the substance are reasonably free from other substances. This test fails to indicate the nature of the impurity.

(iii) **Humidity/Moisture Content:** The amount of moisture content in medicinal substance is determined to estimate the content of water of recrystallisation if present in the compound. It give idea about storage condition of certain drugs like ergot, digitalis.

(iv) **Insoluble Constituents:** The compound which is soluble in water gives a turbid solution if soluble matter is present. The turbidity is due to insoluble material or constituents present in the watersoluble compound. The measurement of turbidity or opalescence helps to indicate the extent of insoluble constituents present as an impurity in the compound.

(v) Organic impurities: These may be from raw material or intermediate products or by products in reaction. Therefore, for some of these objectionable organic impurities the tests are prescribed in official books.

(vi) Acidity and Alkalinity: Excess of acidity and alkalinity has effect on keeping qualities of the compounds as well as the compounds with which they may be mixed.

(vii) Anions: Acids like H_2SO_4 and HCl are widely used in the manufacture of medicinal substances. Therefore, the chloride and sulphate ions are commonly present as impurity in many of the medicinal substance. Hence test for anions like Cl^-, $SO4^{2-}$ is prescribed in official books.

(viii) Cations: Tests for cation include for sodium, potassium ammonium radical and for heavy metal like iron, lead, copper etc. These impurities are toxic in nature and controlled by performing the limit test for Lead and Arsenic.

(ix) Ash: Residue remaining after incineration is the ash content of the drugs, which represents the inorganic salts naturally occuring in the drugs. Determination of ash value is performed to have the idea about content of foreign cations and heavy metals. In organic compounds, the alkali salts are generally present as impurities. In such a case the determination of ash value is preferable. It is also useful to judge the identity or purity of crude drugs.

(x) Loss on Drying (LoD): In this test, absorbed water or water of hydration is determined by drying under specified conditions. Loss in weight due to drying also represents the residual volatile constituents including organic solvents as well as water.

(xi) Loss on Ignition (LoI): This type of test is applied to stable substances which are liable to contain thermolabile impurities. This is applied to two classes of substances,

- Those which are completely volatile when ignited and
- Those which undergo a major decomposition leaving a resistance of definite composition.

Effect of impurities: The impurities present in the pharmaceutical substance may,
- Have toxic effect if present beyond the limits.
- Change the physical and chemical properties of the drug making it unsuitable for medicinal use.
- Be incompatible with other substance.
- Lower the shelf life of the substance.
- Cause technical difficulties in the formulation.
- Cause change in colour, taste, odour etc. making the substance unhygienic.

Types of impurities: Following types of impurities are commonly present in the pharmaceutical substance or preparations.

(i)   The impurities which produce toxic effect on body, if present beyond the prescribed limit e.g. Lead and Arsenic impurities.

(ii) Impurities which are harmless but if present beyond the limit in pharmaceutical substances, lower the active strength of that substance e.g. Impurities of sodium salts in potassium salts.

(iii) Impurities which, if present beyond the limit affect the storage property of the pharmaceuticals e.g. presence of moisture beyond the limit, may loose the free flowing property of substance or may decompose the substance.

(iv) Impurities causing technical difficulties while using the substance in which it is present e.g. presence of carbonate impurity in ammonia solution.

(v)   Impurities such as taste, odour, colour or appearance which are easily detectable by the senses and make the substance unaesthetic or unhygienic. e.g. phenolic impurities present in sodium salicylate alters its odour.

Traces of magnesium salts in sodium chloride renders it damp and changing its appearance.

Factors to be considered while fixing the limit of impurities:

(i)   Use of the substance for which the limit of impurities is to be fixed.

(ii) Minimum quantities of impurities likely to be harmful or to cause undesirable results in dispensing in keeping qualities.

(iii) Practicability of getting the particular limit or particular standard of quality.

(iv) Harmfulness of impurity.

Sources of Impurities

1. **Raw Materials:** If the impurities are present in the raw material, it may come in the final product through the manufacturing processes. e.g. Sodium chloride prepared from rock salt contains traces of calcium and magnesium compounds & Zinc oxide prepared from zinc metal may contain traces of copper, magnesium, nickel, iron and arsenic.

2. **Methods used in manufacture:** There are different number of methods available to manufacture. Some impurities may come into final product during manufacturing processes. So, to avoid impurities, suitable manufacturing process should be adopted.

3. **Intermediate Product:** The intermediate product may come along the process in the final product as impurities. e.g. In the preparation of potassium iodide from potassium hydroxide and iodine, potassium iodate is an intermediate product which is sometimes found in the final product.

4. **Material of the plant:** The vessels used in the manufacturing process are generally made up of metals like iron, copper, zinc, nickel, aluminium, steel etc. Due to solvent action on the material of the plant the traces of metals as a impurities may come in the product. For example, water pipe may contain lead which may accompany the final product.

5. **Impurities in atmosphere:** The atmospheric contaminants like dust, arsenic, carbon dioxide, water vapours etc. may contaminate the substances which are affected by their action.

6. **Adulteration:** Some pharmaceutical products may be adulterated with cheaper substances. e.g. Potassium bromide may be adulterated with sodium bromide. Therefore, it is advisable to purchase drugs from reputed manufacturer.

7. **Defective storage of final products (Adequate storage):** If there is improper storage of pharmaceutical products, same may undergo chemical decomposition. e.g. Iodine react with cork, rubber and some metals therefore it should be stored in glass bottles fitted with glass stoppers & Potassium hydroxide absorbs CO_2 on exposure to air and has effect on lead glass. Therefore, it should be stored in stoppered green glass bottle which is lead free.

8. **Solvent:** Water is mainly used as a solvent in various pharmaceutical product. Water contains various ions like calcium, magnesium, chloride etc. These impurities come along with water in the final product.

9. **Reagents used in the manufacturing:** If the reagents are impure, the impurity may come in the final product. If sulphuric acid is prepared by lead chamber process it contains traces of lead which may come in the final product as an impurity.

10. **Reagents used to remove impurities:** Potassium bromide is used to remove excess of sulphate, but potassium bromide may contain traces of barium which may contaminate the product.

Limit Test

Limit test are quantitative or semi-quantitative tests designed to identify and control small quantities of impurities which are likely to be present in pharmaceutical substance. These limit tests involve simple comparison of opalescence, turbidity or colour with standards prescribed in pharmacopoeias. The standard for opalescence, colour, turbidity is fixed.

In the limit tests, the extent of turbidity, opalescence or colour produced is influenced by the presence of other impurities present in the substance and also by the variations in time and method of performance of the tests and hence, the pharmacopoeias don't prescribe numerical values for the limit tests.

Thus, the limit tests are performed to know whether the impurities in the substance are below the limit or beyond the limit.

Tolerable Limit: It is the value upto which the impurity is accepted and is permissible in the pharmaceutical preparation or substance.

Limit Test for Chloride

Principle: It is based on the reaction between silver nitrate and soluble chloride resulting in formation of opalescence of silver chloride insoluble in dilute nitric acid.

$$Cl + AgNO_3 \xrightarrow{\text{dil. HNO}_3} AgCl \downarrow + NO_3$$

The extent of opalescence formed depends upon the amount of silver chloride formed and therefore, on the amount of chloride impurity present in the substance under test. The opalescence produced by a given amount of the substance is compared with the standard opalescence produced by adding silver nitrate into a standard solution. If the opalescence from the sample is less than the standard opalescence the sample passes the limit test and vice versa.

The principle according to I.P. 1985 is similar to that I.P. 66. But in I.P. 1985, in the preparation of standard opalescence instead of 0.01 N HCl, the use of 0.05845% w/v solution of sodium chloride is recommended.

Procedure

(i) **For test solution:** Prepare solution of given sample as directed in I.P. and transfer it in Nessler's cylinder. Add to it 10 ml of dilute HNO_3. Dilute to 50 ml with water. Add 1 ml of 5% silver nitrate solution and stir immediately and allow to stand for five minutes.

(ii) **For standard solution:** Take 1ml of 0.05845% w/v solution of sodium chloride by pipette in Nessler's cylinder. Add 10 ml of dilute Nitric acid in it. Dilute to 50 ml with water. Add 1ml of 5% silver nitrate solution. Stir immediately with a glass rod and allow to stand for five minutes.

Procedure for Test solution of Potassium permanganate as per IP 1996:

(a) Weigh accurately 1.5 gm of potassium permanganate and transfer it to 250 ml conical flask.

(b) Add 50 ml of distilled water, heat in water bath.

(c) Add gradually 6ml of 95% ethanol and cool.

(d) Dilute to 60 ml with distilled water and filter, the filtrate is colourless.

(e) Take 40 ml of above filtrate in a labelled Nessler's Cylinder (T).

(f) Add 10 ml of dilute HNO_3.

(g) Add 1 ml of 0.1 M silver nitrate solution.

(h) Stir immediately with glass rod and allow to stand for 5 minutes, protect from light.

(i) View transversely against a black background.

(j) Compare the opalescence produced with that of standard solution.

Modification Done (For coloured substance) e.g. KMnO₄: Since the $KMnO_4$ is violet colour substance. Its original violet colour modifies the opalescence, colour, turbidity produced in the test. Therefore, such compounds are decolorized first and then used in the test. The solution of $KMnO_4$ is first decolorized by boiling with alcohol and filtering the coloured matter, manganese dioxide is produced.

Limit Test for Sulphate

Principle: Limit test for sulphate is based on the reaction between barium chloride and soluble sulphates in the presence of dilute hydrochloric acid.

$$SO_4 + BaCl_2 \xrightarrow{\text{dil. HCl}} BaSO_4 \downarrow + 2Cl^-$$

The turbidity produced by given amount of substance is due to the precipitation of $BaSO_4$ which is compared with that produced standard solution. In I.P. 1985 instead of Barium chloride solution Barium sulphate reagent (B.S.R.) is used.

B.S.R. Contains:

- **Barium Chloride solution:** It act as seeding agent for the precipitation of barium sulphate if the given sample contains sulphate ions.
- **Sulphate free alcohol:** Prevents supersaturation and helps to form uniform turbidity.
- **Potassium Sulphate:** Increases the sensitivity of the test.

The ionic concentration of BSR is adjusted such that the solubility products of barium sulphate exceed. In sulphate limit test I.P. 1985, in the preparation of standard turbidity instead of 0.01N, H_2SO_4, the use of 0.1089% w/v solution of potassium sulphate is recommended.

Procedure (I.P. 1985):

Test Solution: Prepare solution of the given substance as directed in I.P. 85 and transfer it in Nessler's cylinder. Add to it 2 ml of dil. HCl. Dilute to 45 ml with water and add 5 ml of barium sulphate reagent (B.S.R.). Stir immediately and allow to stand for five minutes.

Standard Solution: Take 1ml of 0.1089 % w/v solution of potassium sulphate in Nessler's cylinder. Add to it 2 ml dilute hydrochloric acid. Dilute it to 45 ml with water. Add 5 ml of Barium Sulphate reagent. Stir immediately and allow to stand for five minutes. Compare turbidity produced by test solution with that of standard solution.

Procedure for Sulphate limit test I.P. 96: To 1.0 ml of a 2.5% w/v solution of barium chloride in Nessler's cylinder add 1.5 ml of ethanolic sulphate standard solution (10 ppm SO_4) mix and allow to stand for 1 minute. Add 15 ml of the solution prepared as directed in the individual monograph or a solution of specified quantity of the substance being examined in 15 ml of water and 0.15 ml of 5M acetic acid. Add sufficient water to produce 50 ml, stir immediately with glass rod and allow to stand for 5 minutes. When viewed transversely against black background only, opalescence produced is more intense than that obtained by treating in the same manner 15 ml of sulphate standard solution (10 ppm SO_4) in place of solution being examined.

Note: The solution used for this test should be prepared with distilled water.

Limit Test of Iron

Principle: It is based upon the reaction of iron with thioglycollic acid, in ammonical solution in presence of citric acid, to produce pale pink to deep reddish purple colour. The colour produced is due to formation of ferrous compound, ferrous thioglycollate which is stable in absence of air but fades in air due to oxidation. The purple colour is developed only in alkaline medium so ammonia solutions are used. But ammonia reacts with iron forming precipitate, citric acid prevents precipitate of iron with ammonia by forming a complex with it.

Fe^{3+} (ferric) form is reduced to (ferrous) Fe^{2+}.

$$2HSCH_2COOH + Fe^{2+} \longrightarrow Fe(SHCH_2COO)^-_2 + 2H^+$$

OR

$$\begin{array}{ccc} CH_2\,SH & & O\,CO \\ | & \diagdown\diagup & | \\ | & Fe & | \\ COO & \diagup\diagdown & HS\,CH_2 \end{array}$$

(Ferrous thioglycollate complex)

Preparation of standard solution of Iron:

As per I.P. 1996: (Iron standard solution 20 ppm Fe)

Dilute 1 volume of a 0.1726 % w/v solution of ferric ammonium sulphate in 0.05m sulphuric acid to 10 volumes with water contain iron in ferric state.

Procedure:

Test solution: Dissolve the specified weight of substance in 40 ml water or prepare a solution as per I.P. Add 2 ml of 20% w/v solution of Iron free citric acid in water and

2 drops of thioglycollic acid, mix, make alkaline with iron free solution of ammonia, dilute to 50 ml with water and allow to stand for 5 minutes.

Standard solution: Dilute 2 ml of standard solution of iron with 40 ml of water, add 2 ml of 20% w/v solution of iron free citric acid in water and drops of thioglycollic acid, mix make it alkaline with iron free solution of ammonia, dilute to 20 ml with water and allow to stand for five minutes. If the colour produced by test solution is less than that of standard, the sample passes the limit test for iron and vice versa.

Limit Test for Heavy Metal: The I.P. 1985 describes three methods for limit test for Heavy metals.

Method A:

For colourless substance:

Principle: The test is based on the reaction between hydrogen sulphide and certain heavy metals (such as lead, copper, nickel, cobalt, bismuth) leading to the formation of sulphides of respective metals in the presence of dilute acetic acid.

$$\text{Heavy Metals} + H_2S \xrightarrow[\text{Acid}]{\text{Acetic}} \text{Sulphides of Heavy metal} + 2H^+$$

Acetic acid is added to maintain pH 3 to 4. Therefore the sulphide formed are distributed in colloidal state and produce brownish coloured solution.

Procedure:

Test: Place 25 ml of solution prepared according to I.P. in 50 ml Nessler's cylinders. Adjust with dilute acetic acid or ammonia to a pH between 3 to 4, dilute with distilled water to 35 ml and mix. Add 10 ml of freshly prepared saturated solution of hydrogen sulphide. Dilute to 50 ml with distilled water. Stir with glass rod and allow it to stand for 5 min.

Standard: Place 2 ml of standard lead solution in a 50 ml Nessler's cylinder and dilute to 25 ml with distilled water. Adjust with dilute acetic acid or ammonia to a pH between 3-4. Dilute with distilled water to 35 ml and mix.

Add 10 ml of freshly prepared saturated solution of hydrogen sulphide. Dilute to 50 ml with distilled water. Stir with glass rod and allow it to stand for 5 min.

Compare the colour of sample and standard.

Method B: For coloured substance:

It is similar to method A, only difference is test (sample) is given special treatment (with sulphuric acid, ignition nitric acid, ignition HCl and finally digestion with water etc.) to make it colourless before preparing its solution.

Method C: Used for substance which forms clear colourless solution with NaOH.

Principle: It is based on the reaction of heavy metals with sodium sulphide in an alkaline medium leading to formation of heavy metal sulphides.

$$\text{Heavy metals} + Na_2S \xrightarrow[\text{medium}]{\text{alkaline}} \text{Sulphide of heavy metals}$$

Procedure:

Test: Take 25 ml sample solution prepared as per IP in Nessler's cylinder. Add 5 ml of dilute NaOH solution. Dilute to 50 ml with distilled water. Add 5 drops of sodium sulphide solution.

Stir with glass rod and allow it to stand for 5 min.

Standard: Take 2 ml of standard lead solution in a Nessler's cylinder and dilute it with distilled water to 25 ml. Add 5 ml of dilute sodium hydroxide solution. Dilute to 50 ml with distilled water. Add 5 drops of sodium sulphide solution. Stir with glass rod and allow it to stand for 5 minute. Compare the colour of sample and standard.

Limit test for Lead: As per I.P. and USP it, is based upon the reaction between lead and diphenylthio-carbazone (Dithizone). Dithizone in chloroform, extracts lead from alkaline aqueous solution and lead Dithizone complex. (Red Colour).

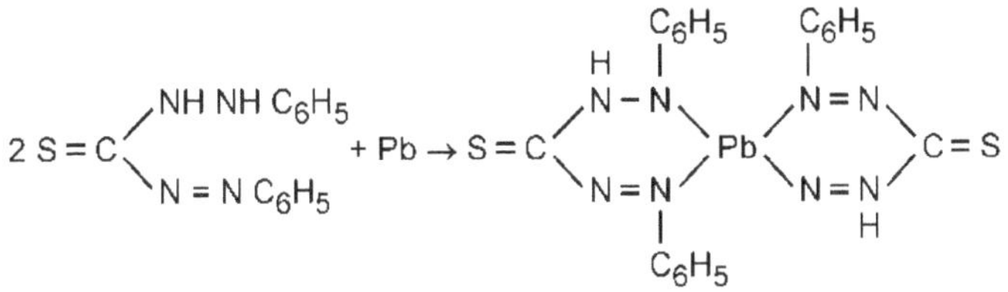

$$2\,S{=}C\underset{N=N\,C_6H_5}{\overset{NH\ NH\ C_6H_5}{{<}}} + Pb \rightarrow S{=}C \cdots Pb \cdots C{=}S$$

The original dithizone has green colour in chloroform thus the lead-dithizone shows a violet colour. The intensity of colour of complex depends upon the amount of lead in solution. The colour of lead dithizone complex in chloroform is compared with a standard volume of lead solution, treated in same manner.

Importance of Potassium Cyanide: The interference and influence of other metal ions etc. is eliminated by adjusting the optimum pH for the extraction by using ammonium nitrate, potassium cyanide, hydroxylamine hydrochloride reagents etc.

P.P.M. (Parts Per Million): It may be defined as the number of parts by weight of a impurity present in one million parts by weight of substance under test.

Limit Test for Arsenic:

Principle and Reactions: It is based upon the conversion of arsenic if present in the sample to the arsine gas with the help of reducing agents. First of all the arsenic present is converted to Arsenic acid in acidic medium.

$$As^{5+} \xrightarrow[\text{medium}]{\text{Acidic}} H_3AsO_4 \quad \text{Arsenic acid}$$

The arsenic acid is then reduced to Arsenious acid with the help of reducing agents.

$$H_3AsO_4 \xrightarrow[\text{KI}]{\text{SnCl}_2} H_3AsO_3 \quad \text{Arsenious Acid}$$

The arsenious acid is further reduced to arsine gas by Nascent hydrogen (which is produced by zinc and hydrochloric acid)

$$H_3AsO_3 + \underset{\substack{\text{Nascent} \\ \text{Hydrogen}}}{6[H]} \xrightarrow[\text{HCl}]{\text{Zn}} \underset{\text{Arsine gas}}{AsH_3 + 3H_2}$$

The arsine gas produced reacts with mercuric chloride paper to produce a yellow stain of mercuric arsenide.

$$\underset{\substack{\text{Arsine} \\ \text{gas}}}{2\,AsH_3} + \underset{\substack{\text{Mercuric} \\ \text{chloride}}}{HgCl_2} \longrightarrow Hg \underset{\substack{\text{Mercuric} \\ \text{arsenide}}}{\overset{AsH_2}{\underset{AsH_2}{<}}} + 2\,HCl$$

The stain produced by sample is compared with stain produced by standard.

Use of Reagents:
- HCl and Zn produce Nascent hydrogens.
- Potassium iodide reduces pentavalent arsenic to trivalent.
- Stannous chloride gives complete evolution of Arsine gas.
- Lead acetate cotton plug prevent the formation of black stain to mercuric chloride paper produced by sulphide impurities which are present in zinc.
- It also trap the impurities evolved along with Arsine gas.
- Granulated zinc helps in steady and prolong evolution of nascent hydrogen.

Procedure:
- Test (sample): Take 50 ml of distilled water in the bottle of arsenic test apparatus.
- Add 2.5 gm of ammonium chloride sample to this.
- Add 10 ml of stannated HCl acid.
- Add 1 gm of stannated KI.
- Add 10 mg of granulated zinc.
- Allow the reaction to proceed for 40 minutes.

Standard:

- Take 50 ml of distilled water in the bottle of another arsenic test apparatus.
- Add 1 ml of dilute arsenic solution to this.
- Add 10 ml stannated HCl acid.
- Add 1 gm of KI.
- Add 10 mg of granulated zinc.
- Allow the reaction to proceed for 40 minutes.
- The apparatus used to perform the limit test of Arsenic is called as GUTZEIT Apparatus.
- It consist of wide mouth glass bottle having capacity of 120 ml and mouth diameter 2.5 cm.
- The mouth of bottle is fitted with rubber bung through which passes a glass tube of length 200 mm, having internal diameter 6.5 mm and outer diameter 8 mm. The lower end of tube is constricted to about 1mm and have a hole not less than 2 mm in diameter to provide alternate passage for arsine gas.
- The other end of glass tube is cut smooth and carries rubber bungs. (25 × 25mm).

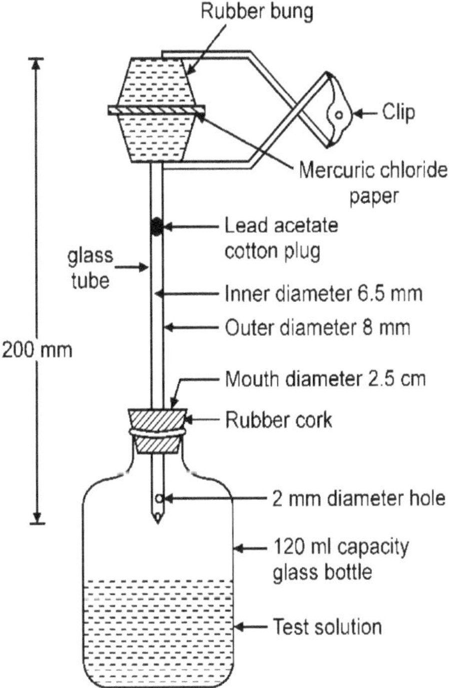

Fig. 1.1 GUTZEIT apparatus

- Mercuric chloride paper is sandwitched between the rubber bungs. The rubber bungs are held in place by means of clip.
- The borings of the two bungs meet to form a true tube of 6.5 mm diameter by a diaphragm of mercuric chloride paper.
- A cotton wool moistened with lead acetate solution and dried, is kept in glass tube.
- When the reaction starts, the arsine gas is formed which goes upward through glass tube. The impurities present with arsine gas are trapped by lead acetate cotton plug. The arsine gas passes through lead acetate cotton plug and reacts with mercuric chloride paper to form yellow stain.

Points to Remember

- Error refers to the difference in the standard values and the true value.
- Common sources of error include instrumental, environmental, procedural, and human.
- The accuracy represents the proximity between the standard reference and the observed value during analysis.
- The precision is the closeness of results obtained from analysis of the same sample repetitively.
- Impurity is a substance which is not part of the drug or medicinal substance. It is foreign substance present in the formulation other than the drug.
- Limit test are quantitative or semi-quantitative tests designed to identify and control small quantities of impurities which are likely to be present in pharmaceutical substance.
- Limit test of chloride is based on the reaction between silver nitrate and soluble chloride resulting in formation of opalescence of silver chloride insoluble in dilute nitric acid.
- Limit test for sulphate is based on the reaction between barium chloride and soluble sulphates in the presence of dilute hydrochloric acid.
- Limit test for iron is based upon the reaction of iron with thioglycollic acid, in ammonical solution in presence of citric acid, to produce pale pink to deep reddish purple colour.
- Limit test for heavy metals is based on the reaction between hydrogen sulphide and certain heavy metals (such as lead, copper, nickel, cobalt, bismuth) leading to the formation of sulphides of respective metals in the presence of dilute acetic acid.
- Limit test for lead is based upon the reaction between lead and diphenylthio-carbazone (Dithizone). Dithizone in chloroform, extracts lead from alkaline aqueous solution and lead Dithizone complex.

- Limit test for arsenic based upon the conversion of arsenic if present in the sample to the arsine gas with the help of reducing agents.
- Pharmaceutical Chemistry is the most important branch of Pharmaceutical Sciences. It includes everything about the processes of drug development and distribution.

Multiple Choice Questions

1. The limit test for heavy metals does not include the following:
    (A) Lead
    (B) Copper
    (C) Nickel
    (D) Selenium

2. Lead discovery is responsible under which sub-area of pharmaceutical chemistry?
    (A) Analytical Chemistry
    (B) Organic Chemistry
    (C) Computational Chemistry
    (D) None of these

3. Which is not a source of impurities?
    (A) Finished Goods
    (B) Raw Mater0069als
    (C) Intermediate Product
    (D) Methods used in manufacture

4. The limit test for lead is based upon the reaction between lead and which component?
    (A) Silver nitrate
    (B) Dithizone
    (C) Sodium thioglycollate
    (D) Arsine

5. Which is not a component in the limit test of arsenic?
    (A) Stannated HCl acid
    (B) Stannated KI
    (C) Citric acid
    (D) Granulated zinc

6. Which is not a type of error?
    (A) Instrumental
    (B) Environmental
    (C) Chemical
    (D) Human

7. The apparatus used to perform the limit test of Arsenic is called
    (A) Gutzeit Apparatus
    (B) Clevenger's Apparatus
    (C) Soxhelet Apparatus
    (D) Franz Apparatus

8. Ferrous thioglycolate complex is formed in which limit test?
    (A) Iron
    (B) Lead
    (C) Arsenic
    (D) Chloride

9. Which is not a key subject of pharmaceutical chemistry?
   - (A) Analytical Chemistry
   - (B) Computational Chemistry
   - (C) Organic Chemistry
   - (D) Explosive Chemistry

10. The area where pharmaceutical chemistry professionals are not have desired scope
    - (A) Food industries
    - (B) Printing
    - (C) Health Centers
    - (D) Product marketing agencies

11. Impurities in pharmaceutical products come from different sources like
    - (A) Raw material
    - (B) Manufacturing process
    - (C) Chemical instability
    - (D) All of the above

12. In limit test for sulphates, which acid in diluted form is used?
    - (A) Sulfuric acid
    - (B) Hydrochloric acid
    - (C) Nitric acid
    - (D) Perchloric acid

13. When iron reacts with thioglycollic acid in the presence of citric acid, what color appears?
    - (A) Pale pink to deep reddish purple
    - (B) Orange to Red
    - (C) Blue to Black
    - (D) Green to Violet

14. What is the role of citric acid in the limit test of iron?
    - (A) Helps enhancing solubility
    - (B) Helps precipitation of iron
    - (C) Helps reducing turbidity
    - (D) All of these

15. In limit test for chlorides, which acid in diluted form is used?
    - (A) Sulfuric acid
    - (B) Hydrochloric acid
    - (C) Nitric acid
    - (D) Perchloric acid

16. Limit tests are performed in
    - (A) Flask
    - (B) Test tube
    - (C) Measuring cylinder
    - (D) All of these

17. In limit test for heavy metals, which acid in diluted form is used?
    - (A) Acetic acid
    - (B) Hydrochloric acid
    - (C) Nitric acid
    - (D) Perchloric acid

18. Citric acid forms a soluble complex with iron and prevents its precipitation by ammonia as
    - (A) Ferrous hydroxide
    - (B) Ferrous chloride
    - (C) Ferrous sulphate
    - (D) Ferrous nitrate

19. In limit test for heavy metals, the reaction between the heavy metals occurs with
  (A) Thioglycollic acid
  (C) Hydrogen sulphides
  (B) Citric acid
  (D) None of them

20. If the opalescence in the sample is less than the standard in limit test for chloride, what does it indicate?
  (A) Sample passed
  (C) Sample reaction occurs
  (B) Sample failed
  (D) No conclusion

CHAPTER 2
Volumetric Analysis

Introduction

The chapter specifically focuses on: Fundamental concept of volumetric analysis, Basics aspects of Acid-base titrations; Basics aspects of Non-aqueous titrations; Basics aspects of Precipitation titration; Basics aspects of Complexometric titration; Basics aspects of Redox titration; and Basics aspects of Gravimetric analysis.

Volumetric Analysis

Volumetric analysis is a widely used method for quantitative analysis of unknown solutions. As the name suggests, this method involves measurement of the volume of a solution whose concentration is known and applied to determine the concentration of the analyte.

In other words, measuring the volume of a second substance that combines with the first in known proportions is known as Volumetric analysis or titration. It is the method of quantitative analysis that allows us to determine the concentration of the analyte.

Procedure for Volumetric Analysis

The procedure can be understood from underline points:

1. A typical titration starts with a beaker or flask containing a precise volume of the analyte and small amount of indicator placed underneath a calibrated burette or pipette containing the titrant.
2. The solution that needs to be analyzed needs to have an accurate weighed in the sample of +/- 0.0001g of the material to be analyzed.
3. Choosing the right kind of material to be analyzed is also very important, as choosing the wrong type of titrant will give us the wrong results. A substance that reacts rapidly and completely to produce a complete solution is chosen.

4. Small quantities of titrant are added to the analyte and indicator till the indicator changes colour in reaction at the endpoint of the titration.
5. The titration has to be continued up until the reaction is complete and the amount of reactant added is exactly the amount that is needed to complete the reaction.
6. Another important step is in measuring the right volume of the standard solution since molarity is a standard metric to calculate the number of moles present in a solution.
7. Based on the desired endpoint, single drops or less than a drop of the titrant makes a difference between a permanent and temporary change in the indicator.
8. If the reagent or reactant that we use is to be made into a standard solution then we can weigh and dissolve the reagent into a solution, so that it is in a definitive volume within a volumetric flask

Basic concept of Volumetric analysis:

The concept can be understood from following points:
1. The solution to be analyzed contains an unknown amount of chemicals.
2. The reagent of unknown concentration reacts with a chemical of an unknown amount in the presence of an indicator (mostly phenolphthalein) to show the end-point. It's the point indicating the completion of the reaction.
3. The volumes are measured by titration which completes the reaction between the solution and reagent.
4. The volume and concentration of reagent which are used in the titration show the amount of reagent and solution.
5. The amount of unknown chemical in the specific volume of solution is determined by the mole fraction of the equation.

When the endpoint of the reaction is reached, the volume of reactant consumed is measured and applied to carry volumetric analysis calculations of the analyte by the following formula,

$$C_a = C_t\, V_t\, M\, /\, V_a$$

Where,

C_a is the analyte concentration, typically in molarity.

C_t is the titrant concentration, typically in molarity.

V_t is the volume of the titrant which is used, typically in liters.

M is the mole ratio of the analyte and reactant from the balanced equation.

V_a is the volume of the analyte, typically in liters.

Many non-acid-base titrations are needed a constant pH throughout the reaction. Therefore, a buffer solution can be added to the titration chamber to maintain the pH value.

Acid-Base titration: An acid-base titration is an experimental technique used to acquire information about a solution containing an acid or base. An acid-base titration involves strong or weak acids or bases. Specifically, an acid-base titration can be used to figure out the following.

1. The concentration of an acid or base
2. Whether an unknown acid or base is strong or weak.
3. pK_a of an unknown acid or pK_b of the unknown base.

Let us consider acid-base reaction which is proceeding with a proton acceptor. In water, the proton is usually solvated as H_3O^+. H_2O is added to the base to lose (OH^-) or gain (H_3O^+). Acid-base reactions are reversible.

The reactions are shown below.

$$HA + H_2O \rightarrow H_3O^+ + A^- \text{ (acid)}$$

$$B^- + H_2O \rightarrow BH + OH^- \text{ (base)}$$

Here $[A^-]$ is the conjugate base, H^+B is conjugate acid. Thus we say

$$\text{Acid + Base} \leftrightharpoons \text{Conjugate base + Conjugate acid}$$

Hence

$$K_A = \frac{[H_3O]^- [A]^-}{[HA]\,[H_2O]}$$

$$K_B = \frac{[HB]^- [OH]^-}{[B]^-}$$

$$K_W = \frac{[H]^+ [OH]^-}{[H_2O]}$$

It is possible to give an expression for $[H^+]$ in terms of K_A, K_R and K_w for a combination of various types of strong and weak acids or bases.

Terminologies associated in Acid-Base titration:

1. Titration – A process where a solution of known strength is added to a certain volume of a treated sample containing an indicator.
2. Titrant – A solution of known strength of concentration used in the titration.
3. Titrand – The titrand is any solution to which the titrant is added and which contains the ion or species being determined.

4. Titration curve – A plot of pH Vs millilitres of titrant showing the manner in which pH changes Vs millilitres of titrant during an acid-base titration.
5. Equivalence point – The point at which just adequate reagent is added to react completely with a substance.
6. Buffer solution – A solution that resists changes in pH even when a strong acid or base is added or when it is diluted with water.

Types of Acid-Base Titration?

Broadly, there are 4 types of Acid-Base Titration:

1. Strong acid-strong base: Hydrochloric acid and sodium hydroxide
2. Weak acid-strong base: Ethanoic acid and sodium hydroxide
3. Strong acid-weak base: Hydrochloric acid and ammonia
4. Weak acid-weak base: Ethanoic and ammonia

Titration Curve & Equivalence Point

In a titration, the equivalence point is the point at which exactly the same number of moles of hydroxide ions has been added as there are moles of hydrogen ions. In a titration, if the base is added from the burette and the acid has been accurately measured into a flask. The shape of each titration curve is typical for the type of acid-base titration.

The pH does not change in a regular manner as the acid is added. Each curve has horizontal sections where a lot of bases can be added without changing the pH much. There is also a very steep portion of each curve except for weak acid and the weak base where a single drop of base changes the pH by several units. There is a large change of pH at the equivalence point.

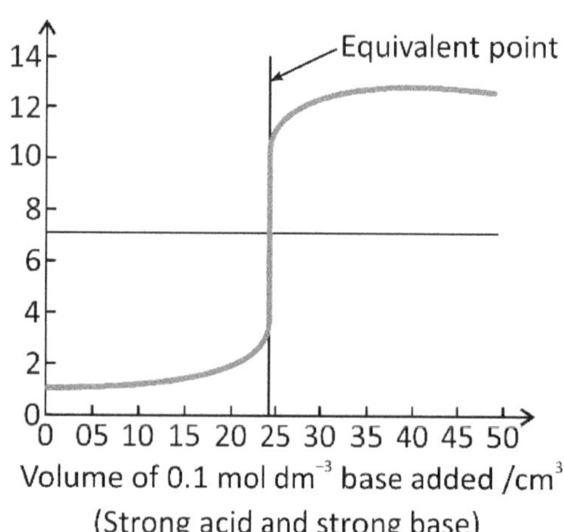

Volume of 0.1 mol dm^{-3} base added /cm^3
(Strong acid and strong base)

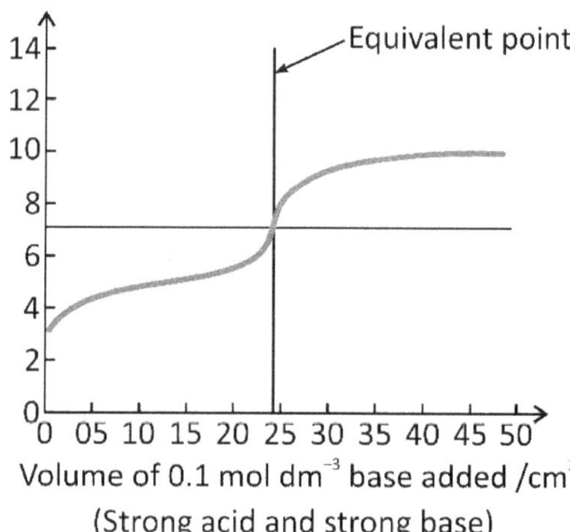

Volume of 0.1 mol dm^{-3} base added /cm^3
(Strong acid and strong base)

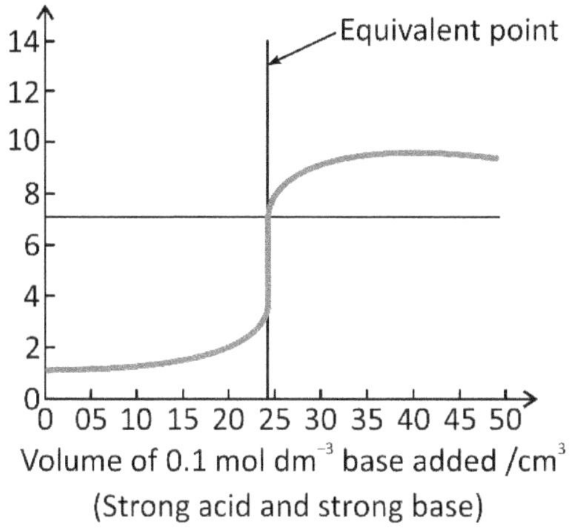

Volume of 0.1 mol dm^{-3} base added /cm^3
(Strong acid and strong base)

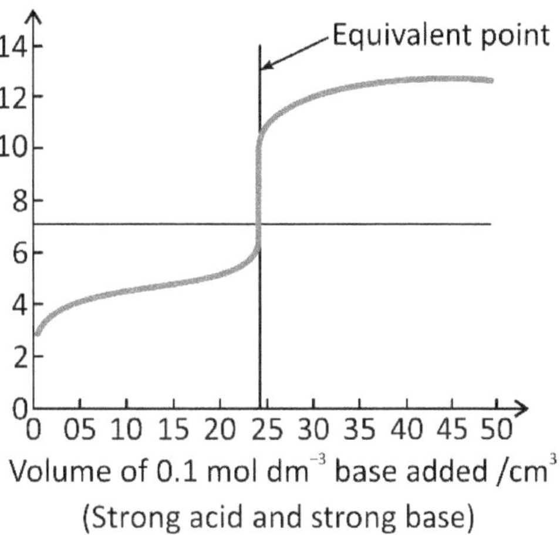

Volume of 0.1 mol dm^{-3} base added /cm^3
(Strong acid and strong base)

Acid-Base indicators

Acid-base indicators are substances which change color or develop turbidity at a certain pH. They locate equivalence point and also measure pH. They are themselves acids or bases are soluble, stable and show strong color changes. They are organic in nature.

A resonance of electron isomerism is responsible for color change. Various indicators have different ionization constants and therefore they show a change in color at different pH intervals.

Acid-base indicators can be broadly classified into three groups.

- The phthaleins and sulphophthaleins (e.g., Phenolphthalein)
- Azo indicators (e.g., Methyl orange)
- Triphenylmethane indicators (e.g., Malachite green)

The two common indicators used in acid-base titration are Phenolphthalein and methyl orange. In the four types of acid-base titrations, the base is being added to the acid in each case. A graph is shown below where pH against the volume of base added is considered. The pH range over which the two indicators change color. The indicator must change within the vertical portion of the pH curve.

The Choice of indicators based on the type of titration:

Strong acid-strong base: Phenolphthalein is usually preferred because of its more easily seen color change.

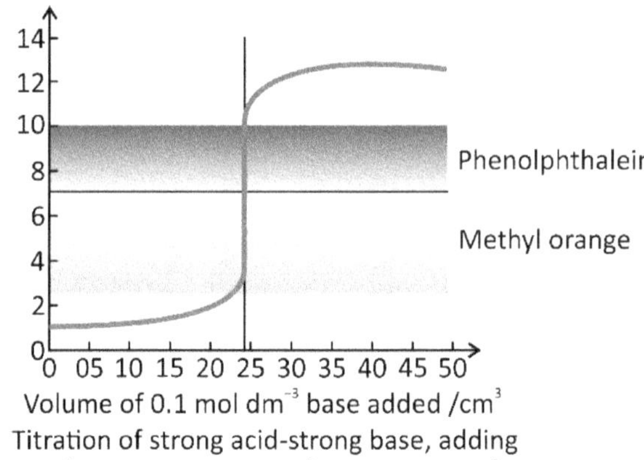

Volume of 0.1 mol dm^{-3} base added /cm^3
Titration of strong acid-strong base, adding
0.1 mol dm^{-3} NaOH(aq) to 25 cm^3 of 0.1 mol dm^{-3} HCL (aq)
(Strong acid and strong base)

Weak acid-strong base: Phenolphthalein is used and change sharply at the equivalence point and would be a good choice.

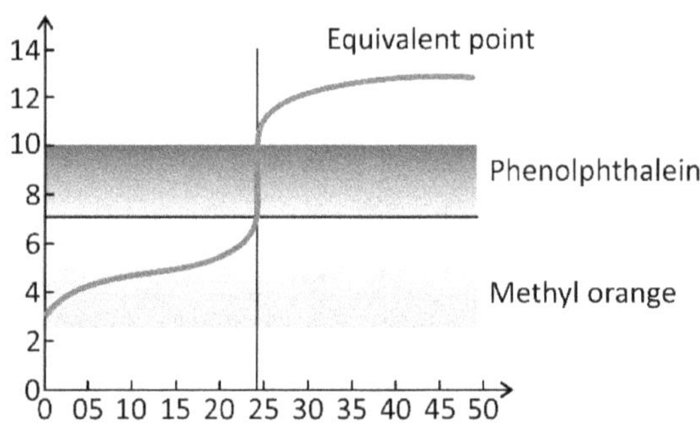

Volume of 0.1 mol dm^{-3} base added /cm^3
Titration of strong acid-strong base, adding
0.1 mol dm^{-3} NaOH(aq) to 25 cm^3 of 0.1 mol dm^{-3} CH$_2$CO$_2$(aq)
(Weak acid and strong base)

Strong acid-weak base: Methyl orange will change sharply at the equivalence point.

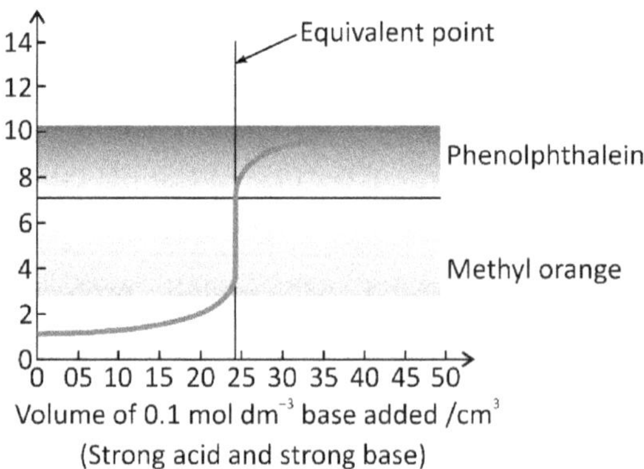

Volume of 0.1 mol dm^{-3} base added /cm^3
(Strong acid and strong base)

Weak acid-weak base: Neither phenolphthalein, not methyl orange is suitable. No indicator is suitable because it requires a vertical portion of the curve over two pH units.

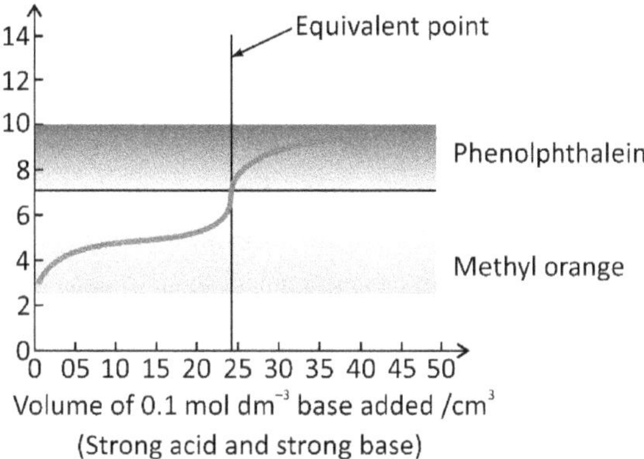

Volume of 0.1 mol dm^{-3} base added /cm^3

(Strong acid and strong base)

Non-aqueous titration: Non-aqueous titration refers to a type of titration in which the analyte substance is dissolved in a solvent which does not contain water. This procedure is a very important one in pharmacopoeial assays. The need for non-aqueous titration arises because water can behave as a weak base and a weak acid as well, and can hence compete in proton acceptance or proton donation with other weak acids and bases dissolved in it. The procedure of non-aqueous titration is very useful because it satisfies two different requirements, namely – suitable titration of very weak acids or bases along with providing a solvent with an ability to dissolve organic compounds.

An example of a reaction in which water is not a suitable solvent is the reaction given by:

$$\textbf{R-NH}_2 + \textbf{H}^+ \rightleftharpoons \textbf{R-NH}_3{}^+$$

which is competed with in an aqueous solvent by the reaction given by:

$$\textbf{H}_2\textbf{O} + \textbf{H}^+ \rightleftharpoons \textbf{H}_3\textbf{O}^+$$

This type of competition provided by water towards weak bases or weak acids makes it difficult to detect the end point of the titration. Therefore, these substances which have very sharp end points when titrated in aqueous solutions due to their weakly basic or weakly acidic nature generally need to be titrated in non-aqueous solvents.

Many reactions which occur in non-aqueous titration procedures can be explained via the Bronsted-Lowry Theory and its definition of acids and bases. Basically, acids can be thought of as proton donors, whereas bases can be thought of as proton acceptors.

It can also be noted that potentially acidic substances can behave as acids only when a base (to which a proton can be donated) is present. The reverse of this statement also true, i.e. potentially basic substances can behave as bases only when an acid (from which a proton can be accepted) is present.

Generally, four types of solvents used in the non-aqueous titration of a given analyte. These are:

1. **Aprotic Solvents** – these solvents are neutral in charge and are chemically inert. They also generally have a low dielectric constant. Examples of these types of solvents include chloroform and benzene.

2. **Protophilic Solvents** – these solvents have a basic character and tend to react with the acids they come in contact with, leading to the formation of solvated protons. Examples of protophilic solvents are ammonia and pyridine.

3. **Protogenic Solvents** – these solvents have a more acidic character and tend to have a levelling effect on the bases they come in contact with. Examples of protogenic solvents used in non-aqueous titration are sulphuric acid and acetic acid.

4. **Amphiprotic Solvents** – these solvents have properties which are protophilic as well as protogenic. Examples of these types of solvents are acetic acid and alcohols.

Thus, the solvents typically used in non-aqueous titrations are described above. The end points of these titrations can also be accurately measured using potentiometric titration procedures.

Titrant for non-aqueous titrations:

Perchloric acid in acetic acid: Amines, amine salts, amino acids, salts of acids

Potassium Methoxide in Toluene-Methanol

Quaternary ammonium hydroxide in Acetonitrilepyridine pyridine, acids, enols, imides & sulphonamides.

Precipitation titration: Precipitation titration is a type of titration which involves the formation of precipitate during the titration technique. In precipitation titration, the titrant reacts with analyte and forms an insoluble substance called precipitate. It continues till the last amount of analyte is consumed. It is used to determine chloride by using silver ions.

The principle of precipitation titration can be shown as follows:

Quantity of added precipitating reagent = quantity of substance being precipitated.

A precipitation titration curve follows the change in either the analyte's or the titrant's concentration as a function of the titrant's volume. As we have done with other titrations, we will show how to calculate the titration curve.

Let's calculate the titration curve for the titration of 50 mL of 0.05 M NaCl with 0.1 M AgNO$_3$. The reaction in this case is

$$Ag^+ (aq) + Cl^- (aq) \rightleftharpoons AgCl(s)$$

Argentometry is derived from a Latin word Argentum which means silver. The most widely applicable precipitation titrations involve the use of silver nitrate with chlorides, bromides, iodides, and thiocyanate. Since silver is always there, precipitation titrations are referred to as Argentometric titrations. According to end point detection method, three main procedures are widely used depending on the type of application. These are:

Mohr's Method: This method utilizes chromate as an indicator. Chromate forms a precipitate with Ag^+ but this precipitate has a greater solubility than that of AgCl, for example. Therefore, AgCl is formed first and after all Cl⁻ is consumed, the first drop of Ag^+ in excess will react with the chromate indicator giving a reddish precipitate.

In this method, neutral medium should be used since, in alkaline solutions pH > 10, silver will react with the hydroxide ions forming AgOH. In acidic solutions, chromate will be converted to $HCrO_4^-$ and the end point is delayed. In other words, silver chromate solubility grows due to the protonation of chromate anions. Therefore, the pH of solution should be kept at about 7. There is always some error in this method because a dilute chromate solution is used due to the intense color of the indicator. This will require additional amount of Ag^+ for the Ag_2CrO_4 to form. This leads to a late equivalent point. To correct for this error, we can determine a blank.

Volhard's Method: This is an indirect method used for determining the anions that precipitate with silver; *e.g.* Cl⁻, Br⁻, and I⁻. For example, an excess amount of standard Ag^+ is added to the chloride unknown solution containing Fe^{3+} as an indicator.

$$Ag^+ + Cl^- \leftrightarrow \textbf{white precipitate of AgCl}$$

The excess Ag+ is then titrated with standard SCN solution

$$Ag^+ + SCN^- \leftrightarrow \textbf{white precipitate of AgSCN}$$

until a reddish color due to $Fe(SCN)^{2+}$ complex formation is obtained which results from the reaction:

$$Fe^{3+} + SCN^- = \textbf{reddish complex Fe (SCN)}^{2+}$$

The indicator system is very sensitive and usually good results are obtained. The medium should be acidic to avoid the formation of Fe (OH)$_3$.

If AgX is less soluble than AgSCN as in the case of I⁻ and Br⁻, the excess Ag^+ can be titrated in the presence of AgX precipitate. But in the case of AgCl when SCN^- is added just after the equivalent point the following reaction will take place:

$$AgCl + SCN^- \leftrightarrow AgSCN + Cl^-$$

This means that SCN instead of reacting with the indicator it will react with the AgCl precipitate. We have two ways to overcome this problem.

The first includes addition of some organic solvent which is heavier and immiscible with water such as nitrobenzene or chloroform, which covers the AgCl precipitate in the bottom of conical flask and shields it from the aqueous medium which contains the excess Ag^+ that can be titrated with SCN^-. The second procedure involves filtration of the precipitate directly after precipitation, which protects the precipitate from coming in contact with the added SCN solution and titrating the excess Ag^+ in the filtrate.

Advantages of Volhard's Method

1. The acidic environment give advantage for halide analysis because anions such as carbonate, oxalate and arsenate that do not form precipitate with silver in acidic medium (but they do in basic medium) will not interfere with halides.
2. Give accurate results due to back titration.

Limitations of Volhard's Method

1. Cannot be used in neutral or basic medium.
2. Time consuming.

Fajan's Method: Fluorescein and its derivatives are adsorbed to the surface of colloidal AgCl. After all chloride is used, the first drop of Ag^+ will react with fluorescein (FI⁻) forming a reddish color.

$$Ag+ + Fl^- = AgF$$

Since fluorescein and its derivatives are weak acids, the pH of the solution should be slightly alkaline to keep the indicator in the anion form but, at the same time, is not alkaline enough to convert Ag^+ into AgOH. Fluorescein derivatives that are stronger acids than fluorescien (like eosin) can be used at acidic pH without problems. This method is simple and results obtained are reproducible.

In the Fajans method for Cl⁻ using Ag^+ as a titrant, for example, the anionic dye dichlorofluoroscein is added to the analyst's solution. Before the end point, the precipitate of AgCl has a negative surface charge due to the adsorption of excess Cl⁻. Because dichlorofluoroscein also carries a negative charge, it is repelled by the precipitate and remains in solution where it has a greenish yellow color. After the end point, the surface of the precipitate carries a positive surface charge due to the adsorption of excess Ag^+. Dichlorofluoroscein now adsorbs to the precipitate's surface where its color is pink. This change in the indicator's color signals the end point.

Complexometric titration: Complexometric titration (sometimes chelatometry) is a form of volumetric analysis in which the formation of a colored complex is used to indicate the end point of a titration. Complexometric titrations are particularly useful for the determination of a mixture of different metal ions in solution. An indicator capable of producing an unambiguous color change is usually used to detect the end-point of the titration.

In theory, any complexation reaction can be used as a volumetric technique provided that:

1. The reaction reaches equilibrium rapidly after each portion of titrant is added.
2. Interfering situations do not arise. For instance, the stepwise formation of several different complexes of the metal ion with the titrant, resulting in the presence of more than one complex in solution during the titration process.
3. A complexometric indicator capable of locating equivalence point with fair accuracy is available.

In practice, the use of EDTA as a titrant is well established.

EDTA, ethylenediaminetetraacetic acid, has four carboxyl groups and two amine groups that can act as electron pair donors, or Lewis bases. The ability of EDTA to potentially donate its six lone pairs of electrons for the formation of coordinate covalent bonds to metal cations makes EDTA a hexadentate ligand. However, in practice EDTA is usually only partially ionized, and thus forms fewer than six coordinate covalent bonds with metal cations. Disodium EDTA is commonly used to standardize aqueous solutions of transition metal cations. Disodium EDTA (often written as Na_2H_2Y) only forms four coordinate covalent bonds to metal cations at pH values ≤ 12. In this pH range, the amine groups remain protonated and thus unable to donate electrons to the formation of coordinate covalent bonds. Note that the shorthand form $Na_{4-x}H_xY$ can be used to represent any species of EDTA, with x designating the number of acidic protons bonded to the EDTA molecule. EDTA forms an octahedral complex with most 2+ metal cations, M^{2+}, in aqueous solution. The main reason that EDTA is used so extensively in the standardization of metal cation solutions is that the formation constant for most metal cation-EDTA complexes is very high, meaning that the equilibrium for the reaction:

$$M^{2+} + H_4Y \rightarrow MH_2Y + 2H^+$$

Carrying out the reaction in a basic buffer solution removes H^+ as it is formed, which also favors the formation of the EDTA-metal cation complex reaction product. For most purposes it can be considered that the formation of the metal cation EDTA complex goes to completion, and this is chiefly why EDTA is used in titrations / standardizations of this type.

Indicators: To carry out metal cation titrations using EDTA, it is almost always necessary to use a complexometric indicator to determine when the end point has been reached. Common indicators are organic dyes such as Fast Sulphon Black, Eriochrome Black T. Color change shows that the indicator has been displaced (usually by EDTA) from the metal cations in solution when the endpoint has been reached. Thus, the free indicator (rather than the metal complex) serves as the endpoint indicator.

Metal ion indicators: The success of an EDTA titration depends upon the precise determination of the end point. The most common procedure utilizes metal ion indicators. The requisites of a metal ion indicator for use in the visual detection of end points include:

    (a) The color reaction must be before the end point, when nearly all the metal ion is complexed with EDTA, the solution is strongly colored.

    (b) The color reaction should be specific or selective.

    (c) The metal-indicator complex must possess sufficient stability, otherwise, due to dissociation, a sharp color change is not attained. The metal-indicator complex must, however, be less stable than the metal-EDTA complex to ensure that, at the end point, EDTA removes metal ions from the metal indicator-complex. The change in equilibrium from the metal indicator complex to the metal-EDTA complex should be sharp and rapid.

    (d) The color contrast between the free indicator and the metal-indicator complex should be readily observed.

    (e) The indicator must be very sensitive to metal ions (*i.e.* to pM) so that the color change occurs as near to equivalence point as possible.

    (f) The above requirements must be fulfilled within the pH range at which the titration is performed.

Titrations: EDTA is a very unselective reagent because it complexes with numerous doubly, triply and quadruply charged cations. When a solution containing two cations which complex with EDTA is titrated without the addition of a complex-forming indicator, and if a titration error of 0.1 % is permissible, then the ratio of the stability constants of the EDTA complexes of the two metals M and N must be such that $K_M/K_N > 10^6$ if N is not to interfere with the titration of M. Strictly, of course, the constants K_M and K_N considered in the above expression should be the apparent stability constants of the complexes. If complex-forming indicators are used, then for a similar titration error $K_M/K_N > 10^8$. The following procedures will help to increase the selectivity:

    (a) **Suitable control of the pH of the solution:** This, of course, makes use of the different stabilities of metal-EDTA complexes. Thus bismuth and thorium can be titrated in an acidic solution (pH = 2) with xylenol orange or methylthymol blue as indicator and most divalent cations do not interfere. A mixture of bismuth and lead ions can be successfully titrated by first titrating the bismuth at pH 2 with xylenol orange as indicator, and then adding hexamine to raise the pH to about 5, and titrating the lead.

(b) Use of masking agents: Masking may be defined as the process in which a substance, without physical separation of it or its reaction products, is so transformed that it does not enter into a particular reaction. Demasking is the process in which the masked substance regains its ability to enter into a particular reaction. By the use of masking agents, some of the cations in a mixture can often be 'masked' so that they can no longer react with EDTA or with the indicator. An effective masking agent is the cyanide ion; this forms stable cyanide complexes with the cations of Cd, Zn, Hg(II), Cu, Co, Ni, Ag, and the platinum metals, but not with the alkaline earths, manganese, and lead. It is therefore possible to determine cations such as Ca^{2+}, Mg^{2+}, Pb^{2+}, and Mn^{2+} in the presence of the above-mentioned metals by masking with an excess of potassium or sodium cyanide. A small amount of iron may be masked by cyanide if it is first reduced to the iron(II) state by the addition of ascorbic acid. Titanium (IV), iron (III), and aluminum can be masked with triethanolamine; mercury with iodide ions; and aluminum, iron(III), titanium(IV), and tin(II) with ammonium fluoride (the cations of the alkaline-earth metals yield slightly soluble fluorides). Sometimes the metal may be transformed into a different oxidation state: thus copper (II) may be reduced in acid solution by hydroxylamine or ascorbic acid. After rendering ammoniacal, nickel or cobalt can be titrated using, for example, murexide as indicator without interference from the copper, which is now present as Cu(I). Iron (III) can often be similarly masked by reduction with ascorbic acid.

(c) Selective demasking: The cyanide complexes of zinc and cadmium may be demasked with formaldehydeacetic acid solution or, better, with chloral hydrate: The use of masking and selective demasking agents permits the successive titration of many metals. Thus, a solution containing Mg, Zn, and Cu can be titrated as follows:

1. Add excess of standard EDTA and back-titrate with standard Mg solution using solo chrome black as indicator. This gives the sum of all the metals present.
2. Treat an aliquot portion with excess of KCN and titrate as before. This gives Mg only.
3. Add excess of chloral hydrate (or of formaldehyde-acetic acid solution, to the titrated solution in order to liberate the Zn from the cyanide complex, and titrate until the indicator turns blue. This gives the Zn only. The Cu content may then be found by difference.

Redox Titration

Redox Titration is a laboratory method of determining the concentration of a given analyte by causing a redox reaction between the titrant and the analyte. These types of titrations sometimes require the use of a potentiometer or a redox indicator.

Redox titration is based on an oxidation-reduction reaction between the titrant and the analyte. It is one of the most common laboratory methods to identify the concentration of unknown analytes.

In order to evaluate redox titrations, the shape of the corresponding titration curve must be obtained. In these types of titration, it proves convenient to monitor the reaction potential instead of monitoring the concentration of a reacting species.

Reduction: A substance can undergo reduction can occur via:

1. The addition of hydrogen.
2. The removal of oxygen.
3. The acceptance of electrons.
4. A reduction in the overall oxidation state.

Oxidation

The following points describe a substance that has undergone oxidation.

1. The addition of oxygen.
2. Removal of hydrogen which was attached to the species.
3. The donation/loss of electrons.
4. An increase in the oxidation state exhibited by the substance.

Thus, it can be understood that redox titrations involve a transfer of electrons between the given analyte and the titrant. An example of a redox titration is the treatment of an iodine solution with a reducing agent. The endpoint of this titration is detected with the help of a starch indicator.

In the example described above, the diatomic iodine is reduced to iodide ions ($I-$), and the iodine solution loses its blue colour. This titration is commonly referred to as iodometric titration.

Examples of Redox titration: An example of a redox titration is the titration of potassium permanganate ($KMnO_4$) against oxalic acid ($C_2H_2O_4$). The procedure and details of this titration are discussed below.

Titration of Potassium Permanganate against Oxalic Acid:

- Prepare a standard Oxalic acid solution of about 250 ml.
- The molecular mass of oxalic acid is calculated by adding the atomic mass of each constituent atom
- The molecular mass of $H_2C_2O_4.2H_2O = 126$

- Since the weight of oxalic acid that is required to make 1000 ml of 1M solution is 126 g. Hence, the weight of oxalic acid needed to prepare 250 ml of 0.1 M solution = 126/1000 x 250 x 0.1 = 3.15 g.

Determining the Strength of KMnO$_4$ using Standard Oxalic Acid Solution: In this titration, the analyte is oxalic acid and the titrant is potassium permanganate. The oxalic acid acts as a reducing agent, and the KMnO$_4$ acts as an oxidizing agent. Since the reaction takes place in an acidic medium, the oxidizing power of the permanganate ion is increased. This acidic medium is created by the addition of dilute sulfuric acid.

$$MnO^-_4 + 8H^+ + 5e^- \rightarrow Mn^{2+} + 4H_2O$$

KMnO$_4$ acts as an indicator of where the permanganate ions are a deep purple colour. In this redox titration, MnO$_4^-$ is reduced to colorless manganous ions (Mn^{2+}) in the acidic medium. The last drop of permanganate gives a light pink color on reaching the endpoint. The following chemical equation can represent the reaction that occurs.

Molecular equation

$$2KMnO_4 + 3H_2SO_4 \rightarrow K_2SO_4 + 2MnSO_4 + 3H_2O + 5[O]$$
$$H_2C_2O_4.2H_2O + [O] \rightarrow 2CO_2 + 3[H_2O] \times 5$$

Complete Reaction

$$\mathbf{2KMnO_4 + 3H_2SO_4 + 5H_2C_2O_4.2H_2O \rightarrow K_2SO_4 + 2MnSO_4 + 18H_2O + 10CO_2}$$

Ionic equation

$$\mathbf{MnO_4^- + 8H^+ + 5e^- \rightarrow Mn^{2+} + 4H_2O] \times 2}$$
$$\mathbf{C_2O_4^{2-} \rightarrow 2CO_2 + 2e^-] \times 5}$$

Complete Reaction

$$\mathbf{2MnO_4^- + 16H^+ + 5C_2O_4^{2-} \rightarrow 2Mn^{2+} + 8H_2O + 10CO_2}$$

From the above-balanced chemical reaction, it can be observed that 2 moles of KMnO$_4$ reacts with 5 moles of oxalic acid.

Gravimetric Analysis: Principle and Method

Gravimetric analysis: Gravimetric analysis is a technique through which the amount of an analyte (the ion being analyzed) can be determined through the measurement of mass. Gravimetric analyses depend on comparing the masses of two compounds containing the analyte. The principle behind gravimetric analysis is that the mass of an ion in a pure compound can be determined and then used to find the mass percent of the same ion in a known quantity of an impure compound. In order for the analysis to be accurate, certain conditions must be met:

1. The ion being analyzed must be completely precipitated.
2. The precipitate must be a pure compound.
3. The precipitate must be easily filtered.

An example of a gravimetric analysis is the determination of chloride in a compound. In order to do a gravimetric analysis, a cation must be found that forms an insoluble compound with chloride. This compound must also be pure and easily filtered. The solubility rules indicate that Ag^+, Pb^{2+}, and Hg_2^{2+} form insoluble chlorides. Therefore, silver chloride could be used to determine % Cl^-, because it is insoluble (that is, about 99.9% of the silver is converted to AgCl) and it can be formed pure and is easily filtered.

In precipitation gravimetry, the analyte is converted to a sparingly soluble precipitate. This precipitate is then filtered, washed free of impurities, converted to a product of known composition by suitable heat treatment, and weighed. For example, a precipitation method for determining calcium in natural waters involves the addition of $C_2O_4^{\ 2-}$ as a precipitating agent:

$$Ca^{2+}\ (aq) + C_2O_4^{\ 2-}\ (aq) \rightarrow CaC_2O_4\ (s)$$

The precipitate CaC_2O_4 is filtered, then dried and ignited to convert it entirely to calcium oxide:

$$CaC_2O_4\ (s) \rightarrow CaO\ (s) + CO\ (g) + CO_2\ (g)$$

After cooling, the precipitate is weighed, and the calcium content of the sample is then computed.

Steps involved in Gravimetric analysis: The steps required in gravimetric analysis, after the sample has been dissolved, can be summarized as follows: preparation of the solution, precipitation, digestion, filtration, washing, drying or igniting, weighing and finally calculation.

1. **Preparation of the Solution:** This may involve several steps including adjustment of the pH of the solution in order for the precipitate to occur quantitatively and get a precipitate of desired properties, removing interferences, etc.

2. **Precipitation:** This requires addition of a precipitating agent solution to the sample solution. Upon addition of the first drops of the precipitating agent, supersaturation occurs, then nucleation starts to occur where every few molecules of precipitate aggregate together forming a nucleus. At this point, addition of extra precipitating agent will either form new nuclei (precipitate with

small particles) or will build up on existing nuclei to give a precipitate with large particles.

3. **Digestion of the Precipitate:** The precipitate is left hot (below boiling) for 30 min to 1 hour in order for the particles to be digested. Digestion involves dissolution of small particles and re-precipitation on larger ones resulting in particle growth and better precipitate characteristics. This process is called Ostwald ripening. An important advantage of digestion is observed for colloidal precipitates where large amounts of adsorbed ions cover the huge area of the precipitate. Digestion forces the small colloidal particles to agglomerate which decreases their surface area and thus adsorption. The precipitate often contains ions that were trapped when the precipitate was formed. This is mostly a problem for crystalline precipitates. If the trapped ions are not volatile, then their presence will corrupt the weighing step. Concentration of interfering species may be reduced by digestion. Unfortunately, post-precipitation as we will see later will increase during digestion.

4. **Washing and Filtering:** Problems with surface adsorption may be reduced by careful washing of the precipitate. With some precipitates, peptization occurs during washing. Each particle of the precipitate has two layers, in primary layer certain ions are adsorbed and in the outer layer other ions of opposite charge are adsorbed. This situation makes the precipitate settle down. If the outer layer ions are removed then all the particles will have the same charge so the particles will be dissonant. This is called peptization. This results in the loss of part of the precipitate because the colloidal form may pass through on filtration, in case of colloidal precipitates we should not use water as a washing solution since peptization would occur. In such situations dilute volatile electrolyte such as nitric acid, ammonium nitrate, or dilute acetic acid may be used. Usually, it is a good practice to check for the presence of precipitating agent in the filtrate of the final washing solution. The presence of precipitating agent means that extra washing is required. Filtration should be done in appropriate sized Goosh or ignition ashless filter paper. After the solution has been filtered, it should be tested to make sure that the analyte has been completely precipitated. This is easily done by adding a few drops of the precipitating reagent to the filtrate; if a precipitate is observed, the precipitation is incomplete.

The common ion effect can be used to reduce the solubility of the precipitate. When Ag+ is precipitated out by addition of Cl^-

$$\textbf{Ag}^+ + \textbf{Cl}^- \rightarrow \textbf{AgCl (s)}$$

The (low) solubility of AgCl is reduced still further by the excess of Ag^+ which is added, pushing the equilibrium to the right. It important to know that the excess of the precipitating agent should not exceed 50% of its equivalent amount, otherwise the precipitating agent may form a soluble complex with the precipitate:

$$AgCl + Cl^- \rightarrow AgCl^{2-} \text{ (soluble complex)}$$

5. **Drying and Ignition:** The purpose of drying (heating at about 120-150°C in an oven) is to remove the remaining moisture while the purpose of ignition in a muffle furnace at temperatures ranging from 600-1200°C is to get a material with exactly known chemical structure so that the amount of analyte can be accurately determined. The precipitate is converted to a more chemically stable form. For instance, calcium ion might be precipitated using oxalate ion, to produce calcium oxalate (CaC_2O_4) which is hydrophil, therefore it is better to be heated to convert it into $CaCO_3$ or CaO. It is vital that the empirical formula of the weighed precipitate be known, and that the precipitate be pure; if two forms are present, the results will be inaccurate.

6. **Weighing the precipitate:** The precipitate cannot be weighed with the necessary accuracy in place on the filter paper; nor can the precipitate be completely removed from the filter paper in order to weigh it. The precipitate can be carefully heated in a crucible until the filter paper has burned away; this leaves only the precipitate. (As the name suggests, "ashless" paper is used so that the precipitate is not contaminated with ash.). If you use Goosh crucible then after the precipitate is allowed to cool (preferably in a desiccator to keep it from absorbing moisture), it is weighed (in the crucible). The mass of the crucible is subtracted from the combined mass, giving the mass of the precipitated analyte. Since the composition of the precipitate is known, it is simple to calculate the mass of analyte in the original sample.

Impurities in Gravimetric Precipitates

There are two types of impurities

A. **Co-precipitation:** This is anything unwanted which precipitates with the analyte during precipitation. Co-precipitation occurs to some degree in every gravimetric analysis (especially barium sulfate and those involving hydrous oxides). You cannot avoid it all what you can do is minimize it by careful precipitation and thorough washing:

1. **Surface adsorption:** Here, the unwanted material is adsorbed onto the surface of the precipitate. Digestion of a precipitate reduces the amount of surface area and hence the area available for surface adsorption. Washing can also remove surface material.

2. **Occlusion:** This is a type of co-precipitation in which impurities are trapped within the growing crystal and can be reduced by digestion and re-precipitation.

B. Post-precipitation: Sometimes a precipitate standing in contact with the mother liquor becomes contaminated by the precipitation of an impurity on top of the desired precipitate. To reduce post-precipitation filter as soon as the precipitation is complete and avoid digestion.

Precipitating agents: Ideally, a gravimetric precipitating agent should react specifically or at least selectively with the analyte. Specific reagents which are rare, react only with a single chemical species. Selective reagents which are more common, react with a limited number of species. In addition to specificity and selectivity, the ideal precipitating reagent would react with analyte to give a precipitate. There are 2 types of precipitating agents:

Inorganic precipitating agents: The inorganic precipitants e.g. S^{2-}, CO_3^{2-}, PO_4^{3-}, etc are usually not selective compared to the organic precipitants but it give precipitates with well known formula.

Organic precipitating agents: The organic precipitants such as dimethglyoxime and 8-hydroxyquinoline are more selective than inorganic precipitants. They produce with the analyte less soluble precipitate (small Ksp). They also have high molecular weight so that the weighing error is reduced. The disadvantage of organic precipitants is that they usually form with the analyte a precipitate of unknown formula, therefore the precipitate is burned to the metal oxide.

Calculation of Gravimetric Analysis

The results of a gravimetric analysis are generally computed from two experimental measurements: the weight of sample and the weight of a known composition precipitate. The precipitate we weigh is usually in a different form than the analyte whose weight we wish to find. The principles of converting the weight of one substance to that of another depend on using the stoichiometric mole relationships. We introduced the gravimetric factor (GF), which represents the weight of analyte per unit weight of precipitate. It is obtained from the ratio of the formula weight of the analyte to that of the precipitate, multiplied by the moles of analyte per mole of precipitate obtained from each mole of analyte, that is:

$$GF = \frac{\text{MW of analyte (g / mole)}}{\text{MW of precipitation (g / mole)}} \times R$$

Where, R is the number of moles of analyte in one mole of precipitate.

Points to Remember

- Volumetric analysis is a quantitative analytical method which involves measurement of the volume of a solution whose concentration is known and applied to determine the concentration of the analyte. In other words, measuring the volume of a second substance that combines with the first in known proportions is known as Volumetric analysis or titration.
- An acid-base titration is an experimental technique used to acquire information about a solution containing an acid or base. An acid-base titration involves strong or weak acids or bases.
- Non-aqueous titration refers to a type of titration in which the analyte substance is dissolved in a solvent which does not contain water.
- Precipitation reaction is a type of reaction in which the analyte and titrant form an insoluble precipitate also can serve as the basis for a titration.
- Complexometric titration (sometimes chelatometry) is a form of volumetric analysis in which the formation of a colored complex is used to indicate the end point of a titration. Complexometric titrations are particularly useful for the determination of a mixture of different metal ions in solution.
- Redox titration is based on an oxidation-reduction reaction between the titrant and the analyte. It is one of the most common laboratory methods to identify the concentration of unknown analytes.
- In precipitation gravimetry, the analyte is converted to a sparingly soluble precipitate. This precipitate is then filtered, washed free of impurities, converted to a product of known composition by suitable heat treatment, and weighed.
- A gravimetric precipitating agent reacts specifically or at least selectively with the analyte. Specific reagents which are rare, react only with a single chemical species. Selective reagents are more common, react with a limited number of species.

Multiple Choice Questions

1. The ideal indicator for the titration of strong acid and weak base should have pH range between

   (A)   5-8   (B)   4-6   (C)   8-10   (D)   7-8

2. Which of the following is a buffer solution?

   (A) $H_2SO_4 + CuSO_4$ (B) $CH_3COOH + CH_3COONH_4$

   (C) $NaCl + NaOH$ (D) $CH_3COONa + CH_3COOH$

3. Which of the following titrations will have the equivalence point at a pH more than 8?
   (A) HCl and NH_3 (B) CH_3COOH and NH_3
   (c) HCl and NaOH   (D) CH_3COOH and NaOH

4. Which of the following is used as an indicator in the titration of a strong acid and a weak base?
   (A) Phenolphthalein   (B) Thymol blue
   (C) Fluorescein   (D) Methyl orange

5. Which of the following is used as an indicator in the titration of a weak acid and a strong base?
   (A) Bromothymol blue (6 to 7.5)   (B) Methyl orange (3 to 4)
   (C) Methyl red (5 to 6)   (D) Phenolphthalein (8 to 9.6)

6. A difference between strong and weak acid is
   (A) Presence and absence of halogen ions
   (B) Negative and positive pH
   (C) Complete and partial ionization
   (D) Proton donation and electron acceptance

7. Which of the following is used as an indicator in the titration of iodine with hypo?
   (A) Methyl red   (B) Methyl orange
   (C) Starch   (D) Potassium ferricyanide

8. What will be the pH at the equivalence point in the titration of a weak acid and a strong base?
   (A) 0   (B) >7   (C) 7   (D) <7

9. On adding a large amount of titrant, an asymptote is obtained in the titration curve, this asymptote represents
   (A) K_a of the initial solution   (B) pH of the initial solution
   (c) pH of the titrant   (D) none of the above

10. The buffer region is represented by
    (A) The concave curve after adding titrant
    (B) The flat curve before the equivalence point
    (C) The flat curve after the cquivalence point
    (D) The steep curve after the equivalence point

11. The pH range of methyl orange as an indicator is
    (A) 3-5   (B) 8-9   (C) 2-4   (D) 6-8

12. The equivalent weight of an acid can be calculated by
    (A) Molecular weight × basicity
    (B) Molecular weight/basicity
    (C) Molecular weight × acidity
    (D) Molecular weight/acidity

13. Which of the following represents the equivalence point in the graph of pH Vs volume of titrant?
    (A) Point at the highest pH
    (B) Point at the greatest magnitude of the slope of the curve
    (C) Point at the lowest pH
    (D) Point at the least magnitude of the slope of the curve

14. Which of the following combinations cannot produce a buffer solution?
    (A) HNO_2 and $NaNO_2$ (B) HCN and $NaCN$
    (C) $HClO_4$ and $NaClO_4$ (D) NH_3 and $(NH_4)_2SO_4$

15. An aqueous solution is prepared by dissolving the salt formed by the neutralization of a weak acid by a weak base. Which statement about the solution is correct?
    (A) The solution is strongly basic.
    (B) The solution is weakly basic.
    (C) The solution is neutral.
    (D) The values for Ka and Kb for the species in solution must be known before a prediction can be made.

16. Consider the following balanced redox reaction

    $$Mn^{2+}(aq) + S_2O_8^{2-}(aq) + 2H_2O(l) \rightarrow MnO_2(s) + 4H+ (aq) + 2SO_4^{2-}(aq)$$

    Which of the following statements is true?
    (A) $Mn^{2+}(aq)$ is the oxidizing agent and is reduced.
    (B) $Mn^{2+}(aq)$ is the oxidizing agent and is oxidized.
    (C) $Mn^{2+}(aq)$ is the reducing agent and is oxidized.
    (D) $Mn^{2+}(aq)$ is the reducing agent and is reduced.

17. Which of the following is a general property of base?
    (A) Taste Sour
    (B) Turn litmus red
    (C) Conduct electric current in solution
    (D) Concentration of H_3O is greater than concentration of OH.

18. A solution of known concentration is the definition of a
    (A) Buffer solution
    (B) Standard solution
    (C) Neutral solutions
    (D) Standard solutions

19. pH of 7 is shown through a color of
    (A) Red
    (B) Blue
    (C) Green
    (D) Yellow

20. Litmus is used to test either the substance is
    (A) Acidic only
    (B) Alkaline only
    (C) Liquid
    (D) Acid and Alkaline

CHAPTER 3
Inorganic Pharmaceuticals

Introduction

The chapter aims at providing the latest and pharmacopoeial information regarding some inorganic pharmaceuticals (Ferrous sulphate, Ferrous gluconate, Aluminium hydroxide gel, Magnesium hydroxide, Hydrogen peroxide, Boric acid, Bleaching powder, Calcium carbonate, Sodium fluoride, Carbon dioxide, Nitrous oxide, and Oxygen) regarding their classification, molecular formula, molecular mass, IUPAC name, formulations, properties, storage conditions, and uses.

Haematinics

Haematinics are the agents used for formation of blood to treat various types of anaemia's. These include: Iron, Vitamin B12 and Folic Acid.

Anaemia

- Decreased capacity of RBCs to carry oxygen to tissues.
- Anaemia occurs when the balance between production and destruction of RBCs is disturbed by:
    (a) Blood loss (acute or chronic)
    (b) Impaired red cell formation due to:
        - Deficiency of essential factors, i.e. iron, vitamin B12, folic acid.
        - Bone marrow depression (hypoplastic anaemia), erythropoietin deficiency.
    (c) Increased destruction of RBCs (haemolytic anaemia)
- Iron deficiency occurs due to:
    1. Malnutrition
    2. Loss
    3. Congenital Atransferrinemia (inability to release iron from transferrin)

Types of Anaemia:

1. Microcytic hypochromic - mainly due to iron deficiency.
2. Macrocytic/megaloblastic - mainly due to deficiency of vitamin B12 and folic acid
3. Haemolytic Anaemia- red blood cells are destroyed faster than they can be made
4. Pernicious Anaemia - decreased intrinsic factor

Ferrous Sulphate

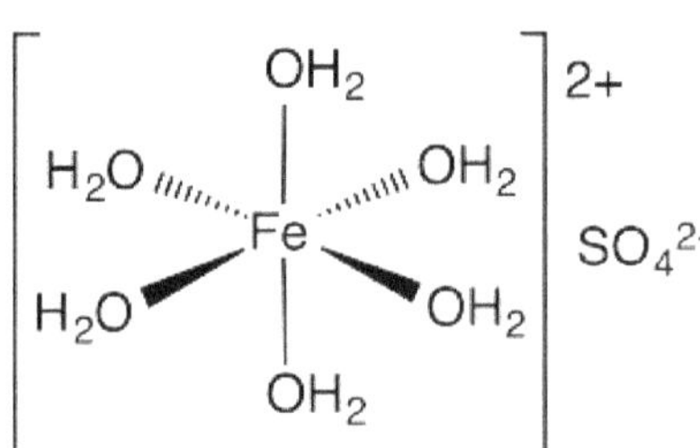

Classification: Nutritional supplement

Chemical Formula: FeO_4S

Molecular weight: 151.91

Synonyms: iron(II) sulfate heptahydrate, Feospan, Hemobion

IUPAC Name: iron(2+); sulfate

Properties

- Ferrous sulfate appears as a greenish or yellow-brown crystalline solid. Melts at 64°C and loses the seven waters of hydration at 90°C.
- White orthorhombic crystals, hygroscopic.
- Odorless; has saline, astringent taste.
- The pH is 3.7 for 10% solution.
- Boiling point of > 300°C and Melting point of 64°C.
- Aqueous solubility of 25.6 g/100 mL (Soluble).
- Practically insoluble in alcohol.
- Density 2.970 Kg/cm^3 at 25 °C; off-white, monoclinic crystals.
- LogP value of -0.84.
- In moist air, ferrous sulfate rapidly oxidizes and becomes coated with brownish-yellow ferric sulfate. The rate of oxidation is increased by the addition of alkali or by exposure to light.

- When heated to decomposition it emits toxic fumes of sulfur oxide.
- Standard molar enthalpy (heat) of formation at 298.15 deg K is -928.4 kJ/mol (crystal)
- Standard molar Gibbs energy of formation at 298.15 deg K is -820.8 kJ/mol (crystal)
- Standard molar entropy at 298.15 deg K is 107.5 J/mol K (crystal)
- Molar heat capacity at constant pressure at 298.15 deg K is 100.6 J/mol K (crystal)
- In moist air, oxidizes to yellow-brown basic iron(III) sulfate. Aqueous solutions tend to oxidize with the rate increasing with increasing pH, temperature, and light.
- Sugar, glycerin, & many organic hydroxy acids hinder precipitation. In neutral solution, soluble carbonates, phosphates, & oxalates produce precipitation.

Pharmaceutical Formulations

- Official USP tablets contain 300 mg iron sulfate. $7H_2O$ or equivalent amount of dried (anhydrous) ferrous sulfate. It is also available as syrup and as elixirs.
- It is usually dispensed as pills or tablets, coated to protect them from moisture. Salt is mixed with glucose or lactose to protect it against oxidation.
- Available in heptahydrate (20% iron) and monohydrate (30% Fe) grades.

Storage Conditions

- Store in a well-ventilated place. Keep cool. Store in a dry area. Store at ambient temperature. Keep container in a well-ventilated place. Meet the legal requirements.
- Keep Substance Away From: Heat sources, oxidizing agents, (strong) bases, and water/moisture.

Uses

- It is used as a hematinic.
- Ferrous sulfate replenishes iron, an essential component in hemoglobin, myoglobin, and various enzymes. It replaces the iron that is usually found in hemoglobin and myoglobin. Iron participates in oxygen transport and storage, electron transport and energy metabolism, antioxidant and beneficial pro-oxidant functions, oxygen sensing, tissue proliferation and growth, as well as DNA replication and repair.
- Nutrient or dietary supplement; trace mineral added to animal feed.
- Astringent.
- Catalysts, pigments, drugs, agriculture, nutrition, metallurgy, and leather tanning.

Ferrous Gluconate

Classification: Nutritional supplement

Chemical Formula: $C_{12}H_{26}FeO_{16}$

Molecular weight: 482.17

Synonyms: Loesferron, Dextriferron, Simron

IUPAC Name: iron(2+);(2R,3S,4R,5R)-2,3,4,5,6-pentahydroxyhexanoate;dehydrate

Properties

- Pale greenish-yellow to yellowish-grey powder or granules, which may have a faint odor of burnt sugar.
- The color of /ferrous gluconate/ solution depends on pH; they are light yellow at pH 2, brown at pH 4.5, and green at pH 7. The iron rapidly oxidizes at higher pH.
- The melting point for *D*-gluconic acid, ferrous salt dihydrate (98%) is 188°C, decomposes. The specific optical rotation is +6.7 deg at 25°C (c=1, H_2O).
- Soluble with slight heating in water. Practically insoluble in ethanol. Soluble in glycerin. Solubility increased by addition of citric acid or citrate ion.
- Aqueous solutions are stabilized by the addition of glucose. Affected by light & ferrous ion slowly oxidizes on exposure to air. Approx neutral solutions undergo rapid oxidation. Oxidation retarded and stability improved by buffering to pH of 3.5 to 4.5 with citrate buffer. When heated to decomposition it emits acrid smoke and irritating fumes.
- The pH lies between 4 and 5,5 (10 % solution).
- Ascorbic acid and aminoacetic acid cause dark coloration; with pyridoxine, green color produced.
- Yellowish-gray or pale greenish-yellow powder. Slight odor of caramel. Soluble in water; practically insoluble in alcohol. Aqueous solutions are stabilized by addition of glucose.
- Ferrous gluconate is affected by light and the ferrous iron slowly oxidizes to ferric on exposure to air.
- Approximately neutral solutions undergo rapid oxidation; oxidation is retarded and stability improved by buffering to a pH of 3.5 to 4.5 with citrate buffer. Glycerin also retards oxidation.

- Sugar, glycerin, & many organic hydroxy acids hinder precipitation. In neutral solution, soluble carbonates, phosphates, & oxalates produce precipitation.

Pharmaceutical Formulations

- Capsules 435 mg (equivalent to 50 mg of elemental iron)
- Elixir 300 mg (equivalent to 37.5 mg of elemental iron)/5 mL
- Tablets 320 mg (equivalent to 40 mg of elemental iron)

Storage Conditions

- Store in original container, tightly sealed container, protected from direct sunlight, in a dry and well-ventilated area, away from incompatible materials. Store in accordance with local regulations. Eliminate all ignition sources.
- Separate from oxidizing materials. Containers that have been opened must be carefully resealed and kept upright to prevent leakage. Do not store in unlabelled containers. Use appropriate containment to avoid environmental contamination. Preserve in tight containers.

Uses

- It is used as a hematinic.
- Nutrient or dietary supplement; trace mineral added to animal feed
- Ferrous Gluconate is a form of mineral iron for oral administration, Ferrous Gluconate is absorbed in the stomach and small intestine and combines with apoferritin to form ferritin, which is stored in the liver, spleen, red bone marrow, and intestinal mucosa. Important in transport of oxygen by hemoglobin to the tissues, iron is also found in myoglobin, transferrin, and ferritin, and is as a component of many enzymes such as catalase, peroxidase, and cytochromes.

Ferrous Fumarate

- Ferrous fumarate is the fumarate salt form of the mineral iron. Administration of ferrous fumarate results in elevation of serum iron concentration, which is then assimilated into hemoglobin, required for the transport of oxygen, or trapped in the reticuloendothelial cells for storage. This agent is used as a dietary supplement, and to prevent or treat iron deficiency related syndromes.
- Iron is an essential heavy metal that is included in many over-the-counter multivitamin and mineral supplements and is used therapeutically in higher doses to treat or prevent iron deficiency anemia. When taken at the usual recommended daily allowance or in replacement doses, iron has little or no adverse effect on the liver. In high doses and in intentional or accidental overdoses, iron causes serious toxicities, one component of which is acute liver damage.

Pharmaceutical Formulations

Ferrous fumarate and folic acid (combination) tablets are used to treat anaemia that is caused by an iron deficiency. Ferrous fumarate has an iron content of 32.87% and is poorly soluble in water, soluble in dilute acid (such as gastric acid) and is well absorbed as ferrous sulphate.

Market preparations: Anemifer, Aritoferon, Bioron, Ferrosi, Iron-200, Jeferin, Kdiron, Tibilin, Vitafer-Fol

Storage conditions: Store in a clean, dry warehouse in the original unopened containers. Store in a well- ventilated place. Keep cool.

Uses: Ferrous fumarate is a medicine used to treat and prevent iron deficiency anaemia. Iron helps the body to make healthy red blood cells which carry oxygen around the body. Some things such as blood loss, pregnancy or too little iron in your diet can make your iron supply drop too low, leading to anaemia.

Ferric Ammonium Citrate

- Ferric ammonium citrate is a yellowish brown to red solid with a faint odor of ammonia. It is soluble in water. The primary hazard is the threat to the environment. Immediate steps should be taken to limit its spread to the environment. It is used in medicine, in making blueprints, and as a feed additive.

$$\left[\text{citrate}^{3-} \right] \left[Fe^{3\oplus} \right]_x \left[\overset{\oplus}{N}H_4 \right]_y$$

- **Pharmaceutical formulations:** Ammonium ferric citrate (brown) contains about 9% ammonia, 16.5-18.5% iron, and about 65% hydrated citric acid; Ammonium ferric citrate, green contains about 7.5% ammonia, 14.5-16% iron, and about 75% hydrated citric acid.
- **Market preparations:** Ammonium iron(III) citrate, 1185-57-5, Ferric ammonium citrate (Brown), Ammonium iron (lll) citrate (Green)
- **Storage conditions:** Keep well closed and protected from light.
- **Uses:** Source of iron in treating iron-deficiency anemias. It is less constipating than inorganic forms of iron. It is free from astringent & irritant properties. However, ferric ion is less well absorbed than ferrous ion, so that its supposed advantages are outweighed by its lesser efficacy, and it is considered to be an obsolete preparation. In the forms presently marketed, a unit dose provides only the recommended daily allowance of iron (15 mg).

Ferrous Ascorbate

Folic acid plays a crucial role in the production of red blood cells in the body that contain oxygen. It is also important in pregnancy because of its role in the brain and spinal cord development of the unborn baby. In various biochemical reactions in our body, Ferrous ascorbate acts as a catalyst, stimulates the transport and use of oxygen, and helps in cell growth and proliferation. This increases red blood cell production and hemoglobin production. Ferrous ascorbate medicine is an iron supplement that is used to treat or avoid low iron levels in the blood. The absorption of iron from the stomach is increased by ascorbic acid (vitamin C). For the treatment and prevention of iron deficiency anemia, ferrous ascorbate is used when the amount of iron taken from the diet is not adequate. It is also used for the treatment of anemia due to chronic kidney failure. This drug is only used to treat iron deficiency-related hemoglobin disorders.

Pharmaceutical formulations: Ferinext syrup (Ferrous ascorbate, folic acid, ZINC and Vitamin B12 syrup)

Market preparations: Ferrous ascorbate, Ferrous cevitamate, Iron(2+) L-ascorbate, L-Ascorbic acid, iron complex, (+)-Iron(II) L-ascorbate, DB14490, J-015682

Storage conditions: Keep well closed and protected from light.

Uses: Ferrous Ascorbate is used in the treatment of iron deficiency anemia and anemia due to chronic kidney disease. Ferrous Ascorbate is a combination of of iron and vitamin C. Iron works by replenishing the iron stores in your body and corrects iron deficiency anemia.

Carbonyl Iron

- Carbonyl iron is an iron replacement product. You normally get iron from the foods you eat. Iron helps your body produce red blood cells that carry oxygen through your blood to tissues and organs.

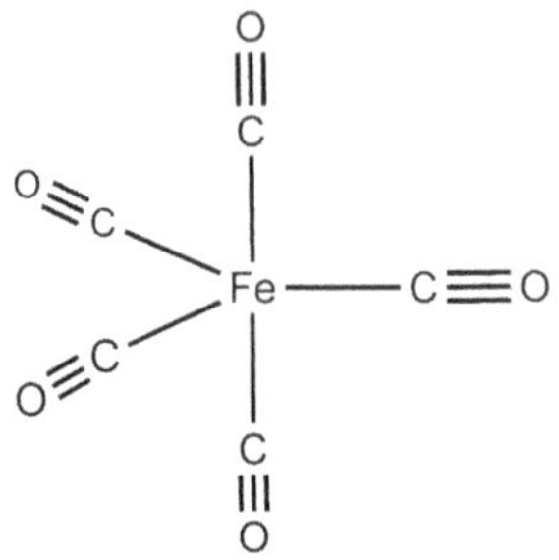

$$\text{(CO)}_5\text{Fe}$$

Pharmaceutical formulations: Tablet-45 mg (Feosol), 66 mg (Ircon); Oral Suspension-15mg/1.25mL (Icar Pediatric); Tablet, Chewable-15mg (Icar Pediatric, Wee Care); Tablet with Vitamin C-100mg iron/250mg vitamin C (Icar C)

Market preparations: Feosol (Carbonyl Fe), Icar C, Icar Pediatric, and Irco.

Storage conditions: Store it in room temperature and in an airtight container.

Uses: This medication is an iron supplement used to treat or prevent low blood levels of iron (such as those caused by anemia or pregnancy). Iron is an important mineral that the body needs to produce red blood cells and keep you in good health.

Antacids

Antacids (anti - against; acidus - acid) are weak alkaline compounds used to neutralize hydrochloric acid in the stomach.

- Antacids are the substances which reduce gastric acidity resulting in an increase in the pH of stomach and duodenum.

  Gastric acidity occurs due to excessive secretion of HCl in stomach due to various reasons.

- The pH of the stomach is 1.5-2.5 when empty and raises to 5-6 when food is ingested.

- Low pH is due to the presence of endogenous HCl, which is always present under physiological conditions.

When hyperacidity occurs the result can range from:

(i) Gastritis (a general inflammation of gastric mucosa)

(ii) Peptic ulcer or oesophageal ulcer (lower end of oesophagus)

(iii) Gastric ulcer (stomach)

(iv) Duodenum ulcers

Criteria of an ideal antacid preparation:
- The antacid should not be absorbable or cause systemic alkalosis
- The antacid should not be a laxative or causes constipation
- The antacid should exert its effect rapidly and over a long period of time
- The antacid should buffer in the pH 4-6 range
- The reaction of the antacid with gastric HCl acid should not cause a large evolution of gas
- The antacid should probably inhibit pepsin

Indications and principles of clinical use:
- Gastro Esophageal Reflux Disease (GERD) Antacids neutralize hydrochloric acid, inactivate pepsin, absorb bile acids, stimulate the synthesis of bicarbonates and raise the tone of the lower esophageal sphincter.
- Gastric and duodenal ulcers
- Acute and Chronic gastritis / gastroduodenitis
- Gastropathy caused by nonsteroidal anti-inflammatory drugs (NSAIDs - gastropathy): Antacids can be taken alone or in addition to anti-secretory drugs in order to prevent gastro- and duodenopathies affected by the administration of nonsteroidal anti-inflammatory drugs (NSAIDs).
- Antacids are recommended for healthy people with discomfort or epigastric pain.
- Antacids are used in the intensive care units to prevent so-called "stress ulcers".

Aluminium Hydroxide Gel

Classification

Antacids

Chemical Formula

$Al(OH)_3$

Molecular weight

78.004

Synonyms

Hydrated Alumina; Alumina, Hydrated; Alhydrogel

IUPAC Name

Aluminum; trihydroxide

Properties

- White, odorless, amorphous powder.
- The melting point is 300°C.
- Insoluble in water; soluble in alkaline solutions, acid solutions.
- Practically insoluble in water, but soluble in alkaline aqueous solutions or in HCl, H_2SO_4 and other strong acids in the presence of some water. Readily soluble in both acids and strong bases.
- The density is 2.42 g/cm^3.
- Forms gels on prolonged contact with water; absorbs acids, carbon dioxide. Less sensitive than trialkylaminums to oxidation upon exposure to air.
- Aluminum hydroxide is capable of reacting as either an acid or a base.

Pharmaceutical Formulations

- Aluminum hydroxide gel is white, viscous suspension contains equivalent of 3.6-4.4% aluminum oxide in form of aluminum hydroxide and hydrated oxide.
- Aldrox; ALternaGEL; Aludyal; Amphojel; Cremorin; Pepsamar; Uracid. White, viscous suspension. May also be used as the dried gel. So-called aluminum hydroxide is actually a mixture of aluminum hydroxide and aluminum oxide hydrates and it usually contains some fixed carbon dioxide.

Storage Conditions

- Store in general storage area with other items with no specific storage hazards. Store in a cool, dry, well-ventilated, locked store room away from incompatible materials.

Uses

- Aluminum hydroxide is an inorganic compound containing aluminum. Used in various immunologic preparations to improve immunogenicity, aluminum hydroxide adjuvant consists of aluminum hydroxide gel in a saline solution. In vaccines, this agent binds to the protein conjugate, resulting in improved antigen processing by the immune system.
- Aluminum hydroxide is an inorganic salt used as an antacid. It is a basic compound that acts by neutralizing hydrochloric acid in gastric secretions. Subsequent increases in pH may inhibit the action of pepsin. An increase in bicarbonate ions and prostaglandins may also confer cytoprotective effects.
- Gastric-peptic disease occurs as a result of an imbalance between protective factors, such as mucus, bicarbonate, and prostaglandin secretion, and aggressive factors, such as hydrochloric acid, pepsin, and *Helicobacter pylori*. Antacids work by restoring acid-base balance, attenuating the pepsin activity and increasing bicarbonate and prostaglandin secretion.

Magnesium Hydroxide

$$Mg^{2+}\left[\quad OH^-\quad\right]_2$$

Classification

Antacids

Chemical Formula

$Mg(OH)_2$

Molecular weight

58.320

Synonyms

Magnesium Hydrate, Brucite

IUPAC Name

magnesium; dihydroxide

Properties

- Dry Powder; Wet Solid; Liquid; Other Solid.
- Odourless, white bulky powder
- Amorphous powder to Granules
- White, hexagonal crystals
- Odorless
- Melts at 350°C (decomposes)
- Practically insoluble in water and in ethanol
- White, friable masses or bulky, white powder; at about 700°C is converted to MgO; solubility in about 3,300 parts CO_2-free water; more solubility in water containing CO_2; soluble in dilute acids with effervescence; insoluble in alcohol, soluble in dilute acids.
- Density is 2.36 g/mL.
- The pH is 9.5-10.5 (aqueous slurry).
- Index of refraction: 1.559, 1.580
- Imparts slight alkaline reaction to water; absorbs CO_2 in the presence of water.
- Opaque, more or less viscous suspension from which water usually separates on standing; alkaline to litmus and phenolphthalein.
- Decomposes on heating above 120°C.
- Heat of formation: -924.54 kJ/mol
- Free energy of formation: -833.58 kJ/mol
- Heat capacity: 77.03 J/mol-K

- Mohs' hardness; 2.5
- Heat of Formation = -1096 kJ/mol

Pharmaceutical Formulations

- Milk of magnesia USP, is an aqueous suspension of magnesium hydroxide containing 7.0-8.5% of $Mg(OH)_2$. Each milliliter is capable of neutralizing approx 2.7 meq of acid. Magnesium hydroxide is also avail as magnesia tablets...generally contain 325 mg each, which can neutralize 11.2 meq of acid.
- USP; 250 ml & 500 ml Bottles with Aluminum Hydroxide Gel; 250 ml, 375 ml, 500 ml & 1 L Bottles.
- Suspension of 30% magnesium hydroxide in water: hydro-magma.
- Available generically: powder; tablets 300 mg & 600 mg.

Storage Conditions

- Store in a dry place. Keep container tightly closed. Protect from freezing and physical damage. Recommended storage temperature: $15-25°C$.

Uses

- Magnesium Hydroxide is a solution of magnesium hydroxide with antacid and laxative properties. Milk of magnesium exerts its antacid activity in low doses such that all hydroxide ions that enter the stomach are used to neutralize stomach acid. This agent exerts its laxative effect in higher doses so that hydroxide ions are able to move from the stomach to the intestines where they attract and retain water, thereby increasing intestinal movement (peristalsis) and inducing the urge to defecate.
- Magnesium dihydroxide is a magnesium hydroxide in which the magnesium atom is bound to two hydroxide groups. It has a role as an antacid and a flame retardant.
- Magnesium hydroxide is an inorganic compound. It is naturally found as the mineral brucite. Magnesium hydroxide can be used as an antacid or a laxative in either an oral liquid suspension or chewable tablet form. Additionally, magnesium hydroxide has smoke suppressing and flame retardant properties and is thus used commercially as a fire retardant. It can also be used topically as a deodorant or for the relief of canker sores (aphthous ulcers).

Magaldrate

Magaldrate is used to treat heartburn, sour stomach, acid indigestion, hyperphosphatemia, and magnesium deficiency. Magaldrate is used off-label to treat gastric and duodenal ulcers and gastroesophageal reflux disease (GERD).

Pharmaceutical formulations: Oral Suspension:540mg/5mL

Market preparations: Riopan, Iosopan, Lowsium, Maoson

Storage conditions: STORAGE: Store tablets and capsules at room temperature between 59- and 86-degrees F (15 to 30 degrees C) away from heat and light. The liquid form of this medication may be stored in the refrigerator to improve taste.

Uses: Magaldrate is an antacid. It neutralizes and reduces stomach acid relieving heartburn and indigestion. It is used to treat an upset stomach, ulcers, hiatal hernia and other digestive disorders.

Sodium Bicarbonate

Sodium bicarbonate is an antacid used to relieve heartburn and acid indigestion. It makes your blood or urine less acidic in certain conditions. This medication is sometimes prescribed for other uses; ask your doctor or pharmacist for more information

Pharmaceutical formulations: The bicarbonate of commerce is about 99.8% pure. Tablets found in 325 mg as Soda Mint (CMC). Parenteral Injection found as 5% (0.595 mEq/mL) (297.5 mEq) where Sodium Bicarbonate Injection (Available from one or more manufacturer, distributor, and/or repackager by generic (nonproprietary) name)

Market preparations: Sobicarwyn 500mg Tab, Nodosis Tab, Acidose Tab, Diosis 500mg Tab

Storage conditions: Stable in dry air, but slowly decomposes in moist air

Uses: Sodium bicarbonate is used in the treatment of metabolic acidosis associated with many conditions including severe renal disease (e.g., renal tubular acidosis), uncontrolled diabetes (ketoacidosis), extracorporeal circulation of the blood, cardiac arrest, circulatory insufficiency caused by shock or severe dehydration, ureterosigmoidostomy, lactic acidosis, alcoholic ketoacidosis, use of carbonic anhydrase inhibitors, and ammonium chloride administration. In metabolic acidosis, the principal disturbance is a loss of proton acceptors (e.g., loss of bicarbonate during severe diarrhea) or accumulation of an acid load (e.g., ketoacidosis, lactic acidosis, renal tubular acidosis).

Calcium Carbonate

Calcium carbonate appears as white, odorless powder or colorless crystals. Practically insoluble in water. Occurs extensive in rocks world-wide. Ground calcium carbonate (CAS: 1317-65-3) results directly from the mining of limestone. The extraction process keeps the carbonate very close to its original state of purity and delivers a finely ground product either in dry or slurry form. Precipitated calcium carbonate (CAS: 471-34-1) is produced industrially by the decomposition of limestone to calcium oxide followed by subsequent recarbonization or as a by-product of the Solvay process (which is used to make sodium carbonate). Precipitated calcium carbonate is purer than ground calcium carbonate and has different (and tailorable) handling properties.

Pharmaceutical formulations: dispersible, nonwettable. Found in: Tums, 500 mg; Tums-Extra strength, 750 mg. Both natural ground or precipitated calcium carbonate are available as dry products. Calcium carbonate slurry, primarily used in the paper industry, is typically >70% solids by weight for ground products and 20-50% solids by weight for precipitated. Some grades are surface coated to improve handling and dispersibility in plastics. Agents used for surface treatment used are fatty acids, resins, and wetting agents.

Market preparations: Alfashell, Calcibon (200 ml), AD – 3, M-Cal 500, Nutribone Plus, Calcikav, Calcium Sandoz, Cypacal Forte, Sunmic-OD, Calfit Tablet, Natica OS, Bio -Citral, Abce, Lycal -D 500, Caca, Caltaur (200 ml), Calci-3 (0.25mcg/500mg/7.5mg), Spcal, Calceedol

Storage conditions: Separated from acids, aluminium and ammonium salts.

Uses: Calcium carbonate is a dietary supplement used when the amount of calcium taken in the diet is not enough. Calcium is needed by the body for healthy bones, muscles, nervous system, and heart. Calcium carbonate also is used as an antacid to relieve heartburn, acid indigestion, and upset stomach.

Antimicrobial Agents

Silver Nitrate: Silver Nitrate is an inorganic chemical with antiseptic activity. Silver nitrate can potentially be used as a cauterizing or sclerosing agent. Silver nitrate is an inorganic compound with the chemical formula $AgNO_3$. In its solid form, silver nitrate is coordinated in a trigonal planar arrangement. It is often used as a precursor to other silver-containing compounds. It is used in making photographic films, and in laboratory setting as a staining agent in protein visualization in PAGE gels and in scanning electron microscopy.

Pharmaceutical formulations: Silver nitrate ophthalmic solution USP is solution of silver nitrate in water medium. it contains 0.95-1.05% of agno3. Solution may be buffered by addition of sodium acetate.

Market preparations: Silver Nitrate

Storage conditions: On exposure to air or light in the presence of organic matter, silver nitrate becomes grey or greyish-black. In the presence of a trace of nitric acid, silver nitrate is stable to 350 °C

Uses: Silver nitrate topical (for use on the skin) is used to cauterize infected tissues around a skin wound. Silver nitrate can also help create a scab to help stop bleeding from a minor skin wound. Silver nitrate is also used to help remove warts or skin tags.

Ionic Silver

Ionic silver solutions are not colloids. The silver ions (silver particles missing one outer orbital electron) can only exist in the solute. Once in contact with free ions or when the water evaporates, insoluble and sometimes undesirable silver compounds will form.

Uses: Ionic silver has been used for countless years as the "ultimate" antibiotic, antifungal and antiviral alternative. This natural element is believed to block the respiratory metabolism in bacteria

Chlorhexidine Gluconate

Chlorhexidine Gluconate is the gluconate salt form of chlorhexidine, a biguanide compound used as an antiseptic agent with topical antibacterial activity. Chlorhexidine gluconate is positively charged and reacts with the negatively charged microbial cell surface, thereby destroying the integrity of the cell membrane. Subsequently, chlorhexidine gluconate penetrates into the cell and causes leakage of intracellular components leading to cell death. Since gram positive bacteria are more negatively charged, they are more sensitive to this agent.

Pharmaceutical formulations: Trade names for various chlorhexidine salts and formulations: chlorhexidine: Sterilon, Hibitane, Rotersept; chlorhexidine dihydrochloride: Lisium, Arlacide H, AY-5312; chlorhexidine diacetate: Hibitane diacetate, Novalsan; chlorhexidine digluconate: Abacil, anti-Plaque, Arlacide G, Bacticlens, Chlorhexamed, Disteryl, Orahexal, Septeal, Unisept, Corsodyl, Hibiclens, Hibidil, Hibiscrub, Hibitane, Larylin, Peridex, Plac out, Plurexid, Rotersept, Savacol, Solvahex.

Storage conditions: Stored in a well closed container.

Market preparations: Hexinate, Acwash (60 ml), Tphexid Mouth Wash, Hygeen, Surgidine (100 ml), Mouden, Gluhex, Doff XL, Microshield (100ml), Sense -32, Arofil, A Fresh, Aroma, Dentra, Refresh Mouthwash, Hexin, Clohex, Daxoin, A.M-P.M, Rexidin (1000 ml)

Uses: Chlorhexidine gluconate is a germicidal mouthwash that reduces bacteria in the mouth. Chlorhexidine gluconate oral rinse is used to treat gingivitis (swelling, redness, bleeding gums). Chlorhexidine gluconate is usually prescribed by a dentist.

Hydrogen Peroxide

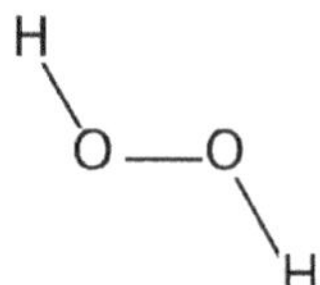

Classification: Microbiocide

Chemical Formula: H_2O_2

Molecular weight: 34.015

Synonyms: Hydroperoxide, Perhydrol, Oxydol

IUPAC Name: hydrogen peroxide

Properties

- Hydrogen peroxide, aqueous solution, stabilized, with more than 60% hydrogen peroxide appears as a colorless liquid. Vapors may irritate the eyes and mucous membranes. Under prolonged exposure to fire or heat containers may violently rupture due to decomposition. Used to bleach textiles and wood pulp, in chemical manufacturing and food processing.
- It is available in Dry Powder; Colorless Liquid with a slightly sharp odor and bitter taste.
- It is slightly acidic in nature.
- The boiling point is 302.4°F at 760 mm Hg.
- The melting point is 31.3°F.
- Soluble in cold water. Very soluble in water. Greater than or equal to 100 mg/mL at 72°F. Soluble in ether; insoluble in petroleum ether. Decomposed into water and oxygen by many organic solvents.
- Density is 1.44 g/cm^3 at 25°C.
- Weak acid; H_2O_2 concentration wt% = 35, 50, 70, 90; corresponding true pH: 4.6, 4.3, 4.4, 5.1
- The dissociation constant (pKa) is 11.62.
- The surface tension is 80.4 dynes/cm at 20°C.
- Vapor density is 1.02.
- Index of refraction: 1.4061 at 28°C.
- Heat of vaporization is 1519 J-g/K at 25°C.
- 1.97 mm Hg at 25°F.
- The logP is -1.36.
- Viscosity is 1.819 cP at 0°C; 1.249 cP at 20°C.
- Solutions of hydrogen peroxide gradually deteriorate and are usually stabilized by the addition of acetanilide or similar organic materials. Hydrogen peroxide

topical solution deteriorates upon standing or upon repeated agitation, undergoes accelerated decomposition when exposed to light or when in contact with many oxidizing or reducing substances, and decomposes suddenly when heated.

Pharmaceutical Formulations

- Valsterane Aseptic 35 Bio (Arkema Inc.): Active ingredient: hydrogen peroxide 35.00%.
- Edelweiss TBC II (Reckitt Benckiser LLC): Active ingredient: hydrogen peroxide 1.2%.
- Spor-Klenz Concentrate (Steris Corporation): Active ingredient: hydrogen peroxide 22.0%.

Storage Conditions

- Store in tightly closed containers in a cool, dry & well-ventilated place. Keep away from sunlight and combustible materials. Keep away from heat, sparks and flames.

Uses

Hydrogen Peroxide is a peroxide and oxidizing agent with disinfectant, antiviral and anti-bacterial activities.

Hydrogen peroxide is a colorless liquid at room temperature with a bitter taste. Small amounts of gaseous hydrogen peroxide occur naturally in the air. Hydrogen peroxide is unstable, decomposing readily to oxygen and water with release of heat. Although nonflammable, it is a powerful oxidizing agent that can cause spontaneous combustion when it comes in contact with organic material.

Hydrogen peroxide is found in many households at low concentrations (3-9%) for medicinal applications and as a clothes and hair bleach. In industry, hydrogen peroxide in higher concentrations is used as a bleach for textiles and paper, as a component of rocket fuels, and for producing foam rubber and organic chemicals.

Hydrogen peroxide, stabilized appears as a crystalline solid at low temperatures.

Some household applications include:
- Auto Products
- Commercial / Institutional
- Home Maintenance
- Inside the Home
- Landscaping/Yard
- Personal Care
- Pet Care

Boric Acid

Classification: Preservative

Chemical Formula: $B(OH)_3$

Molecular weight: 61.84

Synonyms: Boracic acid, Borofax

IUPAC Name: Orthoboric acid

Properties

- Boric acid is an odorless, faintly bitter, white solid. Melting point 171°C. Sinks and mixes with water.
- Dry Powder; Liquid; Other Solid forms are available.
- Colorless, odorless, transparent crystals or white granules or powder; slightly unctuous to the touch; occurs in nature as the mineral sassolite.
- The boiling point is 572°F at 760 mm Hg (decomposes).
- The melting point is 340°F.
- Soluble in hot water, partially soluble in cold water. Slightly unctuous to touch; volatile with steam; solubility in water increased by hydrochloric, citric or tartaric acids. Solubility in water is increased by hydrochloric acid. Solubility: in glycerol 17.5% at 25 °C; ethylene glycol 18.5% at 25 °C; in methanol 173.9 g/L at 25 °C; in ethanol 94.4 g/L at 25 °C; in acetone 0.6% at 25 °C; ethyl acetate 1.5% at 25 °C.
- The density is 1.435 at 68°F.
- The vapor pressure is 1.6×10^{-6} mm Hg at 25 °C.
- The LogP is 0.175.
- The pH is 3.8-4.8 (3.3 % aqueous solution)
- It is stable in air. Boric acid decomposes in heat above 100°C forming boric anhydride and water.

Pharmaceutical Formulations

- Three grades of granular and powdered boric acid are manufactured; technical grade, NF grade, and special quality grade.
- Single Active Ingredient Products: Wettable powder 99.0%; Dust 99.0%, 64.0%, and 65.0%; Liquid Concentrate 26.3%; Ready-to-Use Paste 50.0%; Pelleted/ Tableted 40.0%; Bait Tube 53.3%.
- Harris Famous Roach Tablets, Boric acid 40%.

Storage Conditions

- Keep in a tightly closed container, stored in a cooled, dry, ventilated area. Recommended storage temperature: $15 - 25°C$.

Uses

- Boric acid exhibits minimal bacteriostatic and antifungal activities. Boric acid is likely to mediate antifungal actions at high concentrations over prolonged exposures.
- Boric Acid is a weakly acidic hydrate of boric oxide with mild antiseptic, antifungal, and antiviral properties. The exact mechanism of action of boric acid is unknown; generally cytotoxic to all cells. It is used in the treatment of yeast infections and cold sores.

Bleaching Powder

Classification: Microbiocide

Chemical Formula: $Ca(ClO)_2$

Molecular weight: 142.98

Synonyms: Calcium hypochloride, Hypochlorous acid

IUPAC Name: Calcium; dihypochlorite

Properties

- Calcium hypochlorite appears as a white granular solid (or tablets compressed from the granules) with an odor of chlorine. Toxic, irritating to the skin. Noncombustible, but will accelerate the burning of combustible materials. Prolonged exposure to fire or heat may result in the vigorous decomposition of the material and rupture of the container.
- White solid (Granules or Pellets) in various forms with pungent odor (Strong chlorine odor).
- Decomposes at $100°C$ (melting point / boiling point).
- 21% in water at $25°C$.
- The density is 2.35 g/cm^3.
- All hypochlorite solutions are unstable, especially if acidified; slowly decompose on contact with air. Chlorinated lime is relatively unstable, even in solid form, and loses much of its activity over a period of a year. A complex compound of indefinite composition that rapidly decomposes on exposure to air. The 70% grade may decompose violently if exposed to heat or direct sunlight.
- Index of refraction is 1.545 (alpha); 1.69 (beta).

Pharmaceutical Formulations

- Grades: commercial (70%); high purity (99.2% available chlorine as calcium hypochlorite).
- Chloride of lime (35% calcium chlorine); highest calcium hypochlorite (70% available chlorine).
- Chlorinated lime consists of a mixture of calcium chloride and calcium hypochloride and should contain a minimum of 30% available chlorine.

Storage Conditions

- Keep container tightly closed. Keep in fireproof place.
- Store in a well-ventilated place.

Uses

- Disinfectant for drinking water and swimming pools; algicide; oxidizing agent; as household and industrial bleaching agent and sanitizer.
- Potable-water purification, bleaching agent (paper, textiles).
- Calcium hypochlorite is used to cleanup hydrazine spills.

Dental Products

Calcium Carbonate

Classification: Anti-caking Agent

Chemical Formula: $CaCO_3$

Molecular weight: 100.09

Synonyms: Calcite, Chalk

IUPAC Name: calcium; carbonate

Properties

- Calcium carbonate appears as white, odorless powder or colorless crystals. Practically insoluble in water. Occurs extensive in rocks world-wide. Ground calcium carbonate (CAS: 1317-65-3) results directly from the mining of limestone. The extraction process keeps the carbonate very close to its original state of purity and delivers a finely ground product either in dry or slurry form. Precipitated calcium carbonate (CAS: 471-34-1) is produced industrially by the decomposition of limestone to calcium oxide followed by subsequent recarbonization or as a by-product of the Solvay process (which is used to make sodium carbonate). Precipitated calcium carbonate is purer than ground calcium carbonate and has different (and tailorable) handling properties.

- Dry Powder; Liquid; Other Solid
- White crystalline or amorphous, odorless and tasteless powder.
- Calcium carbonate is soluble in concentrated mineral acids.
- Limestone (calcium carbonate) that has been recrystallized by metamorphism and is capable of taking a polish. Practically insoluble in water.
- White hexagonal crystals or powder (Calcite); white orthrombic crystals or powder (Argonite); colorless hexagonal crystals (vaterite).
- The melting point lies in the range 1517 to 2442 °F (Decomposes).
- Practically insoluble in water and in alcohol. Dissolves with effervescence in diluted acetic acid, in diluted hydrochloric acid and in diluted nitric acid, and the resulting solutions, after boiling, give positive tests for calcium.
- Solubility Product constant: 3.36×10^{-9} at 25°C.
- The density is 2.7 to 2.95 g/cm³.
- Indefinite shelf life. Stable in air. When heated to decomposition it emits acrid smoke and irritating vapors. At about 825 °C it decomposes into calcium oxide and carbon dioxide.
- Non-corrosive.
- The pH lies in range 8 to 9.
- Index of Refraction: 1.7216 (300 nm); 1.6584 (589 nm); 1.6503 (750 nm).
- Vapor pressure is 0 mm Hg.

Pharmaceutical Formulations
- Formulations: dispersible, non-wettable.
- Found in: Tums, 500 mg; Tums-Extra strength, 750 mg.
- Filler grades; USP grades; technical grades; high-purity grades; and specialty grades.
- Both natural ground and precipitated calcium carbonate are available as dry products. Calcium carbonate slurry, primarily used in the paper industry, is typically >70% solids by weight for ground products and 20-50% solids by weight for precipitated. Some grades are surface coated to improve handling and dispersibility in plastics. Agents used for surface treatment used are fatty acids, resins, and wetting agents.

Storage Conditions
- Store in a cool, dry place. Store in a tightly closed container. Protect from moisture.

Uses
- Calcium Carbonate is the carbonic salt of calcium (CaCO3). Calcium carbonate is used therapeutically as a phosphate buffer in hemodialysis, as an antacid in

gastric hyperacidity for temporary relief of indigestion and heartburn, and as a calcium supplement for preventing and treating osteoporosis.

Sodium Fluoride

$$F-Na$$

Classification: Antiplaque

Chemical Formula: NaF

Molecular weight: 41.988

Synonyms: Fluoristat, Ossin, Zymafluor

IUPAC Name: Sodium; fluoride

Properties

- Sodium fluoride is a colorless crystalline solid or white powder, or the solid dissolved in a liquid. It is soluble in water. It is noncombustible. It is corrosive to aluminum. It is used as an insecticide. It is also used to fluorinate water supplies, as a wood preservative, in cleaning compounds, manufacture of glass, and for many other uses.
- Colorless, cubic or tetragonal crystals.
- Odorless with salty taste.
- The boiling point is 3083°F at 760 mm Hg.
- The melting point is 1819°F.
- The solubility is 10 to 50 mg/mL at 73°F. Solubility in water 4.0 g/100 ml water at 15 °C. Solubility in water 4.3 g/100 ml water at 25 °C. Solubility in water 5.0 g/100 ml water at 100 °C. Insoluble in alcohol.
- The density is 2.79 at 68°F.
- The vapor pressure is 1 mm Hg at 1971°F ; 5 mm Hg at 2167°F
- Not flammable
- When heated to decomposition it emits toxic fumes of hydrogen fluoride and disodium oxide.
- Freshly prepared saturated solution is 7.4.
- Index of refraction is 1.336.

Pharmaceutical Formulations

- Commercial grade (purity 93-99%) is used to prepare baits.
- Technical grades are 90% and 95% NaF, light (37 cu in/lb) and dense (23 cu in/lb), and 98%.
- Sodium fluoride solution contains not less than 95% and not more than 105.0% of the labeled amount of sodium fluoride, USP XXI.
- The purity of the commercial material is about 98%.

Storage Conditions

- Keep in a tightly closed container, stored in a cool, dry, ventilated area. Protect against physical damage. Separate from acids and oxidizing materials.

Uses

- Sodium fluoride protects the teeth from acid demineralization while preventing tooth decay by bacteria while strengthening tooth enamel. It is important to note that excess fluoride exposure during tooth mineralization, especially in children 1-3 years old, may cause fluorosis. It is a condition manifested by white lines, pitting, or discoloration of teeth resulting from changes in tooth enamel. The risk of fluorosis can be decreased by the use of a rice-size amount of fluoridated toothpaste in children younger than 3 years old.
- Sodium Fluoride is an inorganic salt of fluoride used topically or in municipal water fluoridation systems to prevent dental caries. Fluoride appears to bind to calcium ions in the hydroxyapatite of surface tooth enamel, preventing corrosion of tooth enamel by acids. This agent may also inhibit acid production by commensal oral bacteria.

Medicinal Gases

Carbon Dioxide

$$\ddot{O} = C = \ddot{O}$$

Classification: Propellant

Chemical Formula: CO_2

Molecular weight: 44.009

Synonyms: Anhydride, Carbonic; Dry ice

IUPAC Name: Dioxide; Carbon

Properties

- Carbon dioxide appears as a colorless, odorless, and faint acid taste gas at atmospheric temperatures and pressures. Relatively nontoxic and noncombustible. Heavier than air and may asphyxiate by the displacement of air. Soluble in water. Forms carbonic acid, a mild acid. Under prolonged exposure to heat or fire the container may rupture violently and rocket.
- CO_2 sublimes at boiling point and melts at -109.3°F. Solubility in water (mL CO2/100 mL H2O at 760 mm Hg): 171 at 0°C; 88 at 20 °C; 36 at 60°C.

- The density is 1.56 at -110.2°F.
- It is 0.2 % soluble at 77°F
- The pH of saturated CO_2 solutions varies from 3.7 at 101 kPa (1 atm) to 3.2 at 2370 kPa (23.4 atm).
- The heat of vaporization is 83.12 g-cal/g.
- The surface tension is 0.0162 Newtons/meter.
- Index of refraction is 1.6630 at 24°C.
- Heat of formation: -393.51 kJ/mol; Entropy: 213.785 J/K-mol.
- Stable under recommended storage conditions.
- Gas is not affected by heat until temp reaches about 2000°C. The substance decomposes on heating above 2000°C producing toxic carbon monoxide.
- The viscosity is 21.29 uPa-sec at 300 K.

Pharmaceutical Formulations
- Grades: Technical, United States Pharmacopeia, commercial and welding, 99.5%, bone dry (99.95%).
- Usually marketed in steel cylinders (under sufficient pressure to keep it liquid) or in solid form as Dry Ice.
- Available in gas, liquid and solid form.
- RADAR aerosol rodenticide containing 2.8 g pressurized CO_2, purity > 99%.

Storage Conditions
- It is stored in porous geological formations that are typically located several kilometers under the earth's surface, with pressure and temperatures such that carbon dioxide will be in the liquid or "supercritical phase".

Uses
- Carbon dioxide is used as a pesticide for insect control in stored grain under modified atmospheres containing approx 60% carbon dioxide.
- Rodenticide (mice and rats).
- Refrigerant; processing of foods; preserving foods; crusting of food; cryogenic freezing of food; production of urea, sodium carbonate (Solvay process), methanol, carbonic acid, lead carbonate, potassium carbonate, potassium bicarbonate, ammonium carbonate, ammonium bicarbonate, sodium salicylate, carbonated petroleum, hydrocarbon products; provides an inert atmosphere for fire extinguishers, refinery products, petroleum products; displacing oxygen to prevent deterioration and flavor loss; in high pressure applications; oil well stimulation; in livestock slaughtering; as fertilizer; hardening of molds for metal castings.

Nitrous Oxide

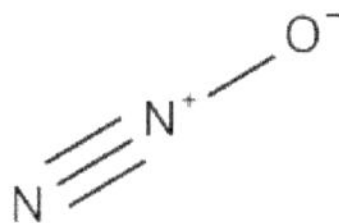

Classification: Propellant

Chemical Formula: N_2O

Molecular weight: 44.013

Synonyms: Dinitrogen oxide, Dinitrogen monoxide

IUPAC Name: Nitrous oxide

Properties

- Nitrous oxide is a colorless, slightly sweetish odor, and sweet-tasting gas. It is also known as "laughing gas". Continued breathing of the vapors may impair the decision making process. It is noncombustible but it will accelerate the burning of combustible material in a fire. It is soluble in water. Its vapors are heavier than air. Exposure of the container to prolonged heat or fire can cause it to rupture violently and rocket.
- The boiling point is -129.1°F at 760 mm Hg.
- The melting point is –131.5°F.
- The aqueous solubility is 130 mL/100 mL water at 0°C, 56.7 mL/100 mL water at 25°C. Soluble in ethanol, ethyl ether. Soluble in alcohol, ether, oils; freely soluble in sulfuric acid.
- The density is 1.266 at -128.2°F.
- The vapor pressure is 51.3 atm.
- The LogP is 0.36.
- 0.0145 cP at 25°C at 101.325 KPa
- Stable under recommended storage conditions. Very stable and rather inert chemically at room temperatures.
- This compound decomposes explosively at high temperatures.

Pharmaceutical Formulations

- Nitrous oxide contains not less than 99.0%, by volume, of nitrous oxide. The remainder is chiefly nitrogen.
- Entonox is a 50:50 combination of nitrous oxide and oxygen.

Storage Conditions

- Store away from direct sunlight in a dry, cool and well-ventilated area, away from incompatible materials.

- Cylinders should be stored upright, with valve protection cap in place, and firmly secured to prevent falling or being knocked over. Cylinder temperatures should not exceed 52 °C (125 °F).

Uses

- Nitrous Oxide is a naturally occurring gas that is colorless and non flammable. It can be manufactured and used for a variety of things such as a pharmacologic agent to produce anesthesia, a food additive as a propellant, and an additive to fuels to increase available oxygen in combustion.

Oxygen

$$\ddot{O} = \ddot{O}$$

Classification: Propellant

Chemical Formula: O_2

Molecular weight: 31.999

Synonyms: Dioxygen; Oxygen-16

IUPAC Name: Molecular oxygen

Properties

- Oxygen is a colorless, odorless and tasteless gas. It will support life. It is non-combustible, but will actively support the burning of combustible materials. Some materials that will not burn in air will burn in oxygen. Materials that burn in air will burn more vigorously in oxygen. As a non-liquid gas it is shipped at pressures of 2000 psig or above. Pure oxygen is nonflammable. Under prolonged exposure to fire or intense heat the containers may rupture violently and rocket. Oxygen is used in the production of synthesis gas from coal, for resuscitation and as an inhalant.
- Liquid; Gas Vapor; Other Solid.
- Colorless, odorless, tasteless, non-flammable gas.
- Turns into slightly bluish liquid at -183°C.
- Boiling point is -297.3°F at 760 mm Hg.
- Melting point is -361°F.
- Solubility is 39mg/L. 1 volume gas dissolves in 32 volume water at 20 °C, in 7 volume alcohol at 20 °C; soluble in other organic liquids and usually to a greater extent than in water.
- The density is 1.14 at -297.4°F.
- LogP is 0.65.

- The viscosity is Gas: 101.325 kPa at 25°C (0.020 75 cP); Liquid: 99.70 K (0.156 cP).
- Liquid: liquid-surface tension: 13.47 dynes/cm= 0.01347 N/m @ -183°C.
- Index of refraction: liquid: 1.2243 at -181°C/D.

Pharmaceutical Formulations

- Liquid: Purity: 99.5+%.
- Grades: low purity; high purity; USP.
- Type I, gas, Grades, O_2 min: A, 99.0%; B, 99.5%; C, 99.5%; D, 99.5%; E, 99.6%; F, 99.995%.
- Type II liquid, grades, O_2 min: A, 99.0%; B, 99.5%; C, 99.5%; D, 99.5%.
- Oxygen is now manufactured in only 2 grades: grade A, aviator's breathing oxygen, and grade B, for industrial or medical purposes.

Storage Conditions

- Oxygen may not be stored with other flammable gases or liquids. Oxygen cylinders must maintain a minimum distance of 20 feet from combustibles (5 feet if room is sprinklered) or be placed within an enclosed cabinet having a fire rating of at least a half hour. Cylinders must be secured in racks or by chains.

Characteristics

- Oxygen is a colorless, odorless and tasteless gas. It will support life. It is non-combustible, but will actively support the burning of combustible materials. Some materials that will not burn in air will burn in oxygen. Materials that burn in air will burn more vigorously in oxygen. As a non-liquid gas it is shipped at pressures of 2000 psig or above. Pure oxygen is nonflammable. Under prolonged exposure to fire or intense heat the containers may rupture violently and rocket. Oxygen is used in the production of synthesis gas from coal, for resuscitation and as an inhalant.
- Oxygen is an element displayed by the symbol O, and atomic number 8. It is an essential element for human survival. Decreased oxygen levels may be treated with medical oxygen therapy. Treatment with oxygen serves to increase blood oxygen levels and also exerts a secondary effect of decreasing blood flow resistance in the diseased lung, leading to decreased cardiovascular workload in an attempt to oxygenate the lungs. Oxygen therapy is used to treat emphysema, pneumonia, some heart disorders (congestive heart failure), some disorders that cause increased pulmonary artery pressure, and any disease that impairs the body's ability to take up and use gaseous oxygen. Higher level of oxygen than ambient air (hyperoxia) can be introduced under normobaric or hyperbaric conditions.

Uses

- Supplemental oxygen is indicated when normal oxygenation is impaired because of pulmonary injury, which may result from aspiration (chemical pneumonitis) or inhalation of toxic gases. The PO_2 should be maintained at 70-80 mm Hg or higher if possible.
- Supplemental oxyugen usually is given empirically to patients with altered mental status or suspected hypoxemia.
- Oxygen (100%) is indicated for patients with carbon monoxide poisoning, to increase the conversion of carboxyhemoglobin and carboxymyoblobin to hemoglobin and myoglobin, and to increase oxygen saturation of the plasma and subsequent delivery to tissues.
- Hyperbaric oxygen (HBO) (100%) oxygen delivered to the patient in a pressurized chamber at 2-3 atm of pressure) may be beneficial for patients with severe carbon monoxide (CO) poisoning. It can hasten the reversal of CO binding to hemoglobin and intracellular myoglobin, can provide oxygen independent of hemoglobin, and may have protective actions in reducing postischemic brain damage.

Points to Remember

- Ferrous sulfate replenishes iron, an essential component in hemoglobin, myoglobin, and various enzymes.
- Ferrous gluconate is used as a hematinic. Iron is an essential heavy metal that is included in many over-the-counter multivitamin and mineral supplements and is used therapeutically in higher doses to treat or prevent iron deficiency anemia. When taken at the usual recommended daily allowance or in replacement doses, iron has little or no adverse effect on the liver. In high doses and in intentional or accidental overdoses, iron causes serious toxicities, one component of which is acute liver damage.
- Aluminum hydroxide gel is white, viscous suspension contains equivalent of 3.6-4.4% aluminum oxide in form of aluminum hydroxide and hydrated oxide.
- Aluminum Hydroxide is an inorganic compound containing aluminum. Used in various immunologic preparations to improve immunogenicity, aluminum hydroxide adjuvant consists of aluminum hydroxide gel in a saline solution. In vaccines, this agent binds to the protein conjugate, resulting in improved antigen processing by the immune system.
- Calcium Carbonate is the carbonic salt of calcium ($CaCO_3$). Calcium carbonate is used therapeutically as a phosphate buffer in hemodialysis, as an antacid in

gastric hyperacidity for temporary relief of indigestion and heartburn, and as a calcium supplement for preventing and treating osteoporosis.
- Sodium fluoride protects the teeth from acid demineralization while preventing tooth decay by bacteria while strengthening tooth enamel. It is important to note that excess fluoride exposure during tooth mineralization, especially in children 1-3 years old, may cause fluorosis.
- Boric acid exhibits minimal bacteriostatic and antifungal activities. Boric acid is likely to mediate antifungal actions at high concentrations over prolonged exposures.
- Nitrous oxide is a colorless, slightly sweetish odor, and sweet-tasting gas. It is also known as "laughing gas".
- Carbon dioxide is used as a pesticide for insect control in stored grain under modified atmospheres containing approx 60% carbon dioxide.
- Supplemental oxygen is indicated when normal oxygenation is impaired because of pulmonary injury, which may result from aspiration (chemical pneumonitis) or inhalation of toxic gases.

Multiple Choice Questions

1. What is the chemical name of bleaching powder?
   (A)   Calcium oxychloride
   (B)   Calcium hydroxide
   (C)   Calcium carbonate
   (D)   Calcium chloride

2. Bleaching powder (chemically known as calcium chloro hypochlorite) is commercially produced by the action of chlorine on?
   (A)   Slaked lime
   (B)   Soda lime
   (C)   Calcium perchlorate
   (D)   None of these

3. Bleaching powder contains?
   (A)   Nitrogen
   (B)   Iodine
   (C)   Chlorine
   (D)   Bromine

4. Aluminium hydroxide is principally used as
   (A)   Antiseptic
   (B)   Anti-oxidant
   (C)   Antacid
   (D)   Diuretic

5. Dried aluminium hydroxide gel contains
   (A)   Hydrated aluminium oxide
   (B)   Small quantities of basic aluminium carbonate and bicarbonate
   (C)   Both A and B
   (D)   None of these

6. The nature of Aluminium hydroxide is
   (A) Basic
   (B) Acidic
   (C) Amphoteric
   (D) None of them

7. Another name for magnesium hydroxide is what?
   (A) Milk of magnesia
   (B) Power of magnesia
   (C) Fruit of magnesia
   (D) Magnolia

8. What is the most common side effect of magnesium hydroxide?
   (A) Diarrhea
   (B) Constipation
   (C) Infrequent urination
   (D) Headaches

9. What is the chemical formula of magnesium hydroxide?
   (A) Mg_2O_2H
   (B) $Mg(OH)_2$
   (C) $MgOH$
   (D) Mg_2OH

10. Aqueous solution of borax is
    (A) Acidic nature
    (B) Basic nature
    (C) Neutral nature
    (D) None of them

CHAPTER 4

Introduction to Nomenclature of Organic Chemical Systems

Introduction

The purpose of the International Union of Pure and Applied Chemistry (IUPAC) system of nomenclature is to establish an international standard of naming compounds to facilitate communication. The goal of this unit is to give each structure a unique and unambiguous name, and to correlate each name with a unique and unambiguous structure. Special emphasis has been provided to organic chemical systems as well as heterocyclic compounds (upto 3-ring systems).

IUPAC system of nomenclature

IUPAC nomenclature is based on naming a molecule's longest chain of carbons connected by single bonds, whether in a continuous chain or in a ring. All deviations, either multiple bonds or atoms other than carbon and hydrogen, are indicated by prefixes or suffixes according to a specific set of priorities.

IUPAC system of nomenclature for Alkanes and Cycloalkanes.

Alkanes are the family of saturated hydrocarbons, that is, molecules containing carbon and hydrogen connected by single bonds only. These molecules can be in continuous chains (called linear or acyclic), or in rings (called cyclic or alicyclic). The names of alkanes and cycloalkanes are the root names of organic compounds. Beginning with the five-carbon alkane, the number of carbons in the chain is indicated by the Greek or Latin prefix. Rings are designated by the prefix "cyclo" (In the geometrical symbols for rings, each apex represents a carbon with the number of hydrogens required to fill its valence).

CH_4	methane	$CH_3[CH_2]_{10}CH_3$	dodecane
CH_3CH_3	ethane	$CH_3[CH_2]_{11}CH_3$	tridecane
$CH_3CH_2CH_3$	propane	$CH_3[CH_2]_{12}CH_3$	tetradecane
$CH_3[CH_2]_2CH_3$	butane	$CH_3[CH_2]_{18}CH_3$	icosane
$CH_3[CH_2]_3CH_3$	pentane	$CH_3[CH_2]_{19}CH_3$	henicosane
$CH_3[CH_2]_4CH_3$	hexane	$CH_3[CH_2]_{20}CH_3$	docosane
$CH_3[CH_2]_5CH_3$	heptane	$CH_3[CH_2]_{21}CH_3$	tricosane
$CH_3[CH_2]_6CH_3$	octane	$CH_3[CH_2]_{28}CH_3$	triacontane
$CH_3[CH_2]_7CH_3$	nonane	$CH_3[CH_2]_{29}CH_3$	hentriacontane
$CH_3[CH_2]_8CH_3$	decane	$CH_3[CH_2]_{38}CH_3$	tetracontane
$CH_3[CH_2]_9CH_3$	undecane	$CH_3[CH_2]_{48}CH_3$	pentacontane

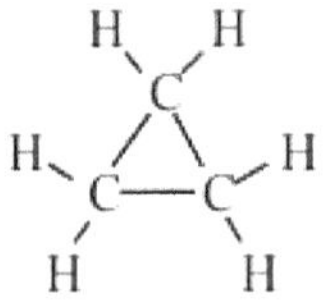

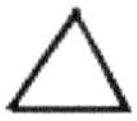

cyclopropane   cyclobutane 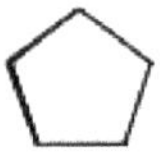   cyclopentane

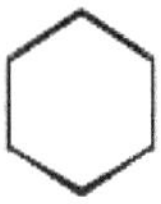

cyclohexane 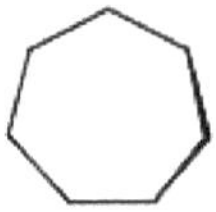   cycloheptane 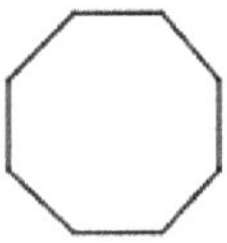   cyclooctane

IUPAC System of Nomenclature for Molecules Containing Substituents and Functional Groups

A. Priorities of Substituents and Functional Groups: Listed here from highest to lowest priority, except that the substituents within Group C have equivalent priority.

Group A - Functional Groups Indicated by Prefix or Suffix

Family of Compound	Structure	Prefix	Suffix
Carboxylic Acid	$R-\overset{\overset{O}{\|\|}}{C}-OH$	carboxy-	-oic acid (-carboxylic acid)
Aldehyde	$R-\overset{\overset{O}{\|\|}}{C}-H$	oxo- (formyl)	-al (carbaldehyde)
Ketone	$R-\overset{\overset{O}{\|\|}}{C}-R$	oxo-	-one
Alcohol	$R-O-H$	hydroxy-	-ol
Amine	$R-N\big\langle$	amino-	-amine

Group B - Functional Groups Indicated By Suffix Only

Family of Compound	Structure	Prefix	Suffix
Alkene	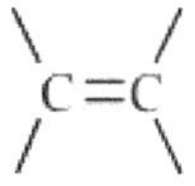 $\diagdown C = C \diagdown$	--------	-ene
Alkyne	$—C\equiv C—$	--------	-yne

Group C - Substituents Indicated by Prefix Only

Substituent	Structure	Prefix	Suffix
Alkyl (see list below)	R—	alkyl-	----------
Alkoxy	R—O—	alkoxy-	----------
Halogen	F —	fluoro-	----------
	Cl —	chloro-	----------
	Br —	bromo-	----------
	I —	iodo-	----------

Miscellaneous substituents and their prefixes

$—NO_2$ $—CH=CH_2$ $—CH_2CH=CH_2$

nitro   vinyl   allyl

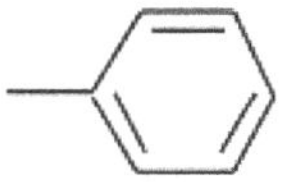

phenyl

Common alkyl groups - replace "ane" ending of alkane name with "yl". Alternate names for complex substituents are given in brackets.

$—CH_3$
methyl

$—CH_2CH_3$
ethyl

$—CH_2CH_2CH_3$
propyl (*n*-propyl)

$—CH_2CH_2CH_2CH_3$
butyl (*n*-butyl)

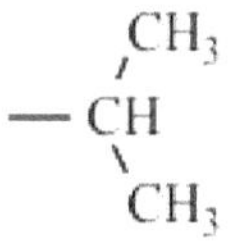

isopropyl
[1-methylethyl]

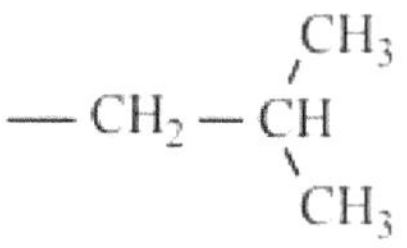

isobutyl
[2-methylpropyl]

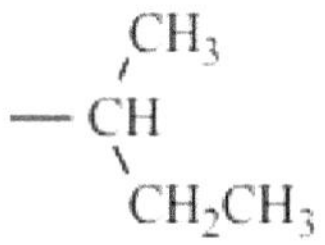

sec-butyl
[1-methylpropyl]

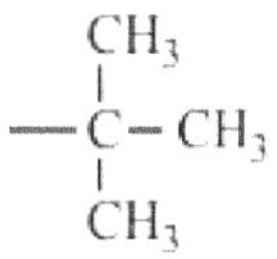

tert-butyl or *t*-butyl
[1,1-dimethylethyl]

B. Naming Substituted Alkanes and Cycloalkanes - Group C Substituents Only

1. Organic compounds containing substituents from Group C are named following this sequence of steps, as indicated on the examples below:

Step 1. Find the longest continuous carbon chain. Determine the root name for this parent chain. In cyclic compounds, the ring is usually considered the parent chain, unless it is attached to a longer chain of carbons; indicate a ring with the prefix "cyclo" before the root name. (When there are two longest chains of equal length, use the chain with the greater number of substituents.)

Step 2. Number the chain in the direction such that the position number of the first substituent is the smaller number. If the first substituents from either end have the same number, then number so that the second substituent has the smaller number, etc.

Step 3. Determine the name and position number of each substituent. (A substituent on a nitrogen is designated with an "N" instead of a number; see Section III.D.1. below.)

Step 4. Indicate the number of identical groups by the prefixes di, tri, tetra, etc.

Step 5. Place the position numbers and names of the substituent groups, in alphabetical order, before the root name. In alphabetizing, ignore prefixes like sec-, tert-, di, tri, etc., but include iso and cyclo. Always include a position number for each substituent, regardless of redundancies.

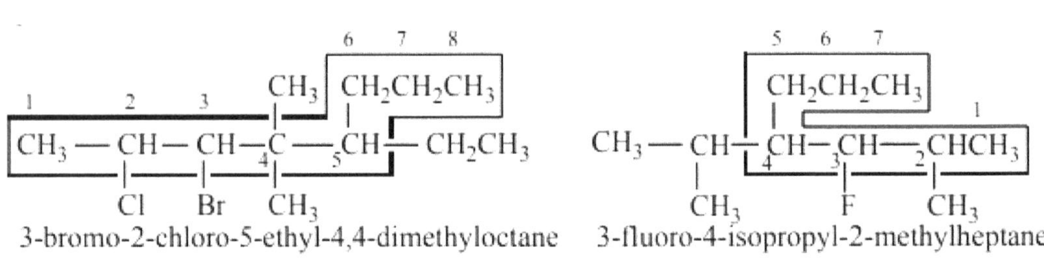

C. Naming Molecules Containing Functional Groups from Group B - Suffix Only

1. Alkenes - Follow the same steps as for alkanes, except:

(a)   Number the chain of carbons that includes the C=C so that the C=C has the lower position number, since it has a higher priority than any substituents;

(b)   Change "ane" to "ene" and assign a position number to the first carbon of the C =C;

(c)   Designate geometrical isomers with a cis, trans or E,Z prefix.

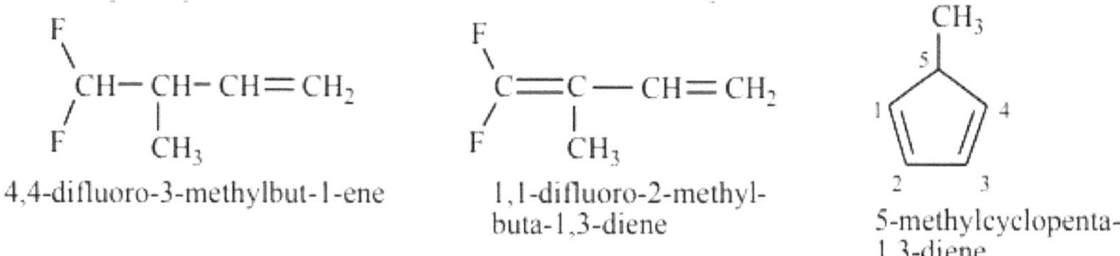

4,4-difluoro-3-methylbut-1-ene

1,1-difluoro-2-methyl-
buta-1,3-diene

5-methylcyclopenta-
1,3-diene

2.   Alkynes - Follow the same steps as for alkanes, except:

(a)   Number the chain of carbons that includes the C=C so that the functional group has the lower position number;

(b)   Change "ane" to "yne" and assign a position number to the first carbon of the C=C.

4,4-difluoro-3-methylbut-1-yne

pent-3-en-1-yne

("yne" closer to end of chain)

pent-1-en-4-yne

("ene" and "yne" have equal priority unless they have the same position number, when "ene" takes the lower number)

D. Naming Molecules Containing Functional Groups from Group A - Prefix or Suffix

In naming molecules containing one or more of the functional groups in Group A, the group of highest priority is indicated by suffix; the others are indicated by prefix, with priority equivalent to any other substituents. Now that the functional groups and substituents from Groups A, B, and C have been described, a modified set of steps for naming organic compounds can be applied to all simple structures:

Step 1. Find the highest priority functional group. Determine and name the longest continuous carbon chain that includes this group.

Step 2. Number the chain so that the highest priority functional group is assigned the lower number.

Step 3. If the carbon chain includes multiple bonds (Group B), replace "ane" with "ene" for an alkene or "yne" for an alkyne. Designate the position of the multiple bond with the number of the first carbon of the multiple bond.

Step 4. If the molecule includes Group A functional groups, replace the last "e" with the suffix of the highest priority functional group, and include its position number.

Step 5. Indicate all Group C substituents, and Group A functional groups of lower priority, with a prefix. Place the prefixes, with appropriate position numbers, in alphabetical order before the root name.

1. Amines: prefix: amino-; suffix: -amine—substituents on nitrogen denoted by "N"

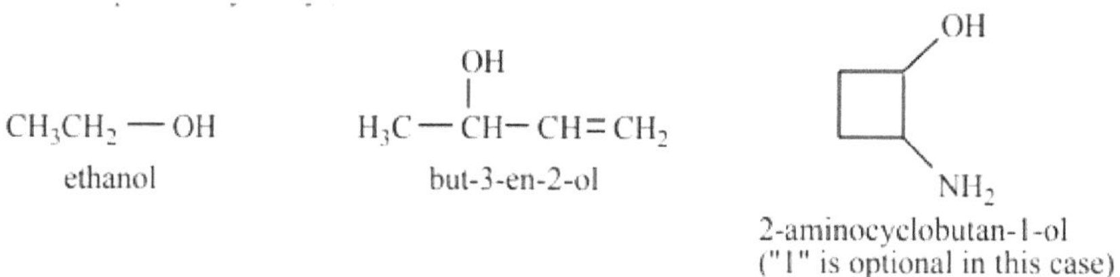

$CH_3CH_2CH_2 - NH_2$

propan-1-amine

3-methoxycyclohexan-1-amine
("1" is optional in this case)

N,N-diethylbut-3-en-2-amine

2. Alcohols: prefix: hydroxy-; suffix: -ol

$CH_3CH_2 - OH$

ethanol

but-3-en-2-ol

2-aminocyclobutan-1-ol
("1" is optional in this case)

3. Ketones: prefix: oxo-; suffix: -one

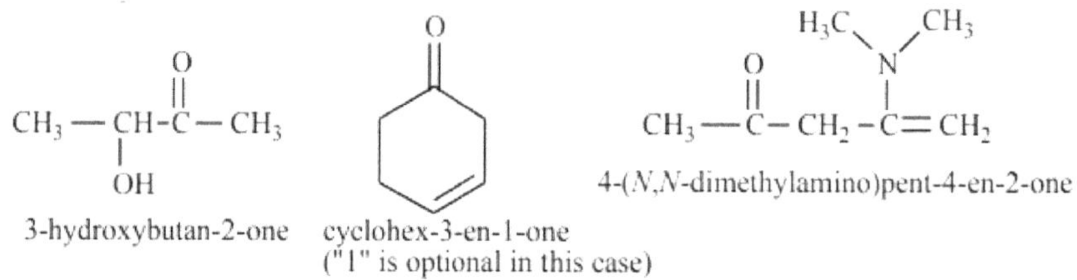

3-hydroxybutan-2-one

cyclohex-3-en-1-one
("1" is optional in this case)

4-(N,N-dimethylamino)pent-4-en-2-one

4. Aldehydes: prefix: oxo-, or formyl- (O=CH-); suffix: -al (abbreviation: — CHO). An aldehyde can only be on carbon 1, so the "1" is generally omitted from the name.

O
||
HCH

methanal;
formaldehyde

O
||
CH₃ — CH

ethanal;
acetaldehyde

OH
|
CH₂ · CH= CH−CH

4-hydroxybut-2-enal

O
||
CH₃CCH₂CH₂ — CH

4-oxopentanal

Special case: When the chain cannot include the carbon of the CHO, the suffix "carbaldehyde" is used:

cyclohexanecarbaldehyde

5. Carboxylic Acids: prefix: carboxy-; suffix: -oic acid (abbreviation: —COOH). A carboxylic acid can only be on carbon 1, so the "1" is generally omitted from the name.

O
||
HC — OH

methanoic acid;
formic acid

O
||
CH₃C — OH

ethanoic acid;
acetic acid

— CH₂ - CH− COH
|
NH₂

2-amino-3-phenylpropanoic acid

O O CH₃
|| || |
HC —C—C— COOH
|
CH₃

2,2-dimethyl-3,4-dioxobutanoic acid

E. Naming Carboxylic Acid Derivatives

1. Salts of Carboxylic Acids: Salts are named with cation first, followed by the anion name of the carboxylic acid, where "ic acid" is replaced by "ate":

acet**ic acid**	becomes	acet**ate**
butano**ic acid**	becomes	butano**ate**
cyclohexanecarboxyl**ic acid**	becomes	cyclohexanecarboxyl**ate**

2. Esters: Esters are named as "organic salts" that is, the alkyl name comes first, followed by the name of the carboxylate anion. (common abbreviation: —COOR)

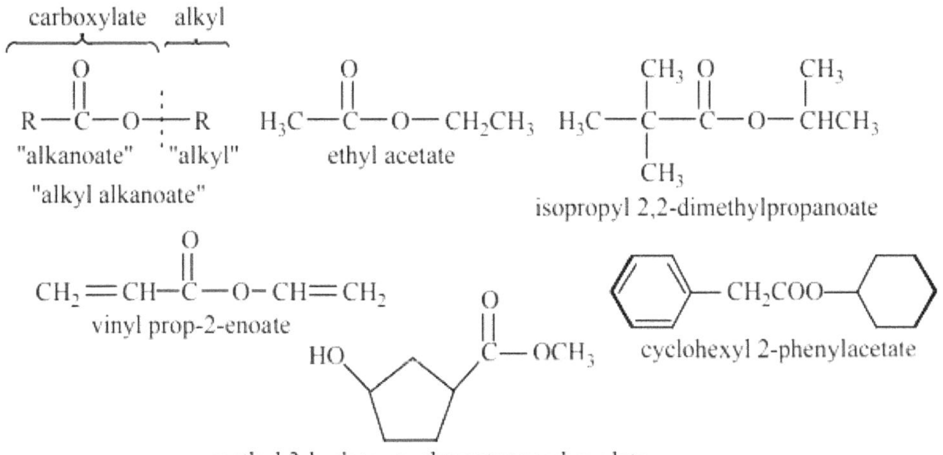

IUPAC System of Nomenclature for Aromatic Compounds

"Aromatic" compounds are those derived from benzene and similar ring systems. As with aliphatic nomenclature described above, the process is: determining the root name of the parent ring; determining priority, name, and position number of substituents; and assembling the name in alphabetical order. Functional group priorities are the same in aliphatic and aromatic nomenclature.

A. Common Parent Ring Systems

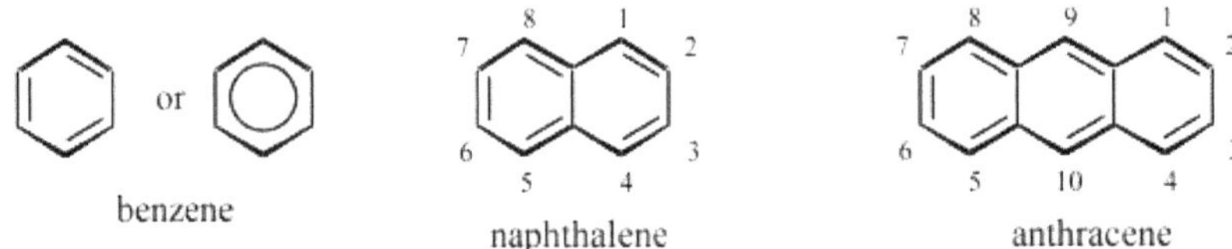

benzene   naphthalene   anthracene

B. Monosubstituted Benzenes

1. Most substituents keep their designation, followed by the word "benzene":

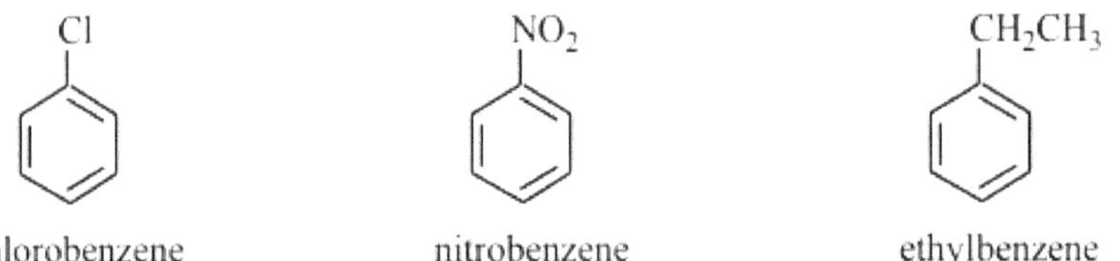

chlorobenzene   nitrobenzene   ethylbenzene

2. Some common substituents change the root name of the ring. IUPAC accepts these as root names, listed here in decreasing priority:

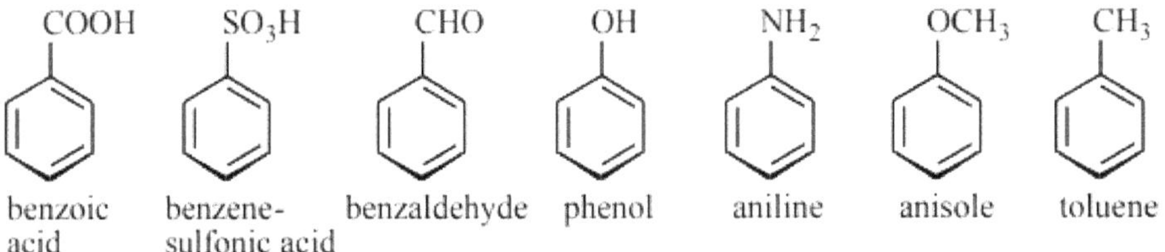

benzoic acid   benzene-sulfonic acid   benzaldehyde   phenol   aniline   anisole   toluene

C. Disubstituted Benzenes

1. Designation of substitution - only three possibilities:

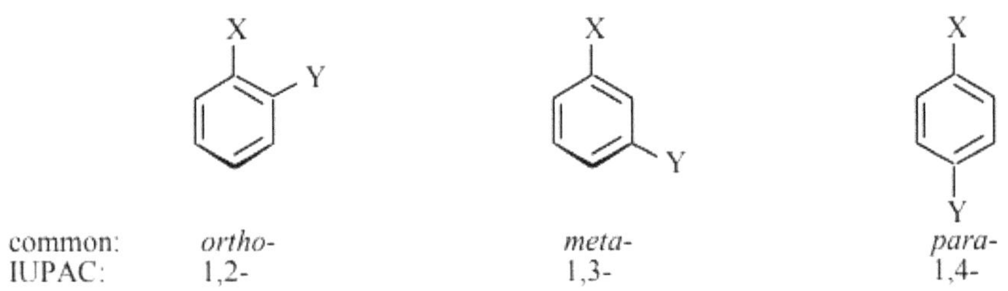

| common: | ortho- | meta- | para- |
| IUPAC: | 1,2- | 1,3- | 1,4- |

2. Naming disubstituted benzenes - Priorities determine root name and substituents

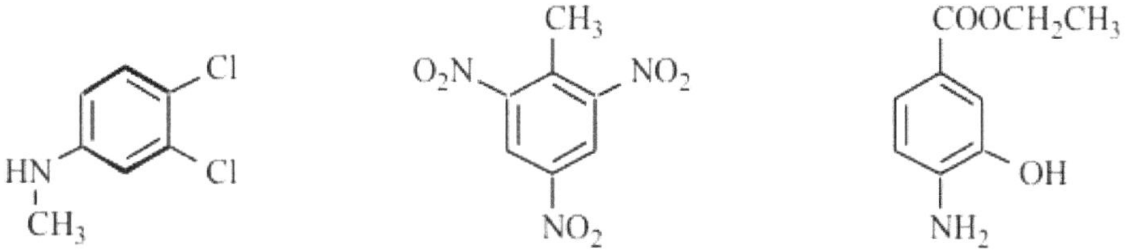

1,4-dibromobenzene   3-aminobenzoic acid   2-methoxybenzaldehyde   3-methylphenol

D. Polysubstituted Benzenes

3,4-dichloro-*N*-methylaniline   2,4,6-trinitrotoluene (TNT)   ethyl 4-amino-3-hydroxybenzoate

E. Aromatic Ketones

A special group of aromatic compounds are ketones where the carbonyl is attached to at least one benzene ring. Such compounds are named as "phenones", the prefix depending on the size and nature of the group on the other side of the carbonyl. These are the common examples:

acetophenone

propiophenone

butyrophenone

benzophenone

Nomenclature of Heterocyclic Compounds

The heterocyclic compounds are the cyclic compounds in which one or more carbon atom is replaced by the atom like N, O, S, P, Si, then such compounds are called as heterocyclic compounds and the atoms like N, O, S, P, Si are known as heteroatoms.

Rules for the nomenclature of heterocyclic compounds:

1. The name of heterocyclic compounds are derived by a prefix indicating the nature of hetero-atoms as

Name	Prefix
Oxygen	oxa
Nitrogen	aza / pyra
Sulphur	thia
Phosphorus	phospha
Silicon	silica

2. Different suffix are used depending on the number of atoms present in the ring as ,

Name	Suffix
3 membered	iridine
4 membered	Edane
5 membered	Ole
6 membered	Ine
7 membered	Epine
8 membered	Ocine
9 membered	Onine

3. The numbering in the heterocyclic compounds are started always from hetero-atom.

4. If more than one heteroatoms are present in the ring, then the sequencing of numbering is done in such a direction that all the heteroatoms are given the lowest possible number (e.g. O,S,N,P etc.)

5. When two or more of the same heteroatoms are present, then prefix di, tri, tetra for 2, 3, & 4 are used respectively.

Five membered heterocyclic compounds with one & two heteroatoms.

Rings	IUPAC Name of heteroatoms	Common Name
	Azole	Pyrrole
	Oxole	Furan
	Thiole	Thiophene

Five membered heterocyclic compounds with two hetero-atoms:

Rings	IUPAC Name of heteroatoms	Common Name
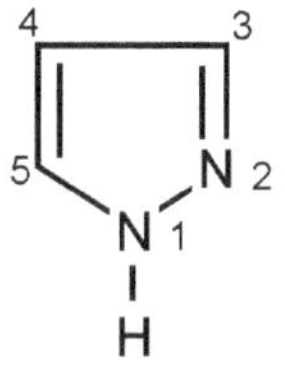	1,2 Diazole	Pyrazole
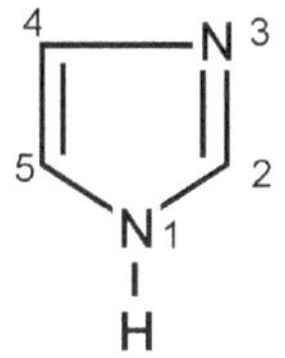	1,3 Diazole	Imidazole
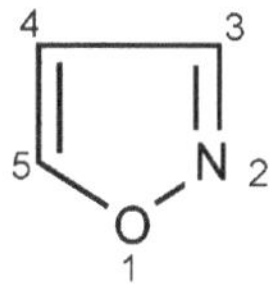	1,2 Oxazole	Isoxazole
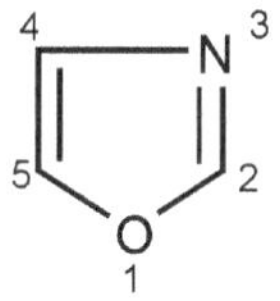	1,3 Oxazole	Oxazole
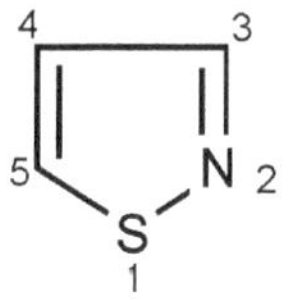	1,2 Thiazole	Isothiazole-

Write the name of following heterocyclic compounds

When only one double bond is present in five-membered ring heterocyclic compound, then suffix `line' is used, and when no double bond is present then suffix "lidine " is used.

Rings	Nomenclature
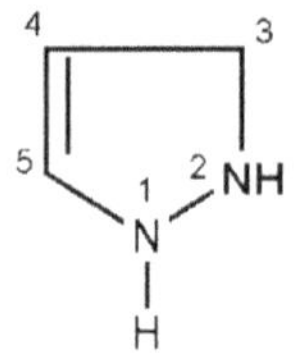	2,3 dihydro pyrazole or (4 Pyrazoline)
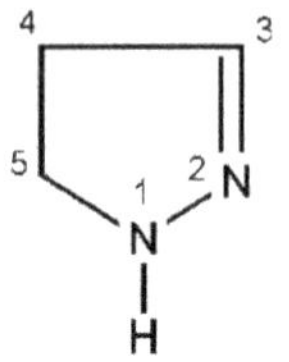	4,5 Dihydro pyrazole or (2 Pyrazoline)
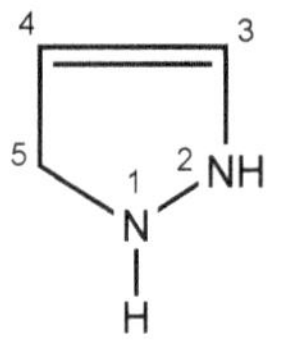	2,5 Dihydro pyrazole or (3 Pyrazoline)
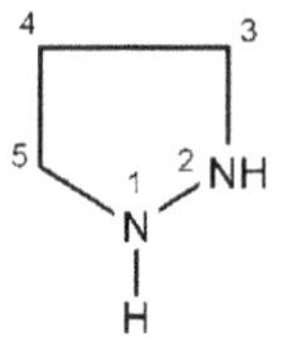	Tetrahydro pyrazole (Pyrazolidine)
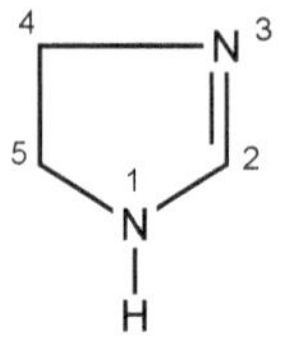	4,5 Dihydro–imidazole (2 Imidazoline)
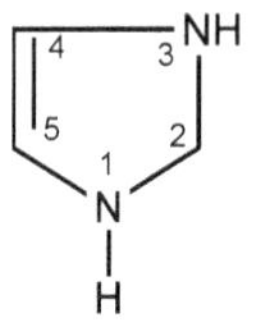	2,3 Dihydro–imidazole (4 Imidazoline)
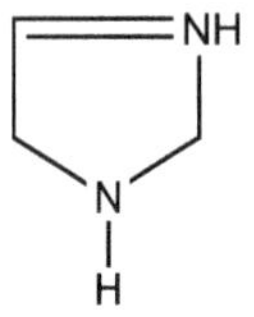	2,5 Dihydro–imidazole (3 Imidazoline)

Contd...

Rings	Nomenclature
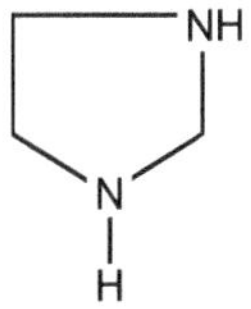	Tetrahydro–imidazole (Imidazolidine)
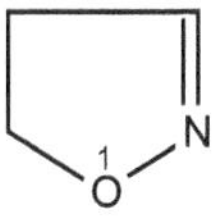	4,5 Dihydro–isoxazole (Isoxazoline)
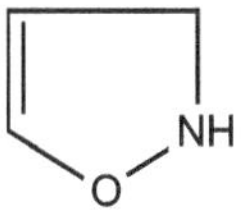	2,3 Dihydro–isoxazole (4 Isoxazoline)
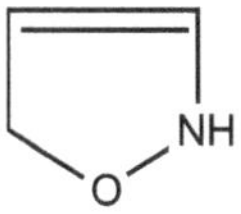	2,5 Dihydro–isoxazole (3 Isoxazoline)
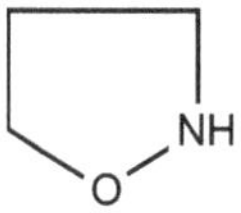	Tetrahydro–isoxazole (Isoxazolidine)
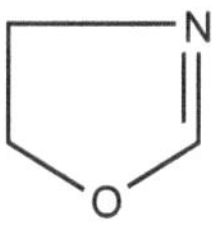	3,4 Dihydro–oxazole (2 Oxazoline)
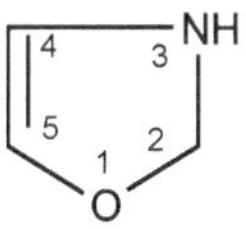	2,3 Dihydro–oxazole (4 Oxazoline)
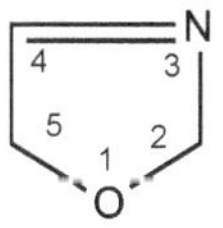	2,5 Dihydro–oxazole (3 Oxazoline)
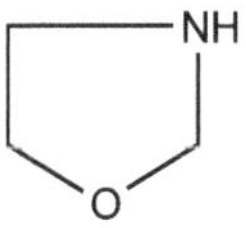	Tetrahydro–oxazole or (Oxazolidine)
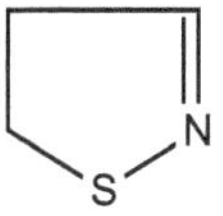	4,5 Dihydro–isothiazole (2 Isothiazoline)

Contd...

Rings	Nomenclature
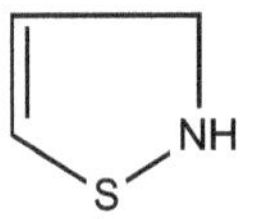	2,3 Dihydro–isothiazole (4 Isothiazoline)
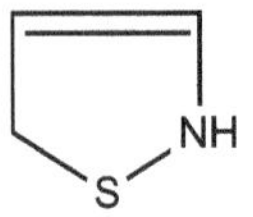	2,5 Dihydro–isothiazole (3 Isothiazoline)
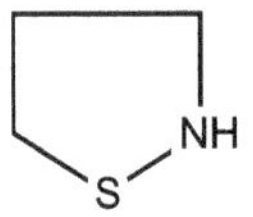	Tetrahydro–isothiazole (Isothiazolidine)
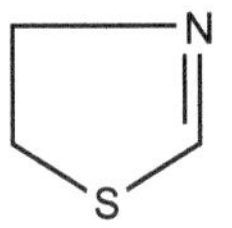	3,4 Dihydro–thiazole (2 Thiazoline)
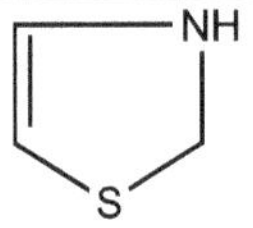	2,3 Dihydro–thiazole (4 Thiazoline)
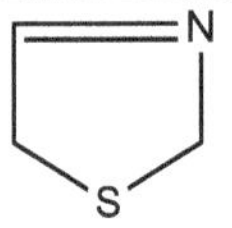	2,5 Dihydro–thiazole (3 Thiazoline)

Fused Ring Heterocyclic Compounds

Rings	Nomenclature
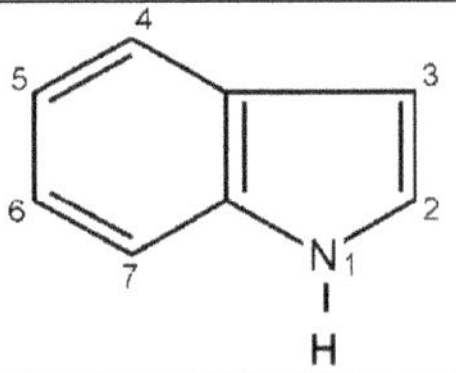	Indole (Benzo-pyrrole)
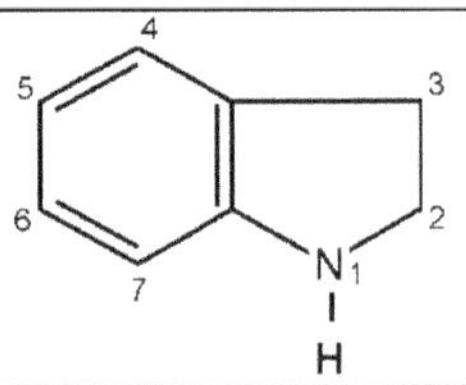	Indoline (Benzo–pyrroline)

Contd...

Rings	Nomenclature
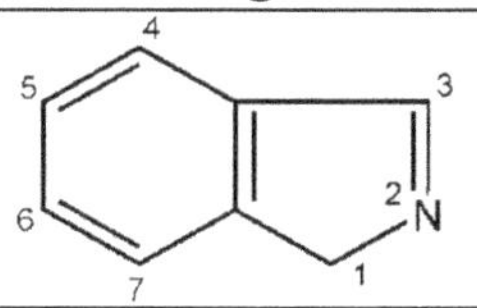 (isoindole structure)	Isoindole
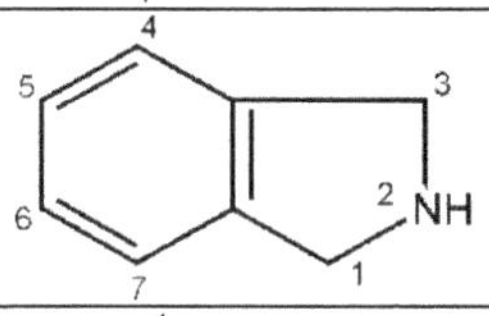 (isoindoline structure)	Isoindoline
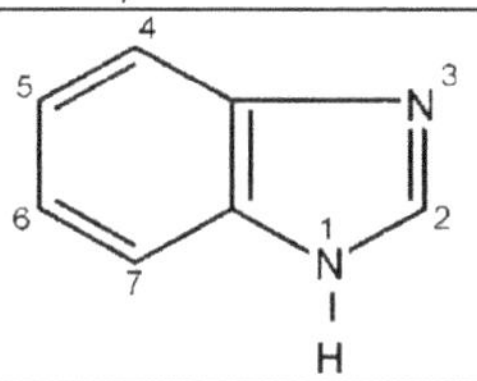 (benzoimidazole structure)	Benzoimidazole

Six-membered Heterocyclic Compounds

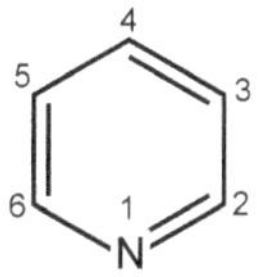 (pyridine structure)	Azine (Pyridine)
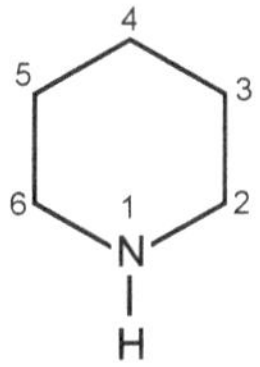 (piperidine structure)	Perhydro-pyridine (Piperidine)
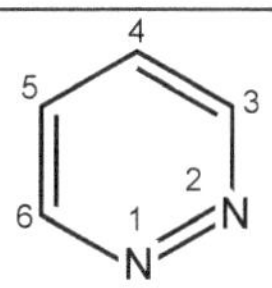 (pyridazine structure)	1,2 Diazine (Pyridazine)
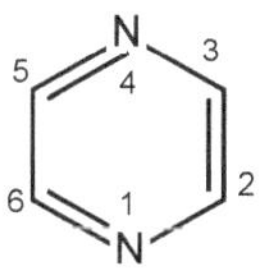 (pyrazine structure)	1,4 Diazine (Pyrazine)
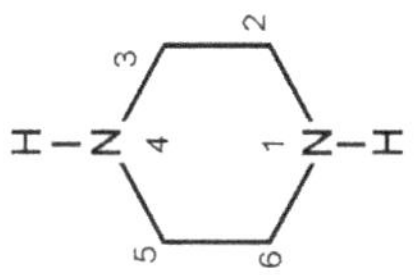 (piperazine structure)	Perhydro-pyrazine (Piperazine)

Points to Remember

- IUPAC nomenclature is based on naming a molecule's longest chain of carbons connected by single bonds, whether in a continuous chain or in a ring.
- Alkanes are the family of saturated hydrocarbons, that is, molecules containing carbon and hydrogen connected by single bonds only. These molecules can be in continuous chains (called linear or acyclic), or in rings (called cyclic or alicyclic).
- In naming molecules containing one or more of the functional groups in Group A, the group of highest priority is indicated by suffix; the others are indicated by prefix, with priority equivalent to any other substituents.
- "Aromatic" compounds are those derived from benzene and similar ring systems. As with aliphatic nomenclature described above, the process is: determining the root name of the parent ring; determining priority, name, and position number of substituents; and assembling the name in alphabetical order.
- A special group of aromatic compounds are ketones where the carbonyl is attached to at least one benzene ring. Such compounds are named as "phenones", the prefix depending on the size and nature of the group on the other side of the carbonyl.
- The heterocyclic compounds are the cyclic compounds in which one or more carbon atom is replaced by the atom like N,O, S, P, Si, then such compounds are called as heterocyclic compounds and the atoms like N, O, S, P, Si are known as heteroatoms.

Multiple Choice Questions

---

1. Saturated hydrocarbons are referred as _______________
   - (A) Alkanes
   - (B) Alkenes
   - (C) Alkynes
   - (D) Alkaloids

2. Identify the correct alkane name for the molecular formula $C_{30}H_{62}$.
   - (A) Propdecane
   - (b) Eicosane
   - (C) Triacontane
   - (d) Dodecane

3. Identify the smallest alkane which can form a ring structure (cycloalkane)?
   - (A) Cyclomethane
   - (B) Methane
   - (C) Cyclopropane
   - (D) Propane

4. In which among the following alkane, a carbon atom is displaced so as to form a compactly structure with the resemblance of a butterfly wing?
   - (A) Cyclopropane
   - (B) Cyclobutane
   - (C) Cyclopentane
   - (D) Cyclohexane

5. The first step in IUPAC nomenclature is to identify the total number of carbon atoms present in the compound.
   (A) True   (B) False

6. The substituent in the chain is named by replacing the "ane" in the alkanes by __________
   (A) ene   (B) ic
   (C) one   (D) yl

7. The C=C bond in the chain of the compound considered is shown by __________
   (A) Specifying the number of carbon atoms associated with the bond
   (B) Specifying the number of carbon atoms at beginning of the C=C bond
   (C) Specifying the number of carbon atoms at end of the C=C bond
   (D) Specifying the number of carbon atoms in the entire chain

8. Dienes are the name given to compounds with __________
   (A) Exactly a double bond   (B) Exactly a triple bond
   (C) Exactly two double bond   (D) More than two double bond

9. Triple bond with two carbon atoms on either side is called __________
   (A) Methnyl group   (B) Ethynyl group
   (C) Propionyl group   (D) Propargyl group

10. The substituent groups that are commonly associated with benzene ring are __________
    (A) Phenyl and benzyl   (B) Propyl and phenyl
    (C) Methyl and benzyl   (D) Butyl and phenyl

11. Which compound is a secondary alcohol?
    (A) Butan-1-ol   (B) Butan-2-ol
    (C) Isobutyl alcohol   (D) 2-methylpropan-2-ol

12. Which compound is different from the others?
    (A) Methyl cthyl kctonc
    (B) Pentan-2-one
    (C) 2-pentanone
    (D) Methyl propyl ketone

13. A molecule with the formula C3H8 is a(n):
    (A) Hexane   (B) Propane
    (C) Decane   (D) Butane

14. The general formula for noncyclic alkenes is:
    (A) C_nH_{2n+2}
    (B) C_nH_{2n}
    (C) C_nH_{2n-2}
    (D) C_nH_{n+2}

15. How many actual double bonds does the benzene ring possess?
    (A) None, carbon-carbon bonds in benzene are delocalized around the ring
    (B) 1 double bond
    (C) 2 double bonds
    (D) 3 double bonds

16. Para-xylene is the same as:
    (A) 1,2-dimethylbenzene
    (B) 1,3-diethylbenzene
    (C) 1,3-dimethylbenzene
    (D) 1,4-dimethylbenzene

17. Which of the following formulas represents an alkene?
    (A) $CH_3CH_2CH_3$
    (B) CH_3CH_3
    (C) $CH_3CH_2CHCH_2$
    (D) CH_3CH_2Cl

18. Which one of the following is a secondary alcohol?
    (A) CH_3CH_2OH
    (B) CH_3OH
    (c) $CH_3CH(OH)CH_3$
    (D) $(CH_3)C_3OH$

19. Select the IUPAC name for: $(CH_3)_2CHCH(OH)CH_2C(CH_3)_3$.
    (A) 2,5,5-trimethyl-3-hexanol
    (B) 1,1,4,4-pentamethylbutanol
    (C) 1,1-dimethylisopentanol
    (D) 2,5-dimethyl-4-hexanol

20. Give the IUPAC name of this compound: CH3OCH2CH3.
    (A) Dimethyl ether
    (B) Methoxyethane
    (C) Methylethyloxide
    (D) Propyl ether

CHAPTER 5

Drugs Acting on Central Nervous System

Introduction

The chapter aims at providing the latest and pharmacopoeial information regarding some Drugs acting on Central Nervous System (Thiopental sodium, Ketamine hydrochloride, Diazepam, Alprazolam, Nitrazepam, Phenobarbital, Chloropromazine hydrochloride, Haloperidol, Droperidol, Risperidone, Sulperide, Phenytoin, Ethosuximide, Carbamazepine, Clonazepam, Primidone, Valproic acid, Gabapentin, Amitriptyline hydrochloride, Imipramine hydrochloride, and Fluoxetine) regarding their classification, chemical name, chemical structure, uses, stability, storage conditions, different types of formulations, and popular brand names.

Drugs acting on Central Nervous System

- Central nervous system agents are medicines that affect the central nervous system (CNS). The CNS is responsible for processing and controlling most of our bodily functions, and consists of the nerves in the brain and spinal cord.
- There are many different types of drugs that work on the CNS, including anesthetics, anticonvulsants, anti-emetics, anti-parkinson agents, CNS stimulants, muscle relaxants, narcotic analgesics (pain relievers), non-narcotic analgesics, and sedatives.

Anaesthetics

- Anesthesia is a medical treatment that keeps you from feeling pain during procedures or surgery. The medications used to block pain are called anesthetics. Different types of anesthesia work in different ways. Some anesthetic medications numb certain parts of the body, while other medications numb the brain, to induce a sleep through more invasive surgical procedures, like those within the head, chest, or abdomen.

- Anesthesia temporarily blocks sensory/pain signals from nerves to the centers in the brain.

The anesthetics are classified into following:

- **Local anesthesia:** This treatment numbs a small section of the body. Examples of procedures in which local anesthesia could be used include cataract surgery, a dental procedure or skin biopsy. You're awake during the procedure.
- **General anesthetics:** These are the drugs, which produce controlled, reversible depression of the functional activities of the central nervous system producing loss of sensation and consciousness.

Stages of General Anesthesia. When an inhalation anesthetic is administered to a patient some of the following well defined stages are produced by increasing the blood concentration of the agent. They are;

- **Stage I (Stage of analgesia):** This is the period from the beginning of anesthetic administration to the loss of consciousness. The patient progressively loses pain. This stage is also called stage of analgesia.
- **Stage II (Stage of delirium):** This period extends from the loss of consciousness through a stage of irregular and specific breathing to the reestablishment of regular breathing. Respiration is normal and regular. The patient may laugh, vomit or struggle and for this reason it is called the stage of excitement.
- **Stage III (Stage of surgical anesthesia):** In this stage excitement is lost and skeletal muscle relaxation is produced. Most types of surgeries are done in this stage.
- **Stage IV (Stage of medullary depression):** Overdose of the anesthetic may bring the patient to this stage. Respiratory and circulatory failure occur in this stage.

Classification

The general anesthetics are classified according to their nature (volatile or non-volatile) at room temperature. They are:

- A. **Volatile Inhalation general anesthetics.** They are administered by inhalation and are further subdivided as;
  - **Gases:** Ex: Cyclopropane: Ethyl chloride, Nitrous oxide
  - **Liquids:** Diethyl ether, Halothane, Chloroform, Trichloroethylene
- B. **Non-Volatile or Intravenous anesthetics.** They are non-volatile at room temperature and are administered by intravenous route. They are;
  - **Barbiturates:** Thiopental sodium, Methohexital sodium.
  - **Non-barbiturates:** Propanidid, Propofol.

Side Effects

Most anesthesia side effects are temporary and go away within 24 hours, often sooner. Depending on the anesthesia type and how providers administer it, you may experience:

- Back pain or muscle pain.
- Chills caused by low body temperature (hypothermia).
- Difficulty urinating.
- Fatigue.
- Headache.
- Itching.
- Nausea and vomiting.
- Pain, tenderness, redness or bruising at the injection site.
- Sore throat (pharyngitis).

Potential complications include:

- **Anesthetic awareness:** For unknown reasons, about one out of every 1,000 people who receive general anesthesia experience awareness during a procedure. You may be aware of your surroundings but unable to move or communicate.
- **Collapsed lung (atelectasis):** Surgery that uses general anesthesia or a breathing tube can cause a collapsed lung. This rare problem occurs when air sacs in the lung deflate or fill with fluid.
- **Malignant hyperthermia:** People who have malignant hyperthermia (MH) experience a dangerous reaction to anesthesia. This rare inherited syndrome causes fever and muscle contractions during surgery.
- **Nerve damage:** Although rare, some people experience nerve damage that causes temporary or permanent neuropathic pain, numbness, or weakness.
- **Postoperative delirium:** Older people are more prone to postoperative delirium. This condition causes confusion that comes and goes for about a week.

Certain factors make it riskier to receive anesthesia, including:

- Advanced age.
- Diabetes or kidney disease.
- Family history of malignant hyperthermia (anesthesia allergy).
- Heart disease, high blood pressure (hypertension) or strokes.
- Lung disease, such as asthma or chronic obstructive pulmonary disease (COPD).
- Obesity (high body mass index or BMI).
- Seizures or neurological disorders.

- Sleep apnea.
- Smoking.

Thiopental Sodium

Classification: Anesthetics, Intravenous

Chemical Name: 5-ethyl-4,6-dioxo-5-pentan-2-yl-1*H*-pyrimidine-2-thiolate

Chemical Structure

Uses

For use as the sole anesthetic agent for brief (15 minute) procedures, for induction of anesthesia prior to administration of other anesthetic agents, to supplement regional anesthesia, to provide hypnosis during balanced anesthesia with other agents for analgesia or muscle relaxation, for the control of convulsive states during or following inhalation anesthesia or local anesthesia, in neurosurgical patients with increased intracranial pressure, and for narcoanalysis and narcosynthesis in psychiatric disorders.

Stability: At 22°C, thiopental remains stable and sterile for 6 days and well beyond 7 days at 3°C.

Storage Conditions

- Store at controlled room temperature 15°C to 30°C (59°F to 86°F).
- Keep reconstituted solution in a cool place.
- When stored in the dry form, thiopental sodium is stable indefinitely.
- Thiopental in pharmacy-filled syringes must be stored at either room temperature or under refrigeration.

Different types of Formulations: Injection, powder, for solution

Popular brand names: Thipen, Thioz, Pentone, Thiosol, Thiowell, Anesthal

Ketamine Hydrochloride

Classification: Anesthetics, Dissociative

Chemical Name: 2-(2-chlorophenyl)-2-(methylamino)cyclohexan-1-one

Chemical Structure

Uses

- Ketamine is indicated as an anesthetic agent for recommended diagnostic and surgical procedures. If skeletal muscle relaxation is needed, it should be combined with a muscle relaxant. If the surgical procedure involves visceral pain, it should be supplemented with an agent that obtunds visceral pain.
- Ketamine can be used for induction of anesthesia prior other general anesthetic agents and as a supplement of low potency agents.
- Reports have indicated a potential use of ketamine as a therapeutic tool for the management of depression when administered in lower doses.

Stability

- Solutions of ketamine are chemically stable for 180 days in polypropylene syringes with storage at room temperature.
- Chemical and physical in-use stability has been demonstrated for 48 hours at 25°C protected from light.

Storage Conditions

- Store between 20°C to 25°C (68° to 77°F).
- Protect from light.
- Do not freeze.

Different types of Formulations

- Injection, solution
- Solution

Popular brand names: Aneket, Ketmin, Hypnoket, Ketajet, Keta, Zokent, Ketajex, Ketamax, Ketanik, Ketriplin

Propofol

Classification: Anesthetics

Chemical Name: 2,6-di(propan-2-yl)phenol

Chemical Structure

Uses

- Propofol is indicated for the induction of general anesthesia.
- It is also indicated for the maintenance of anesthesia utilizing balanced techniques with other appropriate agents such as opioids and inhalation anesthetics.
- Propofol is indicated for the sedation in critically ill patients confined to intensive care units.
- Propofol has successfully controlled seizures in status epilepticus.
- Propofol appears to have significant antiemetic action and is a good choice for sedation or anesthesia in patients at high risk for nausea and vomiting.

Stability

- Propofol has been reported to have high stability in glass and relatively high stability up to 24 hours in polyvinyl chloride-based medical plastics.
- Mixing with propofol substantially increased the pH of the mixture and resulted in significant remifentanil degradation for all reconstitution solutions used, while propofol remained stable (pH 6.5).

Storage Conditions

- Store between 4°C to 22°C (40°F to 72°F); refrigeration is not required.

Different types of Formulations

- Injection, emulsion
- Emulsion

Popular brand names: Fresenius Propoven, Diprivan

Sedatives and Hypnotics

- A sedative drug decreases activity, moderates excitement, and calms the recipient, whereas a hypnotic drug produces drowsiness and facilitates the onset and maintenance of a state of sleep that resembles natural sleep in its electroencephalographic characteristics and from which the recipient can be aroused easily.

- Sedative-hypnotic drug, chemical substance used to reduce tension and anxiety and induce calm (sedative effect) or to induce sleep (hypnotic effect).

- Most such drugs exert a quieting or calming effect at low doses and a sleep-inducing effect in larger doses.

- Sedative-hypnotic drugs tend to depress the central nervous system. Since these actions can be obtained with other drugs, such as opiates, the distinctive characteristic of sedative-hypnotics is their selective ability to achieve their effects without affecting mood or reducing sensitivity to pain.

Classification

Due to chemical differences, the sedative-hypnotics include several related families of drugs having common characteristics but somewhat diverse effects and therapeutic uses. These drugs
are classified as follows ;

1. **Barbiturates:** Ex: Phenobarbitone, pentobarbitone, amobarbitone etc.
2. **Non-barbiturates:** They are further classified as follows;
   (a) **Aldehydes and their derivatives:** Chloral hydrate, paraldehyde, triclofos sodium
   (b) **Piperidine derivatives:** Glutethimide, methyprylone
   (c) **Quinazoline derivatives:** Methaqualone
   (d) **Alcohols and their carbamate derivatives:** Ethchlorvynol, meprobamate, ethinamate
   (e) **Benzodizepine derivatives:** Chlordiazepoxide, diazepam, oxazepam, alprozolam, flurazepam, triazolam, prazepam, halazepam, temazepam, lorazepam

Diazepam

Classification: Anti-Anxiety Agents

Chemical Name: 7-chloro-1-methyl-5-phenyl-3H-1,4-benzodiazepin-2-one

Chemical Structure

Uses

- In general, diazepam is useful in the symptomatic management of mild to moderate degrees of anxiety in conditions dominated by tension, excitation, agitation, fear, or aggressiveness such as may occur in psychoneurosis, anxiety reactions due to stress conditions, and anxiety states with somatic expression.
- Moreover, in acute alcoholic withdrawal, diazepam may be useful in the symptomatic relief of acute agitation, tremor, and impending acute delirium tremens.

Stability

- Diazepam injection is chemically stable as 5-mg doses in disposable glass syringes for 90 days when stored at 4°C or 30°C.

Storage Conditions

- Store at room temperature between 59 and 86 degrees F (15°C - 30°C) away from light and moisture.
- Do not store in the bathroom. Keep all medicines away from children and pets.
- Do not flush medications down the toilet or pour them into a drain unless instructed to do so.

Different types of Formulations: Gel, Emulsion, Tablet, Solution, Injection, solution, Liquid, Spray

Popular brand names: Paxum, Dipax, Anxol, Repam, Equipam, Placidox, Valium, Peacin, Hypose, Calmpose

Alprazolam

Classification: Anti-Anxiety Agents

Chemical Name: 8-chloro-1-methyl-6-phenyl-4*H*-[1,2,4]triazolo[4,3-a][1,4]benzodia-zepine

Chemical Structure

Uses

- Alprazolam is indicated for the management of anxiety disorder, anxiety associated with depression, panic disorder, and panic disorder with agoraphobia.
- Alprazolam may also be prescribed off label for insomnia, premenstrual syndrome, and depression.

Stability

- Product remains stable after being continuously exposed to an elevated temperature of 40°C.
- The mixture stored in the dark remains stable for 60 days at 5°C and 25°C.

Storage Conditions

- Store it in a dry place at room temperature, which is about 68–77°F (20–25°C).
- Do not store in a bathroom, as moisture and humidity can cause the medication to break down sooner.

Different types of Formulations

- Tablet, extended release
- Tablet, orally disintegrating

Popular brand names: Notence, Naztab, Dreamer, Jolistar, Malcoz, Alcalm, Belol, Alora, Manorest, Bliz

Nitrazepam

Classification: Anti-Anxiety Agents

Chemical Name: 7-nitro-5-phenyl-1,3-dihydro-1,4-benzodiazepin-2-one

Chemical Structure

Uses

- Used to treat short-term sleeping problems (insomnia), such as difficulty falling asleep, frequent awakenings during the night, and early-morning awakening.

Stability

- The product remains stable after being continuously exposed to an elevated temperature of 40°C for 7 days.

Storage Conditions

- Store this medication at room temperature between 59°F and 86°F (15°C and 30°C) away from heat and light.
- Protect from direct light.

Different types of Formulations: Tablet

Popular brand names: Baronite, Hypnosed, Nitaz, Nitab, Sopor, Nitravet, Nithra, Nizpam, Nitcalm, Nipam

Phenobarbital

Classification: Hypnotics and Sedatives

Chemical Name: 5-ethyl-5-phenyl-1,3-diazinane-2,4,6-trione

Chemical Structure

Uses

- Phenobarbital is a long-lasting barbiturate and anticonvulsant used in the treatment of all types of seizures, except for absent seizures.

Stability

- The diluted phenobarbital sodium is stable over a four-week period at 4°C without the need for pH adjustment.

Storage Conditions

- Store at controlled room temperature 15 °C - 30°C (59°- 86° F).
- Keep away from children, heat, light and moisture.
- Store unopened vials in the Controlled Drugs Safe.

Different types of Formulations: Tablet, Elixir, Solution

Popular brand names: Barbee, Beetal, Epitan, Fenobarb, Gardenal, Phenetone, Phenobarb, Shinosun, Luminal, Solfoton

Antipsychotics

- Antipsychotic medications are used as short or long-term treatments for bipolar disorder to control psychotic symptoms such as hallucinations, delusions, or mania symptoms. These symptoms may occur during acute mania or severe depression. Some also treat bipolar depression, and several have demonstrated long-term value in preventing future episodes of mania or depression.
- In people with bipolar disorder, antipsychotics are also used "off label" as sedatives, for insomnia, anxiety, and/or agitation. Often, they are taken with a mood-stabilizing drug and can decrease symptoms of mania until mood stabilizers take full effect.
- Some antipsychotics seem to help stabilize moods on their own. As a result, they may be used alone as long-term treatment for people who don't tolerate or respond to lithium and anticonvulsants.
- Antipsychotic drugs help regulate the functioning of brain circuits that control thinking, mood, and perception. It is not clear exactly how these drugs work, but they usually improve manic episodes quickly.
- The newer antipsychotics usually act quickly and can help you avoid the reckless and impulsive behaviors associated with mania. More normal thinking often is restored within a few weeks.
- Older antipsychotic drugs are generally not used as a first-line treatment for bipolar disorder, and they are less established for treating depressive symptoms or preventing episodes during long-term use. However, they may be helpful if a person has troublesome side effects or doesn't respond to the newer drugs.

Older antipsychotics include chlorpromazine (Thorazine), haloperidol (Haldol), and perphenazine (Trilafon). These drugs may cause a serious long-term side effect called tardive dyskinesia, a movement disorder characterized by repetitive, involuntary movement like lip smacking, protruding the tongue, or grimacing. Newer atypical antipsychotics also have the potential to cause this side effect, but have a relatively lower risk than the older conventional antipsychotics.

Classification

The drugs used in the treatment of psychoses are classified as follows ;

1. **Phenothiazine derivatives.** Chlorpromazine, prochlorperazine, trifluoperazine, trifluopromazine, promazine
2. **Butyrophenones.** Haloperidol, droperidol.
3. **Miscellaneous.** Pimozide, molindone.

Chlorpromazine Hydrochloride

Classification: Antipsychotic Agents

Chemical Name: 3-(2-chlorophenothiazin-10-yl)-*N*,*N*-dimethylpropan-1-amine

Chemical Structure

Uses

1. It is used in the management of psychotic conditions. It also controls excitement, aggression and agitation.
2. It has antiemetic, antipruritic, anti-histaminic and sedative properties.

Stability

- The product is stable for at least three months in amber plastic prescription bottles stored at either refrigeration or room temperature.

Storage Conditions

- All dosage forms except Syrup should be stored between 15° and 30°C (59° and 86°F).
- Syrup should be stored below 25°C (77°F).

Different types of Formulations: Tablet, Solution, Drops, Liquid, Syrup

Popular brand names: Clozine, Emetil, Yemetil, Zinetil, Prozen, Prozine, Megatil, Estichlor, Chlorotame, Relitil

Haloperidol

Classification: Antipsychotic Agents

Chemical Name: 4-[4-(4-chlorophenyl)-4-hydroxypiperidin-1-yl]-1-(4-fluorophenyl)butan-1-one

Chemical Structure

Uses

1. Haloperidol is effective in the management of hyperactivity, agitation, and mania.
2. Haloperidol is an effective neuroleptic and also possesses antiemetic properties; it has a marked tendency to provoke extrapyramidal effects and has relatively weak alpha-adrenolytic properties.
3. It may also exhibit hypothermic and anorexian effects and potentiates the action of barbiturates, general anesthetics, and other CNS depressant drugs

Stability

- Haloperidol lactate is chemically stable when stored at 25°C-28°C with and without exposure to light, and at refrigeration temperature over 15 days.
- Haloperidol lacks stability when exposed to elevated temperatures and light.

Storage Conditions

- Store at 20° to 25°C (68° to 77°F) away from heat and moisture.

- Protect from light and do not freeze.
- Do not store in bathroom.

Different types of Formulations: Injection, solution, Liquid, Solution, Tablet

Popular brand names: Halobid, Halidase, Haloxel, Halop, Hypnodol, Ultidol, Hidol, Helinase, Theonase, Qutzal

Risperidone

Classification: Antipsychotic Agents

Chemical Name: 3-[2-[4-(6-fluoro-1,2-benzoxazol-3-yl)piperidin-1-yl]ethyl]-2-methyl-6,7,8,9-tetrahydropyrido[1,2-a]pyrimidin-4-one

Chemical Structure

Uses

- Risperidone is indicated for the treatment of schizophrenia and irritability associated with autistic disorder.
- It is also indicated as monotherapy, or adjunctly with lithium or valproic acid, for the treatment of acute mania or mixed episodes associated with bipolar I disorder.
- Risperidone is additionally indicated in Canada for the short-term symptomatic management of aggression or psychotic symptoms in patients with severe dementia of the Alzheimer type unresponsive to non-pharmacological approaches.
- Risperidone is also used off-label for a number of conditions including as an adjunct to antidepressants in treatment-resistant depression.

Stability

- Risperidone was comparatively stable to the effect of temperature.
- When the drug powder was exposed to dry heat at 80°C for 24 hr 30.09% degradation was observed with corresponding rise to degradants products

Storage Conditions

- The recommended temperature for powder, for suspension is 36 to 46°F (2–8°C).
- Without refrigeration, solution can be stored at temperatures not more than 77°F (25°C) for not more than seven days.

Different types of Formulations: Powder, for suspension, Tablet, orally disintegrating, Kit, Solution, Tablet, film coated

Popular brand names: Respidon, Rispond, Sizodon, Risnia, Riscon, Resque, Riscalm, Regrace, Riscur: e, Rispund

Sulpiride

Classification: Antipsychotic Agents

Chemical Name: *N*-[(1-ethylpyrrolidin-2-yl)methyl]-2-methoxy-5-sulfamoylbenza-mide

Chemical Structure

Uses: Sulpiride is indicated for the treatment of acute and chronic schizophrenia.

Stability: The solution is stable for 7 days when kept in refrigerator.

Storage Conditions: Store in a cool, dry place, away from direct heat and light.

Different types of Formulations: Tablet, Capsule, Solution, Suspension, Suppositories

Popular brand names: Dogmatil, Dolmatil, Eglonyl, Espiride, Modal, Sulpor, Sopid, Sulgin, Sedusen, Betamac

Olanzapine

Classification: Atypical antipsychotic

Chemical **Name:** 2-methyl-4-(4-methylpiperazin-1-yl)-10H-thieno[2,3-b][1,5] benzod-iazepine

Chemical Structure

Uses

- Olanzapine is used to treat certain mental/mood conditions (such as schizophrenia, bipolar disorder). It may also be used in combination with other medication to treat depression.

Stability

- Compatibility and stress stability results demonstrated that tablet formulations of olanzapine are sensitive to temperature and moisture.

Storage Conditions

- Store olanzapine at room temperature between 68°F and 77°F (20°C and 25°C).
- Keep this drug away from light.
- Don't store this medication in moist or damp areas, such as bathrooms.

Different types of Formulations

- Tablet, orally disintegrating
- Tablet
- Powder, for solution
- Injection, powder, for solution
- Injection, powder, for suspension, extended release

Popular brand names: Zyprexa, Dopin, Jolyon, Joyzol, Lanopin, Nexolan, Olace, Odozap, Olandus, Oladay

Quetiapine

Classification: Atypical antipsychotic

Chemical Name: 2-[2-(4-benzo[b][1,4]benzothiazepin-6-ylpiperazin-1-yl)ethoxy]-ethanol

Chemical Structure

Uses

- Quetiapine is used in the symptomatic treatment of schizophrenia. In addition, it may be used for the management of acute manic or mixed episodes in patients with bipolar I disorder, as a monotherapy or combined with other drugs.

Quetiapine is used in combination with antidepressant drugs for the treatment of major depression.

Stability

- Compatibility and stress stability results demonstrated that tablet formulations of olanzapine are sensitive to temperature and moisture.

Storage Conditions

- Store quetiapine at room temperature between 59°F and 86°F (15°C and 30°C).
- Keep this drug away from light.
- Don't store this medication in moist or damp areas.

Different types of Formulations

- Tablet, multilayer, extended release
- Tablet

Popular brand names: Adequet, Placidin, Psyquit, Q-Mind, Q-Pin, Q-Win, Quel, Queine, Queticare, Quser

Lurasidone

Classification: Atypical antipsychotic

Chemical Name: (1S,2R,6S,7R)-4-[[(1R,2R)-2-[[4-(1,2-benzothiazol-3-yl)piperazin-1-yl]methyl]cyclohexyl]methyl]-4-azatricyclo[5.2.1.0^{2,6}]decane-3,5-dione

Chemical Structure

Uses: It is used for the treatment of schizophrenia and lurasidone.

Stability: A shelf-life of 30 months is recommended for expiration dating of the product based on stability data submitted.

Storage Conditions: Store the tablets at 25°C (77°F); excursions permitted to 15° - 30°C (59° -86°F)

Different types of Formulations: Tablet, film coated

Popular brand names: Latuda, Luramax, Luratrend, Lurafic, Lurasid, Tablura, Atlura, Lurace, Alsiva, Lurastar

Anticonvulsants

Anticonvulsants are a diverse group of pharmacological agents used in the treatment of epileptic seizures. Anticonvulsants are also increasingly being used in the treatment of bipolar disorder and borderline personality disorder, since many seem to act as mood stabilizers, and for the treatment of neuropathic pain. Anticonvulsants suppress the excessive rapid firing of neurons during seizures. Anticonvulsants also prevent the spread of the seizure within the brain.

Classification

Barbiturates: phenobarbital

Oxazolidinediones: trimethadione

Succinimides: ethosuximide

Acetylureas: phenacemide

Other: carbamazepine, lamotrigine, vigabatrin,

Phenytoin

Classification: Anticonvulsants

Chemical Name: 5,5-diphenylimidazolidine-2,4-dione

Chemical Structure

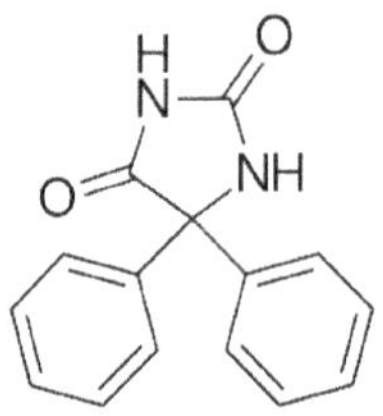

Uses

- Phenytoin is indicated to treat grand mal seizures, complex partial seizures, and to prevent and treat seizures during or following neurosurgery.
- Injectable phenytoin and Fosphenytoin, which is the phosphate ester prodrug formulation of phenytoin, are indicated to treat tonic-clonic status epilepticus, and for the prevention and treatment of seizures occurring during neurosurgery.

Stability: On refrigeration or freezing, a precipitate might form, but this will dissolve when the solution is allowed to stand at room temperature.

Storage Conditions

- Store at 20 to 25°C (68 to 77°F) away from light and moisture.
- Do not freeze.

Different types of Formulations: Injection, Capsule, extended release, Tablet, Suspension

Popular brand names: Eptoin, Epicare, Fentoin, Dilantin, Wyntoin, Celetoin, Epsod, Eptozen, Phalin, Epicent

Ethosuximide

Classification: Anticonvulsants

Chemical Name: 3-ethyl-3-methylpyrrolidine-2,5-dione

Chemical Structure

Uses: For the treatment of petit mal epilepsy.

Stability

- Protect from heat.
- The drug is less stable in dextrose, dextran, or bicarbonate-containing infusion solutions.

Storage Conditions

- Liquid (syrup) should be stored at room temperature.
- Be especially careful to protect it from freezing and keep it away from light and out of the reach of children.
- Ethosuximide is to be stored at room temperature, protected away from light and moisture and keep away from children.
- Store ethosuximide capsules between 15°C and 25°C and protect from heat.
- Store syrup between 15°C and 25°C and protect from freezing and light.

Different types of Formulations: Capsule, Syrup, Capsule, liquid filled, Solution

Popular brand names: Absenz, Zarontin, Arontin

Carbamazepine

Classification: Anticonvulsants

Chemical Name: Benzo[b][1]benzazepine-11-carboxamide

Uses

- Carbamazepine is indicated for the treatment of epilepsy and pain associated with true trigeminal neuralgia.

Chemical Structure

- In particular, carbamazepine has shown efficacy in treating mixed seizures, partial seizures with complex symptoms, and generalized tonic-clonic seizures.
- Carbamazepine is also indicated for the treatment of manic episodes and mixed manic-depressive episodes caused by bipolar I disorder.

Stability: Carbamazepine is stable for at least eight weeks when stored at room temperature in the containers tested.

Storage Conditions

- Store at room temperature away from light and moisture.
- Do not store in the bathroom.
- Keep all medications away from children and pets.

Different types of Formulations

- Tablet, extended release
- Tablet, chewable
- Capsule, extended release
- Suspension
- Injection, powder, for solution

Popular brand names: Carbatol, Mazetol, Zeptol, Mezapin, Tegrital, Carzine, Epnil, Carbadac, Mezocar, Versitol

Clonazepam

Classification: Anticonvulsants

Chemical Name: 5-(2-chlorophenyl)-7-nitro-1,3-dihydro-1,4-benzodiazepin-2-one

Chemical Structure

Uses

- Clonazepam is used to prevent and control seizures. This medication is known as an anticonvulsant or antiepileptic drug. It is also used to treat panic attacks. Clonazepam works by calming your brain and nerves. It belongs to a class of drugs called benzodiazepines.

Stability

- The mixture is stable for 24 hours at room temperature.
- The stability of the diluted clonazepam is maintained for up to 12 hours.

Storage Conditions

- The formulations should be stored at room temperature.
- Keep away from children; Keep in a cool, dry place, away from direct sunlight;
- Do not store in the refrigerator.

Different types of Formulations: Tablet, Wafer

Popular brand names: Clonotril, Clonax, Clonapax, Clonzy, Clonapam, Clonawyn, Clonam, Clozet, Clozep, Clorpam

Valproic Acid

Classification: Anticonvulsants

Chemical Name: 2-propylpentanoic acid

Chemical Structure

Uses

Indicated for:
- Use as monotherapy or adjunctive therapy in the management of complex partial seizures and simple or complex absence seizures.
- Adjunctive therapy in the management of multiple seizure types that include absence seizures.
- Prophylaxis of migraine headaches.
- Acute management of mania associated with bipolar disorder.

Off-label uses include:
- Maintenance therapy for bipolar disorder.
- Treatment for acute bipolar depression.
- Emergency treatment of status epilepticus.

Stability
- Valproic acid is found to be stable at room temperature.
- Valproic acid is a very stable compound. No degradation has been observed by the action of heat, light, and strong aqueous alkali, or acid.

Storage Conditions
- Valproic acid capsules should be stored at 15 to 30°C and freezing should be avoided.
- Keep container tightly closed.

Different types of Formulations
- Injection
- Capsule, liquid filled
- Solution
- Liquid
- Capsule
- Capsule, delayed release
- Tablet, extended release
- Tablet, delayed release
- Tablet, film coated

Popular brand names: Gabantin, Gabator, Laregab, Gabata, Progaba, Gabax, Gabachek, Gabacent, Acegaba, Gabalept

Gabapentin

Classification: Anticonvulsants

Chemical Name: 2-[1-(aminomethyl)cyclohexyl]acetic acid

Chemical Structure

Uses

- Gabapentin is used with other medications to prevent and control seizures. It is also used to relieve nerve pain following shingles (a painful rash due to herpes zoster infection) in adults. Gabapentin is known as an anticonvulsant or antiepileptic drug.

Stability

- Preparations remained stable at least 91 days at 4°C and at least 56 days at 25°C.
- Gabapentin conditioned in low actinic bottles was stable at least 90 days when refrigerated or stored at room temperature.

Storage Conditions

- Keep this medication in the container it came in, tightly closed, and out of reach of children.
- Store the tablets, extended-release tablets, and capsules at room temperature, away from excess heat and moisture (not in the bathroom).
- Store the oral solution in the refrigerator.

Different types of Formulations

- Capsule
- Kit
- Tablet, film coated

Popular brand names: Horizant, Neurontin

Topiramate

Classification: Anticonvulsants

Chemical Name: [(1R,2S,6S,9R)-4,4,11,11-tetramethyl-3,5,7,10,12 pentaoxatricyclo [7.3.0.0^{2,6}] dodecan-6-yl]methyl sulfamate

Chemical Structure

Uses

Topiramate is indicated for the following conditions:

- Monotherapy for partial onset or primary generalized tonic-clonic seizures for patients 2 years of age and above.
- Prophylaxis of migraine in children 12 years of age and older and adults.

Stability

- Topiramate is more stable under acidic degradation conditions than under alkaline degradation conditions.
- Topiramate is unstable under conditions of dry heat at 90°C in an oven for 3 days.

Storage Conditions

- Tablets and extended-release capsules should be stored at room temperature and away from excess heat and moisture (not in the bathroom).
- Sprinkle capsules should be stored at or below 77°F (25°C).
- Never store broken tablets, capsules, or mixtures of sprinkles and soft food.

Different types of Formulations

- Tablet
- Capsule, extended release
- Capsule, coated pellets

Popular brand names: Topirawyn, Topamac, Topirol, Topamed, Ropimate, Leptomate, Topirain, Topitab, Topema, Topival

Vigabatrin

Classification: Anticonvulsants

Chemical Name: 4-aminohex-5-enoic acid

Chemical Structure

Uses

- Vigabatrin is indicated as adjunctive therapy in the treatment of refractory complex partial seizures in patients 2 years of age and older who have had inadequate responses to multiple previous treatments (i.e. not to be used for first-line therapy).
- It is also indicated as monotherapy in the treatment of infantile spasms in patients between 1 month and 2 years of age for whom the potential benefits outweigh the risk of vision loss.

Stability: The drug is stable for at least 4 weeks.

Storage Conditions: Store at 20°C to 25°C (68°F to 77°F).

Different types of Formulations

- Powder, for solution
- Tablet, film coated
- Solution

Popular brand names: Sabril, Vigadrone

Lamotrigine

Classification: Anticonvulsants

Chemical Name: 6-(2,3-dichlorophenyl)-1,2,4-triazine-3,5-diamine

Chemical Structure

Uses

- Lamotrigine is used alone or with other medications to treat epileptic seizures in adults and children. Lamotrigine is also used to delay mood episodes in adults with bipolar disorder (manic depression).

Stability

- Lamotrigine is susceptible to degradation under acidic, basic, neutral and oxidative conditions, among which alkaline-induced hydrolysis had the highest degradative potential.

Storage Conditions

- Keep container tightly closed in a dry and well-ventilated place.
- Recommended storage temperature: 2°C-8°C.
- Keep in a dry place.

Different types of Formulations

- Tablet
- Tablet, chewable
- Tablet, orally disintegrating
- Tablet, extended release
- Tablet, for suspension

Popular brand names: Lamepil, Lamez, Lametec, Lamitor, Lamogine, Favlam, Lamdep, Epilam, Lamocent, Abrolem.

Anti-depressants

Depression is a disease characterized by feelings of sadness and hopelessness, as well as the inability to experience pleasure in usual activities, changes in sleep patterns and appetite, loss of energy, and suicidal thoughts.

Classification of antidepressants:

I. **Monoamine oxidase inhibitors MAO-I:** Phenelzine, Tranylcypromine, Isocarboxazid and Selegiline

II. **Tricyclic antidepressants (TCAs)**

    (A) NA + 5-HT reuptake inhibitors: Imipramine, Amitriptyline, Trimipramine, Doxepin, Dothiepin, Clomipramine

    (B) Predominantly NA reuptake inhibitors: Desipramine, Nortriptyline, Amoxapine, Reboxetine

III. **Selective serotonin reuptake inhibitors (SSRis):** Fluoxetine, Fluvoxamine, Paroxetine, Sertraline, Citalopram, Escitalopram

IV. **Atypical antidepressants** Trazodone, Mianserin, Mirtazapine, Venlafaxine, Duloxetine, Tianeptine, Amineptine, Bupropion and others.

Amitriptyline Hydrochloride

Classification

Antidepressive Agents

Chemical Name: N,N-dimethyl-3-(2-tricyclo[9.4.0.0^{3,8}]pentadeca-1(15),3,5,7,-11,13hexaenylidene)propan-1-amine

Chemical Structure

Uses

This drug in indicated for the following conditions:

- Major depressive disorder in adults
- Management of neuropathic pain in adults
- Prophylactic treatment of chronic tension-type headache (CTTH) in adults
- Prophylactic treatment of migraine in adults

Off-label uses: Irritable bowel syndrome, sleep disorders, diabetic neuropathy, agitation, fibromyalgia, and insomnia.

Stability

- Amitriptyline is reported to be stable in aqueous solution for up to 8 weeks at room temperature if protected from light.
- An oral liquid prepared from crushed tablets of amitriptyline in water may be relatively stable if stored in amber plastic containers and protected from light.

Storage Conditions

- Store amitriptyline at room temperature between 68°F and 77°F (20°C and 25°C).
- It can be kept for brief periods between 59°F and 86°F (15°C and 30°C).
- Keep this drug away from light.

Different types of Formulations

- Tablet, film coated
- Syrup
- Kit

Popular brand names: Amicon, Amitrip, Amilift, Nildep, Amsha, Odep, Sarotena, Amifree, Amitor, Eliwel

Imipramine Hydrochloride

Classification: Antidepressive Agents

Chemical Name: 3-(5,6-dihydrobenzo[b][1]benzazepin-11-yl)-N,N-dimethyl-propan-1-amine

Chemical Structure

Uses

- For the relief of symptoms of depression and as temporary adjunctive therapy in reducing enuresis in children aged 6 years and older.
- May also be used off-label to manage panic disorders with or without agoraphobia, as a second line agent for ADHD in children and adolescents, to manage bulimia nervosa, for short-term management of acute depressive episodes in bipolar disorder and schizophrenia, for the treatment of acute stress disorder and posttraumatic stress disorder, and for symptomatic treatment of postherpetic neuralgia and painful diabetic neuropathy

Stability

- It is relatively stable in the reconstituted extract at 4°C for at least 48 hr. After 48 hr, the concentration of imipramine decreased between 3.9% and 8.0% compared with the corresponding fresh sample concentrations.

Storage Conditions

- Store imipramine at room temperature between 68°F and 77°F (20°C and 25°C).
- Keep this drug away from light.
- Don't store this medication in moist or damp areas, such as bathrooms.

Different types of Formulations

- Tablet, film coated
- Capsule
- Injection, solution

Popular brand names: Amidep, Dimip, Tofranil, Depsol, Deprid, Elamin, Shimin, Impress, Depik, Itca

Fluoxetine

Classification: Antidepressive Agents

Chemical Name: *N*-methyl-3-phenyl-3-[4-(trifluoromethyl)phenoxy]propan-1-amine

Chemical Structure

Uses
- Fluoxetine is a diphenhydramine derivative and selective serotonin reuptake inhibitor with antidepressant, anti-anxiety, antiobsessional, and antibulimic activity and with potential immunomodulating activity.

Stability
- Fluoxetine exhibited good stability at -20°C and 5°C, but is unstable at room temperature under the same conditions.

Storage Conditions
- Store Fluoxetine at room temperature between 59°F and 86°F (15°C to 30°C).
- Keep the drug away from light.
- Keep Fluoxetine bottle closed tightly.
- Keep out of the reach of children.

Different types of Formulations
- Capsule
- Solution
- Tablet, film coated
- Solution
- Liquid
- Capsule, delayed release

Popular brand names: Flutop, Flutine, Flunil, Floatin, Fluoxwyn, Fludac, Flonol, Flumeg, Flugen, Flumod

Venlafaxine

Classification: Antidepressive Agents

Chemical Name: *N*-methyl-3-phenyl-3-[4-(trifluoromethyl)phenoxy]propan-1-amine

Chemical Structure

Uses

- Venlafaxine is indicated in the management of major depressive disorder (MDD), generalized anxiety disorder (GAD), social anxiety disorder (social phobia), and panic disorder with or without agoraphobia.
- Venlafaxine is also used off-label for prophylaxis of migraine headaches, for reduction of vasomotor symptoms associated with menopause, and for management of neuropathic pain (although there is only minimal evidence of efficacy for this condition).
- It is also considered a second-line option for management of obsessive-compulsive disorder (OCD).

Stability

- Venlafaxine hydrochloride liquid formulations (solution and suspension) are chemically stable for 30 days when stored at room temperature and protected from light.

Storage Conditions

- Keep away from children.
- Keep in a cool, dry place, away from direct sunlight.

Different types of Formulations

- Capsule, extended release
- Tablet
- Tablet, extended release

Popular brand names: Veniz, Venfax, Venlor, Venlift, Biofexor, Vanafex, Venjoy, Ventab, Finidep, Flavix

Duloxetine

Classification: Antidepressive Agents

Chemical Name: (3S)-N-methyl-3-naphthalen-1-yloxy-3-thiophen-2-ylpropan-1-amine

Chemical Structure

Uses

Indicated for:

- Management of Major Depressive Disorder.
- Management of Generalized Anxiety Disorder.
- Management of diabetic peripheral neuropathy.
- Management of fibromyalgia.
- Management of chronic musculoskeletal pain.
- Management of osteoarthritis of the knee in adults.
- Management of chronic lower back pain in adults.
- Management of stress urinary incontinence in adult women.

Off-label uses include:

- Management of chemotherapy-induced peripheral neuropathy.
- Management of stress urinary incontinence in adult men after prostatectomy until recovery is complete.

Stability

- The drug was found to be stable on exposure of 30% H_2O_2 for 48 hr.
- It was found to be highly unstable in acidic conditions, as 41.35% degradation was observed in 0.01 N HCl at 40°C after 8 hr.

Storage Conditions

- Store at 25°C (77°F); excursions permitted to 15-30°C (59-86°F).
- Store at room temperature away from light and moisture.
- Do not store in the bathroom.
- Keep all medications away from children and pet.

Different types of Formulations

- Capsule, delayed release pellets
- Capsule, delayed release

Popular brand names: Dulane, Dulopin, Delok, Dulaxus, Dulotin, Duvanta, Ambidext, Sympta, Xeldin, Dulot

Sertraline

Classification: Antidepressive Agents

Chemical Name: (1S,4S)-4-(3,4-dichlorophenyl)-N-methyl-1,2,3,4-tetrahydronaph-thalen-1-amine

Chemical Structure

Uses
- Sertraline is indicated for the management of major depressive disorder (MDD), post-traumatic stress disorder (PTSD), obsessive-compulsive disorder (OCD), panic disorder (PD), premenstrual dysphoric disorder (PMDD), and social anxiety disorder (SAD). Common off-label uses for sertraline include the prevention of post stroke depression, generalized anxiety disorder (GAD), fibromyalgia, premature ejaculation, migraine prophylaxis, diabetic neuropathy, and neurocardiogenic syncope.

Stability: The drug is subjected to alkaline, acidic, oxidative, and photolytic degradation.

Storage Conditions
- Store drug at 20°C to 25°C (68°F to 77°F); excursions permitted to 15°C to 30°C (59°F to 86°F).
- Capsules are packaged in opaque high density polyethylene bottles and are stored at controlled room temperature between 15°C to 30°C.

Different types of Formulations
- Tablet, film coated
- Capsule

Popular brand names: Serlift, Serta, Elesert, Daxid, Sertaj, Serdep, Sermind, Sernext, Sertrax, Serenata

Citalopram

Classification: Antidepressive Agents

Chemical Name: 1-[3-(dimethylamino)propyl]-1-(4-fluorophenyl)-3H-2-benzofuran-5-carbonitrile

Chemical Structure

Uses

- For the treatment of depression, as indicated by the FDA.
- Off-label indications include but are not limited to: treatment of sexual dysfunction, post-stroke behavioral changes, ethanol abuse, obsessive-compulsive disorder (OCD) in children, and diabetic neuropathy

Stability

- The drug is found unstable in hydrolytic and photolytic conditions in all media.
- The drug is stable to heat in solid state.

Storage Conditions

- Store citalopram tablets at room temperature, 77°F (25°C).
- The tablets can temporarily be stored at temperatures between 59°F and 86°F (15°C and 30°C).
- Keep this drug away from high temperatures.

Different types of Formulations

- Tablet, film coated
- Tablet
- Solution

Popular brand names: Citara, Citola, Vocita, Celapram, Citaneo, Citalomine, Citlop, Citox, Celexa, Citalent

Escitalopram

Classification: Antidepressive Agents

Chemical Name: *N*-methyl-3-phenyl-3-[4-(trifluoromethyl)phenoxy]propan-1-amine

Chemical Structure

Uses

- Escitalopram is indicated for both acute and maintenance treatment of major depressive disorder (MDD) and for the acute treatment of generalized anxiety disorder (GAD).
- It is additionally indicated for symptomatic relief of obsessive-compulsive disorder (OCD) in Canada.

Stability

- It degrades under acidic (0.1 M HCL) and oxidative (3% H_2O_2) stress conditions employed.
- It is found to be stable to the alkaline (0.1 M NaOH) and unstable in photo (240 nm) degradation.

Storage Conditions: Store escitalopram at room temperature between 59°F and 86°F (15°C and 30°C).

Different types of Formulations

- Tablet, orally disintegrating
- Tablet, film coated
- Tablet
- Solution

Popular brand names: Ezeepam, Eluga, Galop, Elorpax, Enzycare, Ezvio, Escipix, Escipra, Escigress, Desilam

Fluvoxamine

Classification: Antidepressive Agents

Chemical Name: 2-[(E)-[5-methoxy-1-[4-(trifluoromethyl)phenyl]pentylidene]amino]oxyethanamine

Chemical Structure

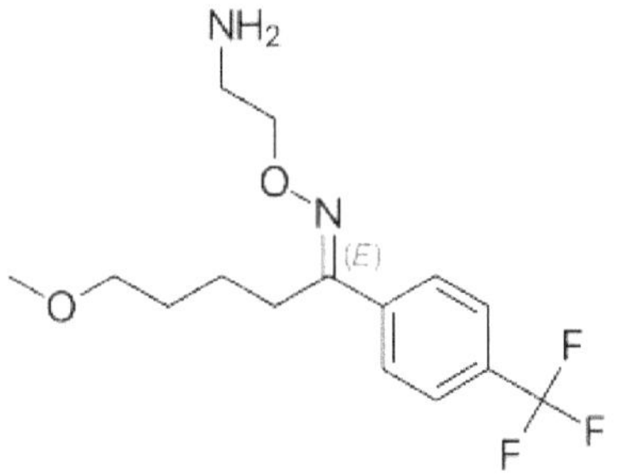

Uses

- Indicated predominantly for the management of depression and for Obsessive Compulsive Disorder (OCD).
- It has also been used in the management of bulimia nervosa.

Stability: Fluvoxamine is relatively unstable under acidic, basic and oxidative conditions and also when exposed to UV radiation.

Storage Conditions

- Store fluvoxamine at room temperature between 59°F and 86°F (15°C and 30°C).
- Keep this drug away from light.

Different types of Formulations

- Tablet, film coated
- Capsule, extended release

Popular brand names: Voxidep, Fluvoxin, Sorest, Frext, Uvox, Floxem, Fluvo, Ambivox, Serovoxin, Voxinix

Paroxetine

Classification: Antidepressive Agents

Chemical Name: 6-(2,3-dichlorophenyl)-1,2,4-triazine-3,5-diamine

Chemical Structure

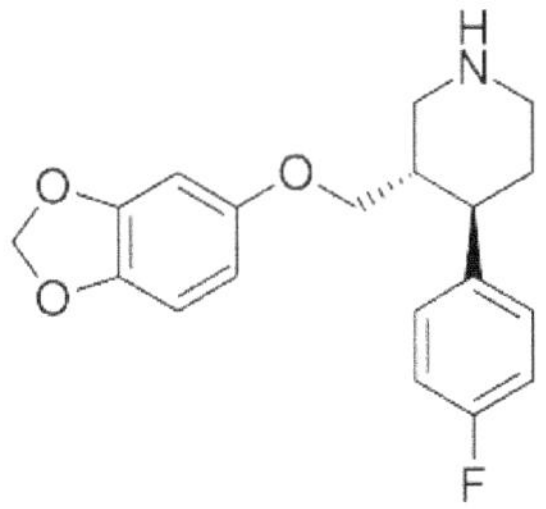

Uses

- Paroxetine is indicated for the management of depression, obsessive-compulsive disorder, panic disorder, social anxiety disorder, generalized anxiety disorder, posttraumatic stress disorder.

Stability

- Paroxetine is degraded completely within 4 day by simulated sunlight in all aqueous media.
- In the dark, paroxetine in all aqueous solutions was found to be stable over 30-days period.

Storage Conditions

- Tablets should be kept at room temperature, $59°F$ - $86°F$ ($15°C$ - $30°C$).
- The suspension and controlled release tablets should be stored at or below $77°F$ ($25°C$).

Different types of Formulations

- Capsule
- Tablet
- Tablet, film coated, extended release
- Suspension

Popular brand names: Pexep, Panex, Oxtus, Parotin, Paroxet, Pirotin, Praxo, Paxit, Xepar, Patix

---

Multiple Choice Questions

1. Which one of the following actions of opioid analgesics is mediated via activation of kappa receptors?
   (a) Cerebral vascular dilation
   (b) Decreased uterine tone
   (c) Euphoria
   (d) Sedation

2. Which of the following antipsychotics (in excess dose) is responsible for cardiac arrhythmias?
   (a) Chlorpromazine
   (b) Clozapine
   (c) Thioridazine
   (d) Haloperidol
   (e) Thiothixene

3. The opiate associated with seizures when given in high doses to patients with renal failure is
   (a) Morphine
   (b) Pethidine
   (c) Methadone
   (d) Fentanyl
   (e) Codeine

4. Which of the following local anaesthetic agents is an ester
   (a) Bupivacaine
   (b) Ropivacaine
   (c) Prilocaine
   (d) Procaine
   (e) Lignocaine

5. The opiate associated with seizures when given in high doses to patients with renal failure is
   (a) Morphine
   (b) Pethidine
   (c) Methadone
   (d) Fentanyl
   (e) Codeine

6. With respect to opioid receptors
   (a) Fentanyl works predominantly at the kappa receptors
   (b) Both U and delta receptors contribute to respiratory depression
   (c) Methadone is used for heroin withdrawal because its actions are predominantly at the delta receptors
   (d) Opioid receptors are coupled to a tyrosine kinase mechanism of action
   (e) Physical dependence and tolerance is caused by the rapid disintegration of receptors

7. Codeine
   (a) Is more potent than fentanyl
   (b) Frequently causes diarrhoea
   (c) Is used to treat nausea caused by morphine
   (d) Occurs in foxglove plants
   (e) Depresses the cough reflex

8. Benzodiazepines
   (a) Increase the duration of GABA gated chloride channel openings
   (b) Will depress (in high doses) the CNS to the point known as stage 3 of general anaesthesia
   (c) Bind to GABAβ receptors
   (d) Have extensive cardiodepressant effects in doses used to cause hypnosis
   (e) Decrease the duration of stage 2 NREM sleep

9. Regarding non-depolarising muscle relaxants
   (a) Pancuronium is eliminated via the kidney
   (b) Roacuronium is an isoquinolone derivative
   (c) Roacuronium undergoes Hoffman elimination
   (d) Vecuronium is eliminated predominantly via the kidney e. Atracurium is eliminated via plasma pseudocholinesterase

10. The main side effect of benztropine is
    (a) Miosis
    (b) Confusion
    (c) Diarrhoea
    (d) GIT haemorrhage
    (e) Bronchorrhoea

CHAPTER 6

Drugs Acting on Autonomic Nervous System

Introduction

The chapter aims at providing the latest and pharmacopoeial information regarding some Drugs acting on Autonomic Nervous System (Nor-epinephrine, Epinephrine, Phenylephrine, Dopamine, Terbutaline, Salmeterol, Salbutamol, Albuterol, Naphazoline, Tetrahydrazoline, Oxymetazoline, Hydroxyamphetamine, Pseudoephedrine, Propylhexadrine, Ephedrine, Metaraminol, Tolazoline, Phentolamine, Phenoxybenzamine, Prazosin, Doxazosin, Propranolol,

Practolol, Acebutolol, Atenolol, Esmolol, Metoprolol, Labetolol, Carvedilol, Acetylcholine, Carbachol, Bethanechol, Methacholine, Pilocarpine, Neostigmine, Pyridostigmine, Edrophonium chloride, Tacrine hydrochloride, Ambinonium chloride, Pralidoxime chloride, Isofluorphate, Echothiophate iodide, Parathion, Malathion, Atropine sulphate, Homatropine hydrogen bromide, Ipratropium bromide, Tropicamide, Cyclopentolate hydrochloride, Clindinium bromide, Dicyclomine hydrochloride, Procylidine hydrochloride, Tridihex ethylchloride, Isopropamide iodide, and Ethopropazine hydrochloride) regarding their classification, chemical name, chemical structure, uses, stability, storage conditions, different types of formulations, and popular brand names.

Sympathomimetic Agents

Sympathetic nervous system is an important regulator of the activities of the vital organs, such as heart and peripheral vasculature, especially in response to stress. The effect of sympathetic stimulation is mediated by the release of norepinephrine from the nerve terminals that serve to activate the adrenoreceptors on postsynaptic sites. Also, in response to a variety of stimuli, such as stress, the adrenal medulla releases epinephrine, and it is transported in the blood to the target tissues.

Drugs that mimic the action of sympathetic system are called sympathomimetic drugs. Like cholinomimetic drugs, the sympathomimetics can be grouped by their mode of action and by the spectrum of receptors. Some of the drugs (e.g. epinephrine, norepinephrine) act by a direct mode, that is, they interact with and activate adrenoceptor. Others act indirectly; their actions are dependent on the release of endogenous catecholamine. These indirect agents may have either of the different mechanisms:

1. Displacement of stored catecholamine from adrenergic nerve ending (e.g. amphetamine and tyramine).
2. By inhibition of reuptake of catecholamine already released (e.g. cocaine and tricyclic antidepressants).
3. Some drugs have both direct and indirect action.

Classification

Adrenergic agents are divided into three classes

I. **Direct-acting adrenergic agonists** They bind to and activate α_1, α_2, β_1, and β_2 receptors. Naturally occurring molecules, which bind to these receptors include NE (a neurotransmitter which binds to $\alpha1$, $\alpha2$, and $\beta1$ receptors), Epinephrine (a hormone produced in and secreted from the adrenal medulla, which binds to $\alpha1$, $\alpha2$, $\beta1$, and $\beta2$ receptors, it is a nonselective adrenergic agonists), and Dopamine (also a neurotransmitter, which binds to $\alpha1$, $\alpha2$, and $\beta1$ receptors).

   Examples of drugs: xylometazoline, phenylephrine, methoxamine.

II. **Indirect-acting adrenergic agonists** They produce NE-like actions by stimulating NE release and preventing its reuptake and produces activation. Example: Tyramine.

III. **Dual-acting adrenergic agonists** These agents act as direct and indirect adrenergic agonists (hence, dual-acting). They bind to adrenergic receptors and stimulate NE release.

   Examples: Ephedrine, Amphetamine, Mephenteramine.

Direct Acting

Norepinephrine

Classification: Adrenergic alpha-Agonists
Chemical Name: 4-[(1*R*)-2-amino-1-hydroxyethyl]benzene-1,2-diol

Chemical Structure

Uses

- Mainly used to treat patients in vasodilatory shock states such as septic shock and neurogenic shock and has shown a survival benefit over dopamine.
- Also used as a vasopressor medication for patients with critical hypotension.

Stability

- Norepinephrine solutions, in concentrations commonly used in the clinical setting, are chemically stable for seven days, at room temperature and under ambient light, when diluted in normal saline.
- It is not stable, and their degradation is favored mainly by the oxidation of catechol moiety.

Storage Conditions

- Injectors should be stored in a cool dark place at room temperature, between 15-25°C, but not refrigerated, as temperatures below 15°C may damage the injector mechanism.

Different types of Formulations: Injection (solution), Solution, Liquid

Popular brand names: Adrenor, Infunor, Noraderin, Noradria, Epinor, Vescue

Epinephrine

Classification: Adrenergic beta-Agonists

Chemical Name: 4-[(1*R*)-1-hydroxy-2-(methylamino)ethyl]benzene-1,2-diol

Chemical Structure

Uses

- Epinephrine injection is indicated in the emergency treatment of allergic reactions as well as idiopathic anaphylaxis or exercise-induced anaphylaxis.
- Epinephrine's cardiac effects may be of use in restoring cardiac rhythm in cardiac arrest.

- Epinephrine is used as a hemostatic agent. It is also used in treating mucosal congestion of hay fever, rhinitis, and acute sinusitis; to relieve bronchial asthmatic paroxysms.
- Epinephrine injection can be utilized to prolong the action of local anesthetics.
- It is also used for the maintenance of mydriasis during intraocular surgery

Stability: Preparations of epinephrine are stable for up to 30 days, with or without refrigeration. Because stability alone does not guarantee bioavailability or efficacy of a drug, future clinical studies are recommended to evaluate the pharmacokinetics and pharmacodynamics of these formulations.

Storage Conditions: Injectors should be stored in a cool dark place at room temperature, between 15-25°C, but not refrigerated, as temperatures below 15°C may damage the injector mechanism.

Different types of Formulations: Injection (solution), Solution, liquid, Spray

Popular brand names: Epipen, Adrenalin, Auvi-Q, Asthimo, Binilon, Cirex, Cinol, Cofwin, Coskap, Franklor.

Phenylephrine

Classification: Adrenergic alpha-1 Receptor Agonists

Chemical Name: 3-[(1R)-1-hydroxy-2-(methylamino)ethyl] phenol

Chemical Structure

Uses

- Phenylephrine injections are indicated to treat hypotension caused by shock or anesthesia, an ophthalmic formulation is indicated to dilate pupils and induce vasoconstriction, an intranasal formulation is used to treat congestion, and a topical formulation is used to treat hemorrhoids.
- Off-label uses include situations that require local blood flow restriction such as the treatment of priapism.

Stability: Phenylephrine is stable for 14 days at room temperature when diluted to 100 and 200 µg/mL in sodium chloride 0.9% in polyvinyl chloride (PVC) bags.

Storage Conditions

- Store injection at 20°C to 25°C (68°F to 77°F), excursions permitted to 15°C to 30°C (59°F to 86°F).

- Protect from light.
- Store in carton until time of use.

Different types of Formulations: Injection (solution), Solution, Drop.

Popular brand names: Phenpres, Paripher, Nefrisol, Frenin, Drosyn, Nefrin, Sunepherine, Deconsal, Histinex, Riyatuss

Dopamine

Classification: Sympathomimetics

Chemical Name: 4-(2-aminoethyl)benzene-1,2-diol

Chemical Structure

Uses: For the correction of hemodynamic imbalances present in the shock syndrome due to myocardial infarction, trauma, endotoxic septicemia, open-heart surgery, renal failure, and chronic cardiac decompensation as in congestive failure.

Stability: Dopamine hydrochloride 0.5 mg/mL in isotonic glucose solution is stable when protected from light for 1 week at 25°C/60% relative humidity and for 3 months at 4°C/ambient humidity.

Storage Conditions: Store injections at 20°C to 25°C (68°F to 77°F); excursions permitted to 15°C to 30°C (59° to 86°F).

Different types of Formulations: Injection(solution), Liquid, Solution

Popular brand names: Cupamin, Domin, Dopacard, Dopacef, Dopan, Dopinga, Dopasol, Dopar, Dopress, Komidop

Terbutaline

Classification: Adrenergic beta-2 Receptor Agonists

Chemical Name: 5-[2-(*tert*-butylamino)-1-hydroxyethyl]benzene-1,3-diol

Chemical Structure

Uses: Terbutaline is indicated for prevention and reversal of bronchospasm in patients at least 12 years old, with asthma and reversible bronchospasm associated with bronchitis and emphysema.

Stability: Terbutaline sulfate in polypropylene syringes is stable for 60 days under refrigeration and at room temperature when protected from light, but substantial degradation and discoloration of the drug can occur when the syringes are not protected from light.

Storage Conditions: Tablets and injection should be stored at room temperature, $15°C - 30°C$ ($59°F - 86°F$).

Different types of Formulations: Tablet, Powder, metered.

Popular brand names: Brethaire, Brethine, Bricanyl, Cosome-A, Cinkof, Resipax, Trucof, Amvoryl, Mucambo-T, Rid-At.

Salmeterol

Classification: Adrenergic beta-2 Receptor Agonists

Chemical Name: 2-(hydroxymethyl)-4-[1-hydroxy-2-[6-(4-phenylbutoxy)hexyl-amino]ethyl]phenol

Chemical Structure

Uses: Salmeterol is indicated in the treatment of asthma with an inhaled corticosteroid, prevention of exercise induced bronchospasm, and the maintenance of airflow obstruction and prevention of exacerbations of chronic obstructive pulmonary disease.

Stability: Salmeterol is prone to alkali hydrolysis, oxidation and thermal degradation.

Storage Conditions

- Salmeterol should be stored from $36°F$ to $86°F$ ($2.2°C$ to $30°C$).
- The canister should be kept away from heat or flame and not punctured; it should not be frozen or placed in direct sunlight.

Different types of Formulations: Aerosol(metered), Powder (metered)

Popular brand names: Seroflo, Flutrol, Salvent, Seretide, Airtec, Forair, Salvent

Salbutamol

Classification: Adrenergic beta-2 Receptor Agonists.

Chemical Name: 4- [2-(*tert*-butyl amino)-1-hydroxyethyl]-2-(hydroxymethyl)phenol

Chemical Structure

Uses: Salbutamol is indicated for:

- The symptomatic relief and prevention of bronchospasm due to bronchial asthma, chronic bronchitis, reversible obstructive airway disease, and other chronic bronchopulmonary disorders in which bronchospasm is a complicating factor.
- The acute prophylaxis against exercise-induced bronchospasm and other stimuli known to induce bronchospasm.

Stability: The decomposition of salbutamol in aqueous solution obeyed apparent first-order kinetics with respect to salbutamol sulphate. The reaction rate increased with increasing initial drug concentration and elevated temperatures. The maximum stability of salbutamol in aqueous solution occurred at a pH of about 3.5.

Storage Conditions: Store at room temperature between 59°F-86°F (15°C-30°C) away from light and moisture.

- It is best to store the inhaler with the mouthpiece down.
- Do not puncture the canister or expose it to high heat or open flame.

Different types of Formulations: Solution, Aerosol (spray), Aerosol (metered), Tablet

Popular brand names: Asthalin, Budesal, Salbair, Servent, Bronosol, Theosalbid, Amrolite, Salmaplon, Lebasma, Ventolin

Albuterol

Classification: Adrenergic beta-2 Receptor Agonists

Chemical Name: 4-[2-(*tert*-butylamino)-1-hydroxyethyl]-2-(hydroxymethyl)phenol

Chemical Structure

Uses

- The symptomatic relief and prevention of bronchospasm due to bronchial asthma, chronic bronchitis, reversible obstructive airway disease, and other chronic bronchopulmonary disorders in which bronchospasm is a complicating factor.
- The acute prophylaxis against exercise-induced bronchospasm and other stimuli known to induce bronchospasm.

Stability

- The drug form has a great impact on the chemical and physical stability of the formulations.
- The sulfate formulations were chemically stable up to 12 months when stored at $30°C$ and 85% relative humidity.

Storage Conditions

- Store nebulizer solution vials in the refrigerator or at room temperature away from excess heat and moisture (not in the bathroom).
- Store the inhaler at room temperature and away from excess heat and moisture (not in the bathroom).

Different types of Formulations: Solution, Aerosol, metered, Aerosol (spray), Inhalant, Powder, Spray.

Popular brand names: Xputum, Respisol, Ventsolv, Somavent, Aerocort, Exiplon, Avasth, Brethmol, Ventirex, Salvent

Naphazoline

Classification: Adrenergic alpha-Agonists

Chemical Name: 2-(naphthalen-1-ylmethyl)-4,5-dihydro-1*H*-imidazole

Chemical Structure

Uses: Naphazoline is indicated for use as OTC eyedrops for ocular vasoconstriction or as a nasal preparation for nasal congestion.

Stability: Naphazoline is degraded up to 94.3% for 240 hr under thermal stress.

Storage Conditions
- Store dropper bottle upright at room temperature between 68-77°F (20-25°C) away from moisture and sunlight.
- Do not store in the bathroom.
- Discard if drops become discolored or cloudy.

Different types of Formulations: Solution, Drops, Liquid, Suspension

Popular brand names: Clearine, E-Line, E-Norm, I-Klean, Efcorlin, N-Cool, Mezol, N-Zolin, Napzol, Niczole

Tetrahydrozoline

Classification: Sympathomimetics

Chemical Name: 2-(1,2,3,4-tetrahydronaphthalen-1-yl)-4,5-dihydro-1*H*-imidazole

Chemical Structure

Uses
- It is indicated for the temporary relief of discomfort and redness of the eye due to minor eye irritations as monotherapy or in combination with other eye lubricants and anti-irritants.
- It is also indicated for decongestion of nasal and nasopharyngeal mucosa.

Stability: Tetrahydrozoline is not stable in acidic and basic solutions.

Storage Conditions
- Tetrahydrozoline ophthalmic solutions should be stored in tight containers.
- Store solutions at room temperature away from moisture and heat. Do not freeze.
- Keep the bottle tightly closed when not in use.

Different types of Formulations: Solution, Drops, Liquid

Popular brand names: Vasozine, Clearview, Vizoline

Oxymetazoline

Classification: Adrenergic alpha-Agonists

Chemical Name: 6-*tert*-butyl-3-(4,5-dihydro-1*H*-imidazol-2-ylmethyl)-2,4-dimethyl-phenol

Chemical Structure

Uses: Oxymetazoline is indicated for the topical treatment of persistent facial erythema associated with rosacea in adults.

- Ophthalmic oxymetazoline is indicated for the treatment of acquired blepharoptosis in adults.

Stability: Oxymetazoline is more stable in aqueous solution in the form of their hydrochloride salts, undesired hydrolytic degradation of the active compounds, in particular due to hydrolytic cleavage of the imidazole ring, does also occur in these on storage, in particular at elevated temperature.

Storage Conditions

- Store the medicine in a closed container at room temperature, away from heat, moisture, and direct light.
- Keep from freezing.

Different types of Formulations: Solution, Cream, Drops, Spray, Liquid, Spray (metered)

Popular brand names: Oxywyn, Oxyspray, Zoamet, Nasivion, Maxtra, Otrivin, Naselin, Breasy, Naso, Nazoden

Indirect acting agents:

Hydroxy Amphetamine

Classification: Sympathomimetics

Chemical Name: 4-(2-aminopropyl)phenol

Chemical Structure

Uses

- Mydriatic agent (eye pupil dilatation) for diagnosis of ophthalmic nerve lesions.
- It is an indirectly acting sympathomimetic agent producing mydriasis for diagnostic purposes.

Stability: Drugs are degraded through oxidation and hydrolytic reactions.

Storage Conditions

- Store between 20°C and 25°C (68°F and 77°F).
- Protect from light.

Different types of Formulations: Tablet, Capsule, Drops

Popular brand names: Paredrine, Paremyd

Pseudoephedrine

Classification: Bronchodilator Agents

Chemical Name: (1*S*,2*S*)-2-(methylamino)-1-phenylpropan-1-ol

Chemical Structure:

Uses: It is an alpha and beta adrenergic agonist used to treat nasal and sinus congestion, as well as allergic rhinitis.

Stability: The drug solutions remain stable for at least 10 days when kept at room temperature.

Storage Conditions:

- The tablets should generally be stored at 15-30°C.
- The freezing of the oral solution should be avoided.

Different types of Formulations: Tablet, film coated, Tablet (extended release), Syrup, Capsule (extended release), Pill, Capsule (gelatin coated), Tablet (sugar coated)

Popular brand names: Cofvyn, Wytuss, Benylin, Licit, Hatric, Verizet, Monlez, Solvin, Allrite, Antizine.

Propylhexedrine

Classification: Alpha adrenergic agonist

Chemical Name: 1-cyclohexyl-*N*-methylpropan-2-amine

Chemical Structure

Uses: It is used to provide temporary symptomatic relief of nasal congestion due to colds, allergies and allergic rhinitis.

Stability: Propylhexedrine (hydrochloride) be stored as supplied at -20°C during shipping. It remains stable for at least two years.

Storage Conditions

- Store at 59°-86° F (15°-30° C).
- Keep inhaler tightly closed.

Different types of Formulations: Inhalant

Popular brand names: Benzedrex, Obesin.

Agents with mixed mechanism:

Ephedrine

Classification: Sympathomimetics

Chemical Name: (1*R*,2*S*)-2-(methylamino)-1-phenylpropan-1-ol

Chemical Structure:

Uses: Ephedrine intravenous injections are indicated to treat hypotension under anesthesia, ephedrine injections by multiple routes are indicated to treat allergic conditions such as bronchial asthma, ephedrine nasal spray is and OTC medication used as a decongestant.

Stability: The injections in polypropylene syringes are stable for up to 60 days at both ambient temperature and at 4°C.

Storage Conditions

- Store this medication at room temperature, between 59°F and 77°F (15°C and 25°C).
- Store away from heat, moisture, and light.
- Do not store in the bathroom.
- Keep ephedrine out of the reach of children and away from pets.

Different types of Formulations: Injection, Injection, solution

Popular brand names: Efipress, Asmapax, Marax, Tedral, Astagon, Asmalax, Cadiphylate

Metaraminol

Classification: Adrenergic alpha-1 Receptor Agonists

Chemical Name: 3-[(1R,2S)-2-amino-1-hydroxypropyl] phenol

Chemical Structure

Uses: For the treatment and prevention of hypotension due to hemorrhage, spinal anesthesia, and shock associated with brain damage.

Stability: Pre-filled syringes are stable for up to 378 days when stored at room temperature.

Storage Conditions

- Stable between 2-8°C for 24-48 hrs. in an intravenous infusion of Sodium Chloride 0.9% Solution or Glucose 5% Solution.
- Do not store above 25°C.
- After dilution, chemical and physical in-use stability has been demonstrated for 48 hours when the diluted product is stored between 2 to 8°C.

Different types of Formulations: Tablet, Capsule, Solution, Suspension

Popular brand names: Aramine, Metaramin, Pressonex.

Adrenergic Antagonists

Adrenergic blockers are also called as antiadrenergic drugs or sympatholytics. Adrenergic blocking agents prevent the response of effector organs to endogenous as well as exogenous adrenaline and noradrenaline. These drugs block the actions of adrenergic drugs at alpha (α) or beta (β) adrenergic receptors. Many types of adrenergic antagonists are used and several of these are clinically useful in medicine, particularly in the treatment of cardiovascular diseases. Drugs that decrease the amount of norepinephrine released as a consequence of sympathetic nerve stimulation as well as drugs that inhibit sympathetic nervous activity by suppressing sympathetic outflow is also widely used in medications. Almost all of these agents are competitive antagonists in their interactions with either α or β adrenergic receptors, and one exception is phenoxybenzamine, an irreversible antagonist that binds covalently to α-adrenergic receptors. These are due to important structural differences among the various types of adrenergic receptors. Selective β1 antagonist drugs are used to act on the heart and selective β2 antagonist drugs are used to act on the respiratory system.

Classification

I. **Alpha receptor blocking agents**
   (a) Beta halo alkyl amines
       (i) Dibenamine
       (ii) Phenoxy benzamine
   (b) Natural and dehydrogenated ergot alkaloids
   (c) Imidazole derivatives
       (i) Tolazoline
       (ii) Phentolamine
   (d) Quinazolines
       (i) Prazosin
       (ii) Terazosin
       (iii) Doxazosin
   (e) Miscellaneous
       (i) Indoramine
       (ii) Yohimbine,
       (iii) Chlorpromazine

II. **Beta-receptor blocking agents**
   (a) β-Blockers with membrane stabilizing activity and intrinsic sympathomimetic property
       (i) Oxprenalol
       (ii) Pindalol
   (b) Specific β-blockers
       (i) Timolol
       (ii) Nodalol
   (c) β-blockers with membrane stabilizing activity
       (i) Propranolol

(d) β-blockers with cardio selective action
- (i) Acebutolol
- (ii) Atenolol
- (iii) Metaprolol
- (iv) Esmolol

(e) β-Blockers with α-blocking property
- (i) Labetolol
- (ii) Carvediol

Alpha Adrenergic Blockers

Q. Write a detailed note on Tolazoline.

Classification: Adrenergic alpha-Antagonists

Chemical Name: 2-benzyl-4,5-dihydro-1*H*-imidazole

Chemical Structure

Uses: For the treatment of pulmonary artery anomalies.

Stability: Tolazoline reconstituted solution is stable for 14 days.

Storage Conditions:
- Protect from light.
- Store at controlled room temperature 15°C to 30°C

Different types of Formulations: Injection, solution.

Popular brand names: Priscoline, Priscol, Priscophen.

Phentolamine

Classification: Adrenergic Alpha-Antagonists

Chemical Name: 3-[*N*-(4,5-dihydro-1*H*-imidazol-2-ylmethyl)-4-methylanilino] phenol

Chemical Structure

Uses

- Used as an aid for the diagnosis of pheochromocytoma, and may be administered immediately prior to or during pheochromocytomectomy to prevent or control paroxysmal hypertension resulting from anesthesia, stress, or operative manipulation of the tumor.
- Phentolamine has also been used to treat hypertensive crisis caused by sympathomimetic amines or catecholamine excess by certain foods or drugs in patients taking MAO inhibitors, or by clonidine withdrawal syndrome.
- Other indications include the prevention of dermal necrosis and sloughing following IV administration or extravasation of norepinephrine, decrease in impedance to left ventricular ejection and the infarct size in patients with MI associated with left ventricular failure, treatment of erectile dysfunction through self-injection of small doses combined with papaverine hydrochloride into the corpus cavernosum, and as an adjunct to the management of cocaine overdose to reverse coronary vasoconstriction following use of oxygen, benzodiazepines, and nitroglycerin.

Stability: Phentolamine is stable in injectable mixtures when stored for up to 30 days at 5°C or 25°C.

Storage Conditions:

- Store injection at 20°C to 25°C (68°F to 77°F). The reconstituted solution should be used upon preparation and should not be stored.
- Do not permit to freeze.

Different types of Formulations: Injection (solution), Solution, Injection (powder, lyophilized, for suspension), Powder (for solution), Injection (powder, for solution)

Popular brand names: Fentanor, Rogitine, Phentosol, Fentosol, Oraverse

Phenoxybenzamine

Classification: Adrenergic alpha-Antagonists

Chemical Name: *N*-benzyl-*N*-(2-chloroethyl)-1-phenoxypropan-2-amine

Chemical Structure

Uses: For the treatment of phaeochromocytoma (malignant), benign prostatic hypertrophy and malignant essential hypertension.

Stability: Phenoxybenzamine hydrochloride 2 mg/mL in 1% propylene glycol and 0.15% citric acid in distilled water is stable for 7 days at 4°C.

Storage Conditions: Rapid degradation takes place in neutral or basic aqueous solutions.

Different types of Formulations: Capsule.

Popular brand names: Fenoxene.

Q. Write a detailed note on Prazosin.

Classification: Adrenergic alpha-1 Receptor Antagonists

Chemical Name: [4-(4-amino-6,7-dimethoxyquinazolin-2-yl)piperazin-1-yl]-(furan-2-yl)methanone

Chemical Structure

Uses

- This drug is indicated for the treatment of hypertension (high blood pressure).
- Prazosin can be given alone or given with other blood pressure-lowering drugs, including diuretics or beta-adrenergic blocking agents.

Stability: Prazosin is more sensitive towards acidic, basic, and oxidative degradation.

Storage Conditions: Prazosin hydrochloride capsules should be stored in well closed, light resistant containers at 15°C - 30°C.

Different types of Formulations: Capsule, Tablet.

Popular brand names: Prozoten, Prazopill, Prazon, Unipraz, Prazopress, Prazowyn, Prazonol, Pracept, Minipress, Renopress.

Q. Write a detailed note on Doxazosin.

Classification: Adrenergic alpha-1 Receptor Antagonists

Chemical Name: [4-(4-amino-6,7-dimethoxyquinazolin-2-yl)piperazin-1-yl]-(2,3-dihydro-1,4-benzodioxin-3-yl)methanone.

Chemical Structure

Uses

- Doxazosin is indicated to treat the symptoms of benign prostatic hypertrophy, which may include urinary frequency, urgency, and nocturia, among other symptoms.
- In addition, doxazosin is indicated alone or in combination with various antihypertensive agents for the management of hypertension.
- Off-label uses of doxazosin include the treatment of pediatric hypertension and the treatment of ureteric calculi.

Stability: Doxazosin mesylate was observed degradation under base hydrolysis and acid hydrolysis.

Storage Conditions: Doxazosin should be stored at room temperature, 15°C - 30°C (59°F - 86°F).

Different types of Formulations: Tablet.

Popular brand names: Doxacard, Duracard, Noksin, Cardura

Q. Write a detailed note on Propranolol.

Classification: Adrenergic beta-Antagonists

Chemical Name: 1-naphthalen-1-yloxy-3-(propan-2-ylamino)propan-2-ol

Chemical Structure

Uses: Propranolol is indicated to treat hypertension.

- Propranolol is also indicated to treat angina pectoris due to coronary atherosclerosis, atrial fibrillation, myocardial infarction, migraine, essential tremor, hypertrophic subaortic stenosis, pheochromocytoma, and proliferating infantile hemangioma.

Stability: Propranolol suspensions stored at 25°C maintained at least 94.7% of their initial concentration for 120 days, and suspensions stored at 4°C maintained at least 93.9% of their initial concentration for 120 days.

Storage Conditions: Tablets and capsules should be stored at room temperature, 15°C to 30°C (59°F to 86°F), in a tightly closed container.

Different types of Formulations: Tablet, Solution, Capsule (extended release), Liquid, injection (solution).

Popular brand names: Prolol, Provanol, Betacap, Inderal, Erolol, Ponol, Kipnol, Capinol, Movalol, Betapill.

Q. Write a detailed note on Practolol.

Classification: Adrenergic beta-1 Receptor Antagonists.

Chemical Name: *N*-[4-[2-hydroxy-3-(propan-2-ylamino)propoxy]phenyl]acetamide

Chemical Structure

Uses: Used in the emergency treatment of cardiac arrhythmias.

Stability: Degradation is observed in acidic solution.

Storage Conditions: Store between 15°C and 30°C.

Different types of Formulations: Tablet, Capsule.

Popular brand names: Eraldin, Dalzic.

Q. Write a detailed note on Acebutolol.

Classification: Adrenergic beta-1 Receptor Antagonists

Chemical   Name: *N*-[3-acetyl-4-[2-hydroxy-3-(propan-2-ylamino)propoxy]phenyl]butanamide

Chemical Structure

Uses: For the management of hypertension and ventricular premature beats in adults.

Stability: Acid induced degradation products have been reported.

Storage Conditions
- Store acebutolol at room temperature between 68°F (20°C) and 77°F (25°C).
- Keep this drug away from light.
- Don't store this medication in moist or damp areas, such as bathrooms.

Different types of Formulations: Tablet, Capsule.

Popular brand names: Sectral, Prent.

Q. Write a detailed note on Atenolol.

Classification: Adrenergic beta-1 Receptor Antagonists

Chemical Name: 2-[4-[2-hydroxy-3-(propan-2-yl amino)propoxy]phenyl]acetamide

Chemical Structure

Uses: Indicated for:
- Management of hypertension alone and in combination with other antihypertensives.
- Management of angina pectoris associated with coronary atherosclerosis.
- Management of acute myocardial infarction in hemodynamically stable patients with a heart rate greater than 50 beats per minutes and a systolic blood pressure above 100 mmHg.
- Off-label uses include:
- Secondary prevention of myocardial infarction.
- Management of heart failure.
- Management of atrial fibrillation.
- Management of supraventricular tachycardia.
- Management of ventricular arrythmias such as congenital long-QT and arrhythmogenic right ventricular cardiomyopathy.
- Management of symptomatic thyrotoxicosis in combination with methimazole.
- Prophylaxis of migraine headaches.
- Management of alcohol withdrawal.

Stability: Atenolol in an oral liquid is stable for up to 40 days when stored at 5°C or 25°C.

Storage Conditions:
- Store this drug at room temperature between 68°F and 77°F (20°C and 25°C).
- Keep the medication tightly closed and in a light-resistant container.
- Store it away from moisture.

Different types of Formulations: Tablet, Tablet (coated)

Popular brand names: Aten, Atecard, Tenormin, Hipres, Atpark, Hypoff, Itel, Ziblok, Atenex, Lonol.

Q. Write a detailed note on Esmolol

Classification: Adrenergic beta-1 Receptor Antagonists.

Chemical Name: methyl 3-[4-[2-hydroxy-3-(propan-2-ylamino)propoxy]phenyl] propanoate

Chemical Structure

Uses
- For the rapid control of ventricular rate in patients with atrial fibrillation or atrial flutter in perioperative, postoperative, or other emergent circumstances where short term control of ventricular rate with a short-acting agent is desirable.
- Also used in noncompensatory sinus tachycardia where the rapid heart rate requires specific intervention.

Stability: Esmolol is stable in the various i.v. fluids for at least 168 hours when stored at 5°C or 23-27°C, for at least 24 hrs, when stored under intense light, and, with one exception, for at least 48 hrs. when stored at 40°C.

Storage Conditions
- Store at 25°C (77°F). Excursions permitted to 15°-30°C (59°-86°F).
- Esmolol hydrochloride concentrate for injection should be stored at 15-30 °C.

- Exposure to temperatures of 40°C or warmer should be avoided; freezing does not adversely affect the concentrate for injection.
- When stored at 15-30 °C, unopened ampoules of the drug have an expiration date of 3 years following the date of manufacture.
- At a concentration of 10 mg/ml, esmolol hydrochloride is chemically and physically stable for at least 24 hours at 15-30 °C or when refrigerated in the following IV solutions.

Different types of Formulations: Injection, Injection (solution)

Popular brand names: Neotach, Clol, Esocard, Esmocard.

Metoprolol

Classification: Adrenergic beta-1 Receptor Antagonists

Chemical Name: 1-[4-(2-methoxyethyl)phenoxy]-3-(propan-2-ylamino)propan-2-ol

Chemical Structure

Uses

- Metoprolol is indicated for the treatment of angina, heart failure, myocardial infarction, atrial fibrillation, atrial flutter and hypertension.
- Some off-label uses of metoprolol include supraventricular tachycardia and thyroid storm.
- All the indications of metoprolol are part of cardiovascular diseases. These conditions correspond to a number of diseases that involve the function of the heart and blood vessels. The underlying causes of these conditions are variable and can be due to genetic disposition, lifestyle decisions such as smoking, obesity, diet, and lack of exercise, and comorbidity with other conditions such as diabetes. The cardiovascular diseases are the leading cause of death on a global scale.

Stability: Metoprolol tartrate injection 1 mg/mL undiluted and 0.5 mg/mL in 0.9% sodium chloride injection and 5% dextrose injection are stable at room temperature for at least 30 hrs.

Storage Conditions

- Store at room temperature between 68°F and 77°F (20°C and 25°C).

- Briefly the drug can be stored at temperatures as low as 59°F (15°C) and as high as 86°F (30°C).
- Keep this drug away from light.

Different types of Formulations: Tablet, extended release, Solution, Tablet, Capsule (extended release), Injection (solution), Tablet (film coated).

Popular brand names: Metoprolite, Supermet, Cord, Velol, Vinicor, Sahamet, Metwyn, Starcad Beta, Metfirst, Metomac.

Labetalol

Classification: Adrenergic beta-Antagonists

Chemical Name: 2-hydroxy-5-[1-hydroxy-2-(4-phenylbutan-2-ylamino)ethyl]benz-amide

Chemical Structure

Uses

- Labetalol injections are indicated to control blood pressure in severe hypertension.
- Labetalol tablets are indicated alone or in combination with antihypertensives like thiazides and loop diuretics to manage hypertension.

Stability

- Labetalol injection has been shown to be incompatible with Sodium Bicarbonate injection BP 4.2% w/v.
- Chemical and physical in-use stability has been demonstrated for 24 hrs at 25°C, 30°C and 40°C.

Storage Conditions: Store at room temperature or under refrigeration (2°C-30°C [36°F-86°F]).

Different types of Formulations: Injection (solution), Tablet, Tablet (film coated), Liquid, Solution.

Popular brand names: Lobet, Labecor, Gravidol, Labol, Eubet, Lebatens, Lexol, Culol, Evabet, Hypobeta.

Carvedilol

Classification: Adrenergic alpha-1 Receptor Antagonists

Chemical Name: 1-(9*H*-carbazol-4-yloxy)-3-[2-(2-methoxyphenoxy)ethylamino] propan-2-ol

Chemical Structure

Uses: Carvedilol is indicated to treat mild to severe heart failure, left ventricular dysfunction after myocardial infarction with ventricular ejection fraction ≤40%, or hypertension.

Stability

- In the alkaline solution, carvedilol was stable during 56 days at 25°C, but only 28 days at 4 and 40°C.
- In the aqueous suspension, carvedilol was stable during 56 days at 4 and 25°C, but only 28 days at 40°C.

Storage Conditions: Store carvedilol tablet at 20°C to 25°C (68°F to 77°F).

- Pediatric oral liquids must be stored in amber glass vials and kept refrigerated (4°C).

Different types of Formulations: Tablet, Tablet (coated), Tablet (film coated), Capsule (extended release).

Popular brand names: Cardilarc, Carca, Conpres, Carvil, Carloc, Cardipure, Carvicare, Carvenol, Carzec, Carvibeta.

Cholinergic Drugs and Related Agents

The nervous system is divided into the somatic nervous system, which controls organs under voluntary control (mainly muscles) and the autonomic nervous system (ANS) which regulates individual organ function and homeostasis, and for the most part is not subject to voluntary control. The autonomic nervous system is also known as the visceral or automatic system. The ANS is predominantly an efferent system transmitting impulses from the central nervous system (CNS) to peripheral organ systems. The autonomic nervous system consists of sensory neurons and motor neurons that innervates between the central nervous system (especially the hypothalamus and medulla oblongata) and various internal organs such as the: heart, lungs, viscera, glands (both exocrine and endocrine). Thus, it is responsible for monitoring conditions in the internal environment and bringing about appropriate changes in them.

The ANS is divided into two separate divisions called the parasympathetic and sympathetic systems, on the basis of anatomical and functional differences. Both of these systems consist of myelinated preganglionic fibres which make synaptic connections with unmyelinated postganglionic fibres, and it is these which then innervate the effector organ. These synapses usually occur in clusters called ganglia. The main nerves of the parasympathetic system are the tenth cranial nerve, the vagus nerve, which originate in the medulla oblongata. Other preganglionic parasympathetic neurons also extend from the brain as well as from the lower tip of the spinal cord. Each preganglionic parasympathetic neuron synapses with just a few postganglionic neurons, which are located near or in the effector organ, a muscle or major gland. Acetylcholine (ACh) is the neurotransmitter of all the pre and many of the postganglionic neurons of the parasympathetic system.

The terms cholinergic and parasympathomimetic are not equivalent but are generally considered as synonyms. Compounds that mimic the action of arch at parasympathetic system are called as cholinergic parasympathomimetic agents. Thus, these drugs stimulate the effect of cells innervated by postganglionic parasympathetic cholinergic nerves. They are classified as directly acting and indirectly acting cholinergic.

Classification

A. Directly Acting Cholinergic Drugs:

I.   Choline Esters

Acetylcholine, Carbachol, Methacholine, Bethanechol

II.   Cholinomimetic Alkaloids

(a)   Mainly Muscarinic Agonists

Muscarine, Pilocarpine, Arecholine, Oxotramorine, Cevimeline

(b)   Mainly Nicotinic Agonists

Nicotine, Lobeline, Dimethyl phenyl piperazinium (DMPP), Varenicline

Tertiary alkaloids

Pilocarpine, Nicotine, Lobeline

Quaternary amines

Muscarine

B. Indirectly Acting Cholinergic Drugs (Anticholinesterases)

I. Reversible

(a) Carbamates

Tertiary amines: Physostigmine

Quaternary Ammonium compounds

Neostigmine, Pyridostigmine, Distigmine, Ambenonium, Demecarium

(b) Alcohols

Edrophonium

(c) Miscellaneous

Tacrine, Donepezil, Galantamine, Rivastigmine

II. Irreversible Anticholinesterases (Organophosphorus Compounds)

1. Therapeutically useful:

   Ecothiophate

2. War Gases:

   Sarin, Tuban, Soman

3. Insecticides: - Parathion, Malathion, DiisopropylFlurophosphate (DFP), Tetramethyl Pyrophosphate (TMPP), Octamethyl Pyrophosphotetraamide (OMPA)

Direct acting agents:

Acetylcholine

Classification: Cholinergic Agonists

Chemical Name: 2-acetyloxyethyl(trimethyl)azanium

Chemical Structure

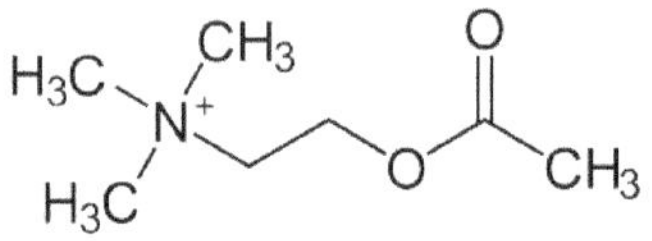

Uses: Used to obtain miosis of the iris in seconds after delivery of the lens in cataract surgery, in penetrating keratoplasty, iridectomy and other anterior segment surgery where rapid miosis may be required.

Stability: ACh solution stored at 25°C was stable for about 28 days, after such time, modest breakdown occurs.

- At a temperature of 50°C, ACh showed a rapid breakdown after 1 day.

Storage Conditions
- Store at Room Temperature.
- Store under desiccating conditions.
- The product can be stored for up to 12 months.

Different types of Formulations: Powder (for solution), Kit.

Popular brand names: Miochol E, Miogan PWS.

Carbachol

Classification: Cholinergic Agonists

Chemical Name: 2-carbamoyloxyethyl(trimethyl)azanium; chloride

Chemical Structure

Uses: Carbamoylcholine is indicated to induce miosis for surgery and to reduce intraocular pressure elevations in the first 24 hours after cataract surgery.

Stability: Stock solutions are stable for up to 6 months at 4°C.

Storage Conditions:
- Store at Room Temperature.
- Store under desiccating conditions.
- The product can be stored for up to 12 months.

Different types of Formulations
- Tablet
- Liquid
- Injection, solution
- Solution

Popular brand names
- Miostat
- Isopto
- Dichol
- Carbastat
- Carboptic

Bethanechol

Classification: Muscarinic Agonists

Chemical Name: 2-carbamoyloxypropyl(trimethyl)azanium

Chemical Structure

Uses: Bethanechol is indicated for the treatment of acute, functional postpartum and postoperative urinary retention.

- It is also indicated for the treatment of neurogenic atony of the bladder with retention.

Stability: Bethanechol chloride oral solution 1 mg/mL in sterile water for irrigation is stable at least 30 days when stored at 4°C.

Storage Conditions

- Store at room temperature between 59°F-86°F (15°C-30°C) away from light and moisture.
- Do not store in the bathroom.
- Keep all medicines away from children and pets.
- Do not flush medications down the toilet or pour them into a drain unless instructed to do so.

Different types of Formulations: Tablet, Liquid

Popular brand names: Urivoid, Bzon, Bethacol, Macpee, Mictuease, Betheran, Urolaxwyn, Rotone.

Methacholine

Classification: Muscarinic Agonists

Chemical Name: 2-acetyloxypropyl(trimethyl)azanium

Chemical Structure

Uses: Methacholine is indicated in adult and pediatric patients aged five years and older without clinically apparent asthma for the diagnosis of bronchial airway hyperactivity via the methacholine challenge test.

Stability: When prepared with saline diluent and stored at 4°C, methacholine solutions of 0.125 mg/ml and greater should be stable for 3 months.

Storage Conditions: Refrigerate the reconstituted solution at 2°C to 8°C.

Different types of Formulations: Powder (for solution), Solution

Popular brand names: Provocholine, Methacholine Omega

Pilocarpine

Classification: Muscarinic Agonists

Chemical Name: (3S,4R)-3-ethyl-4-[(3-methylimidazol-4-yl)methyl]oxolan-2-one

Chemical Structure

Uses: For the treatment of radiation-induced dry mouth (xerostomia) and symptoms of dry mouth in patients with Sjogren's syndrome.

Stability

- Pilocarpine in ophthalmic solutions decomposes fairly rapidly.
- Pilocarpine is not stable at high pH values.

Storage Conditions

- Store at 15°C to 25°C (59°F to 77°F) and protect from freezing.
- The drops must be kept away from children in a cool, dry place, away from direct sunlight.

Different types of Formulations: Solution, Drops, Liquid, Tablet, Implant, Tablet (film coated)

Popular brand names: Carpinol, Aurocarpine, Pilomin, Andre Carpine, Pilocar, Cucarp, Pilagan, Karpine, Piloxine, Pilomax.

Neostigmine

Classification: Cholinesterase Inhibitors

Chemical Name: [3-(dimethylcarbamoyloxy)phenyl]-trimethylazanium

Chemical Structure

Uses: Neostigmine is used for the symptomatic treatment of myasthenia gravis by improving muscle tone.

Stability: The injections in plastic syringes were stable for up to 90 days at both ambient temperature and at 4°C.

- The pH of neostigmine methyl sulfate injection did not change appreciable over the 90-day study period.

Storage Conditions: It should be kept in a cool, dry place where the temperature stays below 25°C and protected from light.

Different types of Formulations: Injection, Injection (solution), Solution

Popular brand names: Neutrum, Neotroy, Neomine, Neotagmin, Myostigmin, Stigmerase, Tilstigmin.

Pyridostigmine

Classification: Cholinesterase Inhibitors

Chemical Name: (1-methylpyridin-1-ium-3-yl) *N,N*-dimethylcarbamate

Chemical Structure

Uses

- Pyridostigmine is indicated for the treatment of myasthenia gravis.
- When administered intravenously, it is indicated for the reversal or antagonism of the neuromuscular blocking effects of nondepolarizing muscle relaxants.
- Pyridostigmine has also been used as a prophylactic agent against irreversible organophosphorus acetylcholinesterase inhibitors, primarily in a military capacity.

Stability: It is stable in acid medium (pH 1.0) at both 25°C and 70°C for 3 hrs.

Storage Conditions

- Tablets and Syrup must be kept at 25°C (77°F) in a dry place with the silica gel enclosed.
- Maximum excursions permitted to 15°C-30°C (59°F-86°F).

Different types of Formulations: Tablet, Tablet (extended release), Injection (solution), Liquid, Solution

Popular brand names: Gravitor, Mustone, Myestin, Pyodistig, Mygris, Yristig, Distinon, Trostigmin

Edrophonium Chloride

Classification: Cholinesterase Inhibitors

Chemical Name: ethyl-(3-hydroxyphenyl)-dimethylazanium

Chemical Structure

Uses: For the differential diagnosis of myasthenia gravis and as an adjunct in the evaluation of treatment requirements in this disease. It may also be used for evaluating emergency treatment in myasthenic crises.

Stability: Alkaline-induced degradation product have been reported.

Storage Conditions: The drug should be stored at controlled room temperature 15°-30°C (59°-86°F).

Different types of Formulations: Injection, Liquid, Injection, solution

Popular brand names: Enlon, Tensilon, Reversol

Tacrine Hydrochloride

Classification: Cholinesterase Inhibitors

Chemical Name: 1,2,3,4-tetrahydroacridin-9-amine

Chemical Structure

Uses: For the palliative treatment of mild to moderate dementia of the Alzheimer's type.

Stability: It is found to be relatively stable at acidic pHs but subjected to a base-catalyzed degradation at the alkaline pHs.

Storage Conditions: Capsules should be stored at room temperature, 15-30°C (59-86°F).

Different types of Formulations: Capsule

Popular brand names: Cognex

Ambenonium Chloride

Classification: Anticholinesterases

Chemical Name: (2-chlorophenyl)methyl-[2-[[2-[2-[(2-chlorophenyl)methyl-diethylazaniumyl]ethylamino]-2-oxoacetyl]amino]ethyl]-diethylazanium

Chemical Structure

Uses: Ambenonium is used to treat muscle weakness due to muscle disease (myasthenia gravis).

Stability: The stability of the drug solutions decreases with rising pH.

Storage Conditions
- Store at room temperature up to 77°F (25°C) away from light and moisture.
- Do not store in the bathroom.
- Keep all medicines away from children and pets.
- Do not flush medications down the toilet or pour them into a drain unless instructed to do so.

Different types of Formulations: Tablet

Popular brand names: Mytelase, Mytelase Chloride.

Pralidoxime Chloride

Classification: Cholinesterase Reactivators

Chemical Name: (*NE*)-*N*-[(1-methylpyridin-1-ium-2-yl)methylidene]hydroxylamine

Chemical Structure

Uses: For the treatment of poisoning due to those pesticides and chemicals of the organophosphate class which have anticholinesterase activity and in the control of overdosage by anticholinesterase drugs used in the treatment of myasthenia gravis.

Stability: Conversion of intramuscular to intravenous pralidoxime results in a stable and sterile solution for up to 28 days under a variety of environmental conditions.

Storage Conditions: Store at 20°-25°C (68°-77°F), excursions permitted to 15°-30°C.

Different types of Formulations: Injection, Powder(for solution), Injection (powder, lyophilized, for solution)

Popular brand names: Clopam, Unipam, Adipam, Elpam, Toxipam, Allpam, Aldopam, Aquapam, Purepam, Neopam.

Isoflurophate

Classification: Cholinesterase Inhibitors

Chemical Name: 2-[fluoro(propan-2-yloxy)phosphoryl]oxypropane

Chemical Structure

Uses: For use in the eye to treat certain types of glaucoma and other eye conditions, such as accommodative esotropia.

Stability: The drug solutions are moderately stable at pH 1–7.

Storage Conditions: The drug solutions should be protected from light and moisture, and stored in airtight bottles.

Different types of Formulations: Solution, Ointment.

Popular brand names: Diflupyl, Dyflos, Floropryl

Echothiophate Iodide

Classification: Cholinesterase Inhibitors

Chemical Name: 2-diethoxyphosphorylsulfanylethyl(trimethyl)azanium

Chemical Structure

Uses: For use in the treatment of subacute or chronic angle-closure glaucoma after iridectomy or where surgery is refused or contraindicated.

Stability: Massive degradation takes place under both acidic and alkaline conditions.

Storage Conditions: The drug solution may be stored at room temperature about 77°F (25°C) for up to 4 weeks. Do not freeze.

Different types of Formulations: Powder (for solution), Solution.

Popular brand names: Echodide, Phospholine Iodide.

Parathion

Classification: Cholinesterase Inhibitors

Chemical Name: diethoxy-(4-nitrophenoxy)-sulfanylidene-λ^5-phosphane

Chemical Structure

Uses: Parathion was used as a chemical warfare agent, most notably by an element of the British South Africa Police (BSAP) attached to the Selous Scouts during the Rhodesian Bush War. They used it to poison clothing that was then supplied to anti-government guerrillas.

Stability: Extreme hydrolysis takes place under acid and alkaline conditions.

Storage Conditions: Store at 20°-25°C (68°-77°F), excursions permitted to 15°-30°C (59°-86°F).

- Parathion may also be stored in fat.

Different types of Formulations: Solution, Suspension, Spray

Popular brand names: Kriss, Niram, Orthophos, Panthion, Paramar, Paraphos, Parathene, Parawet, Phoskil, Rhodiatox.

Malathion

Classification: Cholinesterase Inhibitors

Chemical Name: diethyl 2-dimethoxyphosphinothioylsulfanylbutanedioate

Chemical Structure

Uses: For patients infected with Pediculus humanus capitis (head lice and their ova) of the scalp hair.

Stability: It was found that malathion is more unstable than dichlorvos and diazinon, there was an over 70% loss in 90 days even at –20°C in coarsely chopped form.

Storage Conditions: Store it at room temperature (20° to 25°C).

Different types of Formulations: Lotion, Shampoo

Popular brand names: Ovide

Cholinergic Blocking Agents

Cholenergic antagonists inhibit the actions of endogenous acetyl choline and muscarinic agonists at muscarnic receptor sites in peripheral tissues and in the CNS. These drugs are highly specific reversible competitive antagonists for muscarinic ACh receptors. The pharmacological effects are blockage of parasympathetic stimulation at effector organs. They are rapidly absorbed from the gastrointestinal tract, slowly absorbed when applied locally on eye or skin. The potent anticholinergics are used to control the secretion of saliva and gastric acid, slow down gut motility, and to prevent vomiting. They also have a limited therapeutic use for the treatment of Parkinson's disease.

Solanaceous alkaloids and analogues

Atropine Sulphate

Classification: Parasympatholytic

Chemical Name: [(1S,5R)-8-methyl-8-azabicyclo[3.2.1]octan-3-yl]3-hydroxy-2-phenyl-propanoate.

Chemical Structure

Uses: For the treatment of poisoning by susceptible organophosphorous nerve agents having anti-cholinesterase activity (cholinesterase inhibitors) as well as organophosphorous or carbamate insecticides.

Stability:
- Atropine sulphate should be stored in single or multiple-dose containers, preferably glass, at a temperature of less than 40°C (preferably between 15°C to 30°C).
- It should be protected from light and stored in airtight containers.

Storage Conditions: Faster degradation takes place by addition of an acidic (pH ≈ 1.2).

Different types of Formulations: Injection, Solution, Drops, Ointment, Liquid

Popular brand names: Atrochlor-D, Atrisolon, Atrocin, Atrosun, Atroren-P, Brovon, Topin, Deco-At, Atrover, Lomotil.

Homatropine Hydrogen Bromide

Classification: Parasympatholytic

Chemical Name: [(1R,5S)-8-methyl-8-azabicyclo[3.2.1]octan-3-yl] 2-hydroxy-2-phenylacetate

Chemical Structure

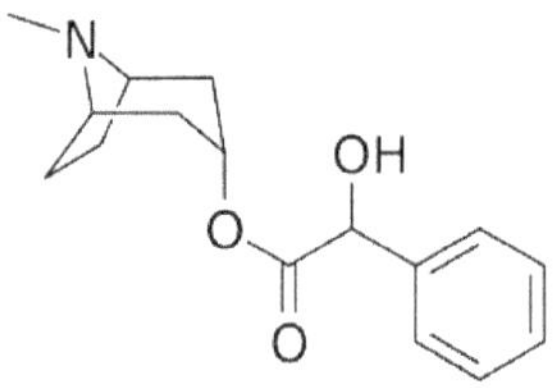

Uses
- Indicated as an overdose-rescuing agent in combination with hydrocodone antitussive.
- Indicated for the induction of mydriasis in ophthalmic solutions.

Stability: It degrades very rapidly at elevated temperature of 50°C.

Storage Conditions
- Store between 46-75°F (8-24°C) away from light and heat.
- Do not freeze.
- Keep all medicines away from children and pets.
- Do not flush medications down the toilet or pour them into a drain unless instructed to do so.
- Properly discard this product when it is expired or no longer needed.

Different types of Formulations: Solution, Drops, Liquid.

Popular brand names: Homide, Mydryn, Homacid, Homat, Homozen, Homabact, Aurohom, Homocid, Homarin, Ha2.

Ipratropium Bromide

Classification: Cholinergic Antagonists

Chemical Name: [(1S,5R)-8-methyl-8-propan-2-yl-8-azoniabicyclo[3.2.1]octan-3-yl] 3-hydroxy-2-phenylpropanoate.

Chemical Structure

Uses

- Inhaled ipratropium is indicated in combination with inhaled beta-agonist systemic corticosteroids for the management of severe exacerbations of asthma flares requiring treatment.
- Ipratropium has also been studied to be used for the treatment of sialorrhea.

Stability

- Admixtures of proprietary ipratropium bromide and salbutamol nebulizer solutions (1:1 v/v) retain greater than 90 percent of their initial concentrations if stored between 4°C and 22°C for periods of up to five days. An expiry period of five days for these admixtures would seem reasonable in practice.
- Ipratropium bromide is fairly stable in neutral and acidic solutions, but is rapidly hydrolyzed in alkaline solution

Storage Conditions

- Do not store above 25°C. Store in the original package.
- The ampoule should be opened immediately before use and any solution remaining after use should be discarded.
- Keep away from light and moisture. Do not store in the bathroom. Keep all medications away from children and pet.

Different types of Formulations: Aerosol (metered), Spray (metered), Solution, Liquid

Popular brand names: Ipravent, Combimist, Salbair, Duolin, Duojet, Duoneb, Iprazo, Iprarite, Salvent, Digihaler

Synthetic cholinergic blocking agents:

Tropicamide

Classification: Muscarinic Antagonists

Chemical Name: *N*-ethyl-3-hydroxy-2-phenyl-*N*-(pyridin-4-ylmethyl)propanamide

Chemical Structure

Uses

- Tropicamide is indicated to induce mydriasis (dilation of the pupil) and cycloplegia (paralysis of the ciliary muscle of the eye) in diagnostic procedures.
- It is used in combination with hydroxyamphetamine for the same indication.

Stability: Tropicamide is stable in aqueous solution; eye-drops prepared from such a solution are stable for no less than 5 years.

Storage Conditions: Tropicamide is stable in aqueous solution; eye-drops prepared from such a solution are stable for no less than 5 years.

Different types of Formulations: Solution, Liquid, Drops.

Popular brand names: Tropico, Tropind, Trophen, Optimide, Tmide, Tropicamet, Tropicacyl Eye, Tropind

Cyclopentolate Hydrochloride

Classification: Muscarinic Antagonists

Chemical Name: 2-(dimethyl amino)ethyl 2-(1-hydroxycyclopentyl)-2-phenylacetate

Chemical Structure

Uses: Used mainly to produce mydriasis and cycloplegia for diagnostic purposes.

Stability: Cyclopentolate eye drops are stable physically and chemically for up to 60 days when stored at refrigeration temperatures (2-8 °C).

Storage Conditions:
- Store at room temperature below 25°C.
- Some brands of cyclopentolate eye drops should be stored in a fridge (2-8°C) where children cannot reach them.
- Do not freeze.
- Protect from light.

Different types of Formulations: Solution, Drops

Popular brand names: Pentol, Cyclogic, Cyclogyl, Cyclomid, Auropent, Thiopent, Locy, Cepenta, Biodyle, Sensiclo

Clidinium Bromide

Classification: Parasympatholytic

Chemical Name: (1-methyl-1-azoniabicyclo[2.2.2]octan-3-yl) 2-hydroxy-2,2-diphenyl-acetate

Chemical Structure

Uses: For the treatment of peptic ulcer disease and also to help relieve abdominal or stomach spasms or cramps due to colicky abdominal pain, diverticulitis, and irritable bowel syndrome.

Stability: Heat and photolytic degradation is common.

Storage Conditions
- Store at room temperature between 59°F-86°F (15°C-30°C) away from light and moisture.
- Do not store in the bathroom.

Different types of Formulations: Capsule, Capsule (gelatin coated), Tablet, coated

Popular brand names: Equilium, Spasmolar, Gutrex, Solibs, Tribs, Odemed, Librax, Spasril, Equirex, Egrex.

Dicyclomine Hydrochloride

Classification: Parasympatholytic

Chemical Name: 2-(diethylamino)ethyl 1-cyclohexylcyclohexane-1-carboxylate

Chemical Structure

Uses: Dicyclomine is indicated for the treatment of functional bowel disorder and irritable bowel syndrome.

Stability: The formulated product is high stable and effective at pH 4.0-5.0.

Storage Conditions

- Store at room temperature, preferably below 86°F (30°C).
- Avoid excessive heat (above 104°F).
- Tablets and capsules should be stored at controlled room temperature (between 68°F and 77°F).

Different types of Formulations: Injection (solution), Capsule, Liquid, Tablet, Syrup, Tablet (extended release).

Popular brand names: Colicure, Balagin, Leospas, Dolospas, Dcmol, Dispas, Baxspas, Colinol, Spasmid, Cyclospa.

Procyclidine Hydrochloride

Classification: Muscarinic Antagonists

Chemical Name: 1-cyclohexyl-1-phenyl-3-pyrrolidin-1-ylpropan-1-ol

Chemical Structure

Uses: For the treatment of all forms of Parkinson's Disease, as well as control of extrapyramidal reactions induced by antipsychotic agents.

Stability: Relevant degradation was found to take place under acidic (0.1 N HCl) and photolytic (visible and long-wavelength UV-light) conditions

Storage Conditions

- Store at room temperature between 68-77°F (20-25°C) away from light and moisture.
- The tablets should be stored at 15–25°C temperature.

Different types of Formulations: Tablet, Elixir

Popular brand names: Modin, Dine, Kemad, Maxidine, Proclid, Floclid, Kemadrin, Sycline, Ultidine, Gemdrin

Tridihexethyl Chloride

Classification: Anticholinergic

Chemical Name: (3-cyclohexyl-3-hydroxy-3-phenylpropyl)-triethylazanium

Chemical Structure

Uses:
- Used as an adjunct in the treatment of peptic ulcer disease and in Acquired nystagmus.
- It has been shown in experimental and clinical studies to have a pronounced antispasmodic and antisecretory effect on the gastrointestinal tract.
- Tridihexethyl is an antimuscarinic, anticholinergic drug.

Storage Conditions: Dry, dark and at 0 - 4°C for short term (days to weeks) or -20°C for long term (months to years).

Different types of Formulations: Tablet

Popular brand names: Hexedyl, Hexylent, Hexyriv-2, Relihex, Ptempt, Parnon, Pacidyl, Parales, Texyl, Trihexy

Isopropamide Iodide

Classification: Anticholinergic

Chemical Name: (4-amino-4-oxo-3,3-diphenylbutyl)-methyl-di(propan-2-yl)azanium

Chemical Structure

Uses: For the treatment of a wide range of gastrointestinal disorders, including such conditions as peptic ulcer, gastritis, hyperchlorhydria, functional diarrhea, irritable or spastic colon, pyloroduodenal irritability, pylorospasm, acute nonspecific gastroenteritis, biliary dyskinesia and chronic cholelithiasis, duodenitis, gastrointestinal spasm; it may also be used to treat genitourinary spasm.

Stability: Hydrogen peroxide induces degradation and degraded products are formed.

Storage Conditions: Isopropamide should be stored at room temperature in well-closed, light-resistant containers away from direct sunlight.

Different types of Formulations: Tablet

Popular brand names: Stelbid, Gastabid, Isorez, Isozex, Spascol

Ethopropazine Hydrochloride

Classification: Muscarinic Antagonists

Chemical Name: *N,N*-diethyl-1-phenothiazin-10-ylpropan-2-amine

Chemical Structure

Uses: For use in the treatment of Parkinson's disease and also used to control severe reactions to certain medicines.

Stability: Hydroperoxides degrades the drug component.

Storage Conditions:

- Stable for 2 years as supplied.
- Solutions in DMSO or distilled water may be stored at -20° for up to 3 months.

Different types of Formulations: Tablet

Popular brand names: Cayman, Parsidol, Parsidan, Parkin, Parsitan

---

Multiple Choice Questions

1. Which of the following agents is a competitive antagonist at the neuromuscular junction nicotinic cholinoceptors?
   - (a) Dantrolene
   - (b) Atracurium
   - (c) Mecamylamine
   - (d) Isoflurophate (DFP)
   - (e) Succinylcholine

2. A drug that stimulates beta1- and beta2-adreneceptors can be expected to cause:
   - (a) A decrease in heart rate
   - (b) A decrease in total peripheral resistance
   - (c) A constriction of airway smooth muscle resistance
   - (d) A decrease in renin release

3. Dantrolene is the drug of choice to treat malignant hyperthermia caused by succinylcholine because:
   - (a) Dantrolene blocks calcium release from SR
   - (b) Dantrolene induces contraction of skeletal muscle
   - (c) Dantrolene increases the rate of succinylcholine metabolism
   - (d) Succinylcholine binding to nicotinic receptors is antagonized by dantrolene
   - (e) Dantrolene acts centrally to reduce fever

4. Hereditary deficiency of which of the following enzymes can lead to prolonged effects of succinylcholine?
   - (a) Glucose-6-phosphate dehydrogenase
   - (b) Plasma cholinesterase
   - (c) Heme oxygenase
   - (d) Cytochrome oxidase
   - (e) Liver transaminase

5. Neostigmine would be expected to reverse which one of the following conditions?
   (a) Paralysis of skeletal muscle induced by a competitive (non-depolarizing) muscle relaxant
   (b) Paralysis of skeletal muscle induced by a depolarizing muscle relaxant
   (c) Cardiac slowing induced by stimulation of the vagus nerve
   (d) Pupillary miosis induced by bright light

6. The direct cardiac effects of dobutamine would be blocked by which of the following agents?
   (a) Atropine (b) Metoprolol
   (c) Clonidine (d) Isoproterenol

7. Topical application of timolol to the eye would be expected to induce which of the following?
   (a) Miosis
   (b) Mydriasis
   (c) Decreased formation of aqueous humor
   (d) Increased outflow of aqueous humor

8. All of the following drugs produce either direct or indirect parasympathomimetic effects, EXCEPT?
   (a) Bethanechol (b) Atropine
   (c) Neostigmine (d) Nicotine

9. Which one of the following drugs generally should NOT be administered to a patient with asthma?
   (a) Atropine (b) Propranolol
   (c) Epinephrine (d) Isoproterenol

10. Tricyclic antidepressant drugs may produce blurred vision, dry mouth, constipation, and difficulty initiating urination because of their blockade of:
   (a) Alpha-adrenergic receptors (b) GABA receptors
   (c) Muscarinic receptors (d) Nicotinic receptors
   (e) Serotonergic receptors

CHAPTER 7

Drugs Acting on Cardiovascular System

Introduction

The chapter aims at providing the latest and pharmacopeial information regarding some Drugs acting on Cardiovascular System (Quinidine sulphate, Procainamide hydrochloride, Verapamil, Diltiazem hydrochloride, Phenytoin sodium, Lidocaine hydrochloride, Tocainide hydrochloride, Mexiletine hydrochloride, Lorcainide hydrochloride, Amiodarone Sotalol, Propranolol, Timolol, Captopril, Lisinopril, Enalapril, Benazepril hydrochloride, Quinapril hydrochloride, Methyldopa hydrochloride, Clonidine hydrochloride, Reserpine, Hydralazine hydrochloride, Nifedipine, Isosorbide dinitrate, and Amyl nitrite) regarding their classification, chemical name, chemical structure, uses, stability, storage conditions, different types of formulations, and popular brand names.

Anti-Arrhythmic Drugs: Antiarrhythmic agents corrects the arrhythmia of the heart. Cardiac arrhythmias are frequent problems in clinical practice, occurring in up to 25% of the patients treated with digitalis, 50% of the anaesthetized patients, and over 8% of the patients with acute myocardial infarction. Many factors can precipitate or exacerbate arrhythmias, ischaemia, hypoxia, acidosis, alkalosis, electrolyte abnormalities, excessive catecholamine exposure, autonomic influences, drug toxicity, over stretching of cardiac fibers, and the presence of any diseased tissue. However, all the arrhythmias results from the following:

1. Disturbances in impulse formation
2. Disturbances in impulse conduction
3. Or both

Classification: Antiarrhythmic drugs are classified into four types, according to their electrophysiological properties. The drugs that are used for arrhythmias are sodium, potassium, and calcium channel blockers. Some have additional or even primary autonomic effects.

Class 1: These have primary action on Na^+ and K^+ across the cell membrane. Procainamide, Quinidine, Mexiletine, Lidocaine, Flecainide, Propafenone

Class 2: These have primary action to suppress adrenergically mediated ectopic activity. Bisoprolol, Carvedilol

Class 3: These are the drugs that prolong the repolarization. Action potential is widened and effective refractory period is increased. Amiodarone, Sotalol

Class 4: Their primary action is to inhibit Ca^{2+} mediated current. Verapamil, Diltiazem

Quinidine Sulphate

Classification: Antiarrhythmics

Chemical Name: (S)-[(2R,4S,5R)-5-ethenyl-1-azabicyclo[2.2.2]octan-2-yl]-(6-methoxy-quinolin-4-yl)methanol

Chemical Structure

Uses: Quinidine is a medication used to restore normal sinus rhythm, treat atrial fibrillation, and flutter, and treat ventricular arrhythmias.

Stability: Quinidine sulfate was reported to be stable for up to 60 days in oral liquid formulations prepared extemporaneously.

Storage Conditions

- Store quinidine at room temperature between 68°F and 77°F (20°C and 25°C).
- Keep the drug away from light and high temperature.

Different types of Formulations: Tablet.

Popular brand names: Cardioquin, Quinaglute, Quinalan, Quinidex.

Procainamide Hydrochloride

Classification: Antiarrhythmics

Chemical Name: 4-amino-N-[2-(diethylamino)ethyl]benzamide

Chemical Structure

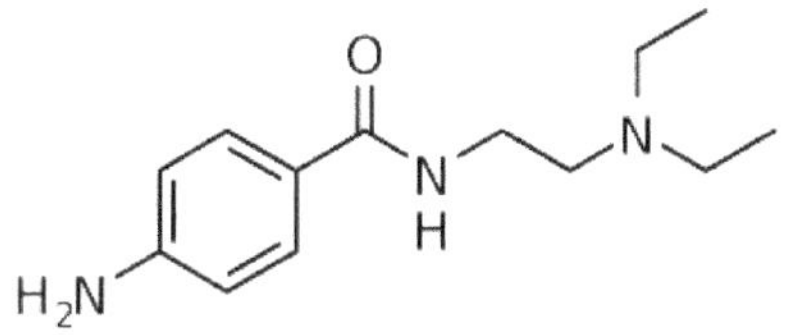

Uses
- Procainamide is a medication used to treat life threatening ventricular arrhythmias.
- Procainamide is an agent indicated for the treatment of ventricular tachycardia occurring during cardiac manipulation, such as surgery or catheterization, or which may occur during acute myocardial infarction, digitalis toxicity, or other cardiac diseases.

Stability: The stability of procainamide hydrochloride, when diluted in 5% dextrose in water (D5W) or normal saline (NS) to 2 to 4 mg/mL, is reported by the manufacturer to be 24 hours at room temperature or 7 days when refrigerated.

Storage Conditions
- Store in airtight containers.
- Store tablets and capsules at room temperature.
- Avoid excessive heat (104° F).
- Protect from moisture.
- Store intact vials at 20°C to 25°C (68°F to 77°F).

Different types of Formulations: Solution, Capsules, Tablet (extended release), Table (film coated).

Popular brand names: Pronestyl, Procan-SR, Procanbid.

Verapamil

Classification: Calcium Channel Blockers.

Chemical Name: 2-(3,4-dimethoxyphenyl)-5-[2-(3,4-dimethoxyphenyl)ethyl-methylamino]-2-propan-2-ylpentanenitrile.

Chemical Structure

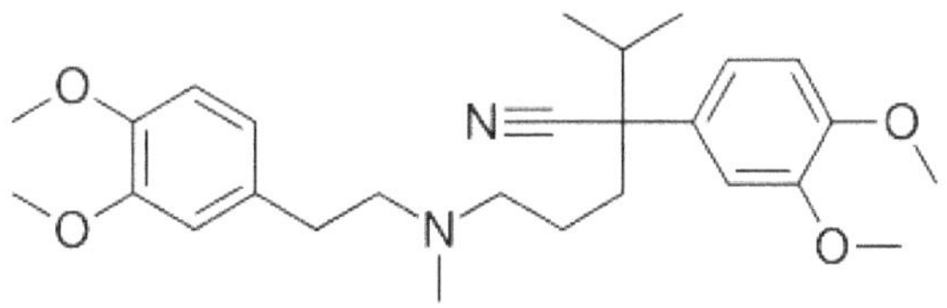

Uses

- Verapamil is a non-dihydropyridine calcium channel blocker used in the treatment of angina, arrhythmia, and hypertension.
- Verapamil is indicated in the treatment of vasopastic (i.e. Prinzmetal's) angina, unstable angina, and chronic stable angina. It is also indicated to treat hypertension, for the prophylaxis of repetitive paroxysmal supraventricular tachycardia, and in combination with digoxin to control ventricular rate in patients with atrial fibrillation or atrial flutter. Given intravenously, it is indicated for the treatment of various supraventricular tachyarrhythmias, including rapid conversion to sinus rhythm in patients with supraventricular tachycardia and for temporary control of ventricular rate in patients with atrial fibrillation or atrial flutter.
- Verapamil is commonly used off-label for prophylaxis of cluster headaches.

Stability: Verapamil hydrochloride is reported to be stable when refluxed under neutral, acidic, and basic aqueous conditions with an optimum pH range for stability of 3.2 to 5.6.

Storage Conditions

- The formulations should be stored at room temperature and protected from light.
- Keep in a cool, dry place, away from direct sunlight.

Different types of Formulations: Tablet (film coated), Tablet (extended release), Liquid, Solution, Injection, Capsule (delayed release pellets), Capsule (extended release).

Popular brand names: Calaptin, Vasopten, Trapmil, Veramil, Isoptin, Verelan, Calan, Bosoptin, Covera, Verap.

Diltiazem Hydrochloride

Classification: Calcium Channel Blockers.

Chemical Name: [(2S,3S)-5-[2-(dimethylamino) ethyl]-2-(4-methoxyphenyl)-4-oxo-2,3-dihydro-1,5-benzothiazepin-3-yl] acetate.

Uses

- Indicated for the management of hypertension, to lower blood pressure, alone or in combination with other antihypertensive agents.
- Indicated for use to improve exercise tolerance in patients with chronic stable angina.
- Indicated for the management of variant angina (Prinzmetal's angina).

Stability: Diltiazem hydrochloride diluted to 1 mg/mL in 5% dextrose injection is stable for 30 days.

Chemical Structure

Storage Conditions
- Injection is to be stored under refrigeration 2 to 8°C (36 to 46°F).
- Do not freeze.
- May be stored at room temperature (25°C (77°F)) for up to 1 month.

Different types of Formulations
- Capsule, extended release
- Tablet, coated
- Injection
- Solution
- Liquid

Popular brand names: Angizem, Dilcor, Dilgard, Dilocor, Eldizem, Dilzewyn, Axzem, Dilrite, Dilsantin, Dilzem.

Phenytoin Sodium

Classification: Antiarrhythmics

Chemical Name: 5,5-diphenylimidazolidine-2,4-dione

Chemical Structure

Uses: It is a potential treatment option for patients with refractory ventricular arrhythmia when other agents have failed or are unavailable. However, phenytoin has a narrow therapeutic range and the potential for multiple drug interactions.

Stability: The drug was generally more stable in plain collection tubes than in SSTs. No degradation occurred in plain red-top tubes or in refrigerated SSTs, but clinically significant degradation was present in SSTs stored at room temperature and at elevated temperature (32°C) 24 h after collection.

Storage Conditions

- Store at 20 to 25°C (68 to 77°F).
- Preserve in tight, light-resistant containers.
- Protect from moisture.

Different types of Formulations: Capsule (extended release), Tablet, Injection, Liquid, Suspension.

Popular brand names: Eptoin, Phenytal, Atoin, Kiptoin, Gradil, Epsod, Protoin, Qtoin, Phalin, Tribarb.

Lidocaine Hydrochloride

Classification: Antiarrhythmics

Chemical Name: 2-(diethylamino)-*N*-(2,6-dimethylphenyl)acetamide

Chemical Structure

Uses

- It has moderate efficacy against ventricular arrhythmias.
- It is particularly useful in the setting of myocardial infarction or ischemia.
- It may be used as an alternative to amiodarone in the management of recurrent or shock refractory ventricular fibrillation/tachycardia.

Stability: Lidocaine hydrochloride injection is chemically stable for up to 120 days at either 30 °C or 4 °C when mixed with 5% dextrose injection in plastic infusion bags.

Storage Conditions: Injections should be stored below 104 °F (40°C) at room temperature, between 59 and 86°F (15-30°C), preferably at 77 °F (25°C).

Different types of Formulations: Injection, Gel, Liquid, Patch, Ointment, Solution, Lotion.

Popular brand names: Xylocaine, Xcin, Gesicain, Lignox, Lidopox, Lidozone, Otogen, Lidophen, Otofast, Lox.

Tocainide Hydrochloride

Classification: Antiarrhythmics.

Chemical Name: 2-amino-*N*-(2,6-dimethylphenyl)propanamide

Chemical Structure

Uses

- It interferes with cardiac sodium channels and typically used to treat ventricular arrhythmias.
- It is an antiarrhythmic agent which exerts a potential-dependent and frequency-dependent block of sodium channels.

Stability: The drug is stable in both alkaline and acidic conditions.

Storage Conditions

- Store below 40°C (104°F); preferably between 15°C and 30°C (59°F and 86°F).
- Store in a well-closed container.

Different types of Formulations: Tablet.

Popular brand names: Tonocard, Tocolol, Tocain.

Mexiletine Hydrochloride

Classification: Antiarrhythmics

Chemical Name: 1-(2,6-dimethylphenoxy)propan-2-amine

Chemical Structure

Uses: For the treatment of ventricular tachycardia and symptomatic premature ventricular beats, and prevention of ventricular fibrillation.

Stability

- Mexiletine was stable in the formulation containing water, stored in plastic prescription bottles for 13 weeks at 4°C and 7 weeks at 25°C.

- It was also stable in the sorbitol formulation but for a shorter period–4 weeks at 4°C and 2 weeks at 25°C.

Storage Conditions
- Store the medicine in a closed container at room temperature, away from heat, moisture, and direct light.
- Store below 40°C (104°F); preferably between 15°C and 30°C (59°F and 86°F).

Different types of Formulations: Capsule.

Popular brand names: Mexohar. Mexitil, Namuscla.

Lorcainide Hydrochloride

Classification: Antiarrhythmics

Chemical Name: N-(4-chlorophenyl)-2-phenyl-N-(1-propan-2-ylpiperidin-4-yl)acet-amide

Chemical Structure

Uses: It is used to help restore normal heart rhythm and conduction in patients with premature ventricular contractions, ventricular tachycardiac, and Wolff-Parkinson-White syndrome.

Stability: The drug is vulnerable to acidic attack.

Storage Conditions
- Store at -20°C temperature under desiccating conditions.
- The product can be stored for up to 12 months.

Different types of Formulations: Tablet, Capsule

Popular brand names: Remivox, Lorcid.

Amiodarone

Classification: Antiarrhythmics

Chemical   Name: (2-butyl-1-benzofuran-3-yl)-[4-[2-(diethylamino)ethoxy]-3,5-diiodophenyl]methanone.

Chemical Structure

Uses:
- It is indicated for the treatment of recurrent hemodynamically unstable ventricular tachycardia and recurrent ventricular fibrillation.
- Off-label indications include atrial fibrillation and supraventricular tachycardia.

Stability: Amiodarone hydrochloride is stable when mixed with either 5% dextrose injection or 0.9% sodium chloride injection in polyvinyl chloride or polyolefin containers alone or with potassium chloride, lidocaine, procainamide, verapamil, or furosemide and stored for 24 hours at 24°C.

Storage Conditions
- Amiodarone diluted in 5% Dextrose Injection is stable at concentrations of 1 to 6 mg/mL for 2 hours in polyvinyl chloride (PVC) and for 24 hours in polyolefin or glass bottles at room temperature.
- Store at room temperature; protect from light and excessive heat.
- Do not refrigerate or freeze.
- Keep the ampoules in the outer carton in order to protect from light.

Different types of Formulations: Tablet, Injection, Solution, Liquid.

Popular brand names: Cordarone, Ritebeat, Duron, Amione, Amiodar, Pacenorm, Amione, Amipace, Tachyra, Eurythmic.

Sotalol

Classification: Beta-Blockers

Chemical Name: *N*-[4-[1-hydroxy-2-(propan-2-ylamino)ethyl]phenyl]methanesulfon-amide.

Chemical Structure

Uses: It is used to treat life-threatening ventricular arrhythmias and to maintain sinus rhythm in atrial fibrillation or flutter.

Stability: Sotalol hydrochloride oral liquid suspensions (5mg/mL) were chemically stable for 12 weeks regardless of storage conditions (room temperature or refrigerated).

Storage Conditions

- Sotalol hydrochloride can be prepared in either of 2 liquid dosage forms and stored in plastic bottles for 13 weeks at 4 to 25°C without substantial loss of potency.
- The drug can be stored at 15°C to 30°C (59°F to 86°F).

Different types of Formulations: Tablet, Solution, Injection

Popular brand names: Solet, Sotalar, Setalol, Sotagard.

Anti-Hypertensive Agents

Antihypertensive drugs are defined as the drugs that are used to decrease the elevated blood pressure (hypertension).

Hypertension: It is one of the common cardiovascular disorders and it is a state of the body in which the systolic blood pressure (BP) is 150 mm Hg or more and diastolic BP is 95 mm Hg or more. Hypertension may be classified into primary and secondary:

Classification

I. **Diuretics**
   (a) Thiazides: Chlorthiazide, Hydrochlorthiazide, Cyclopenthiazide, Bendrofl umethiazide
   (b) Loop diuretics: Frusemide or furosemide, Ethacrynic acid, Bumetanide
   (c) Potassium-sparing diuretics: Triamterene, Spiranolactone (Aldosterone antagonists)

II. **Drugs acting on sympathetic system**
   (a) Centrally acting drugs : Clonidine, α-Methyl dopa, Guanabenz

(b) Catacholamine depletors Reserpine

(c) Adrenergic blockers

    (i) β-adrenergic blockers; Propronolol, Atenolol, Metoprolol, Oxprenolol, Acebutalol, Timolol, Nadolol, Pindolol

    (ii) α-Aderenergic blockers; Phentolamine, Phenoxy benzamine hydrochloride, Tolazoline, Prazosin, Terazosin, Doxazosin

    (iii) Mixed α and β blockers (nonselective): Labetalol, Carvedilol

    (iv) Imidazoline receptor agonist: Moxonidine, Rilmenidine

(d) Aderenergic neuron blockers: Guanethidine, Guanoxan, Debrisoquine, Bethanidine

(e) Ganglion blockers

    (i) Quaternary ammonium compounds: Hexamethonium bromide, Pentolinium tartarate

    (ii) Secondary amines: Mecamylamine HC

    (iii) Tertirary amines: Pempidine, Trimethophan

III. Calcium channel blockers: Verapamil, Nifedipine, Diltiazem, Felodipine, Amlodipine, Nicardipine, Nitrendipine

IV. Drugs acting on renin-angiotensin system

    (a) Drugs that block renin release—Propranolol.

    (b) Drugs that inhibit angiotensin II—Saralasin.

    (c) Drugs that inhibit angiotensin II receptors - Losartan, Irbesartan, Candesartan, Telmiesartan, Valsartan

    (d) Drugs that inhibit aldosterone—Spironolactone e. ACE inhibitors

    (i) Sulphahydryl containing ACE inhibitors Captopril

    (ii) Dicarboxylate containing ACE inhibitors

V. Vasodilators: Hydralazine, Diazoxide, Minoxidil, Sodium Nitroprusside

VI. Miscellaneous: MAO inhibitors—Pargyline, Metyrosine, Pinacidil

Propranolol

Classification: Beta-Blockers

Chemical Name: 1-naphthalen-1-yloxy-3-(propan-2-ylamino)propan-2-ol

Chemical Structure

Uses: Propranolol is also indicated to treat angina pectoris due to coronary atherosclerosis, atrial fibrillation, myocardial infarction, migraine, essential tremor, hypertrophic subaortic stenosis, pheochromocytoma, and proliferating infantile hemangioma.

Stability: Propranolol suspensions 2 mg/mL and 5 mg/mL stored at 25°C maintained at least 94.7% of their initial concentration for 120 days.

Storage Conditions

- Store in a cool, dry place, away from direct sunlight.
- Do not store in the bathroom.
- Keep all medications away from children.

Different types of Formulations: Capsule (extended release), Tablets, Liquid, Solution, Injection.

Popular brand names: Inderal, Mibeta, Erolol, Arminol, Migrabeta, Betapill, Prograin, Capinol, Kipnol, Movalol.

Timolol

Classification: Beta-Blockers

Chemical Name: (2*S*)-1-(*tert*-butylamino)-3-[(4-morpholin-4-yl-1,2,5-thiadiazol-3-yl)oxy] propan-2-ol

Chemical Structure

Uses:

- Ophthalmic timolol is indicated for the treatment of increased intraocular pressure in patients with ocular hypertension or open-angle glaucoma.
- The oral form of this drug is used to treat high blood pressure.
- In certain cases, timolol is used in the prevention of migraine headaches.

Stability: Timolol maleate is stable at room temperature.

Storage Conditions

- Do not store above 25°C. Store the bottle in outer carton properly without moisture.

- Ophthalmic solution should be kept at room temperature, 15°C - 30°C (59°F - 86°F) and must be protected from sunlight.

Different types of Formulations: Liquid, Solution, Drops, Gel forming liquid, extended release, Tablet.

Popular brand names: Glucomol, Timolet, Iotim, Lopres, Akutim, Gluchek, Timolong, Timolen, Timolast, Nyolol.

Captopril

Classification: Angiotensin-Converting Enzyme (ACE) Inhibitors.

Chemical Name: (2S)-1-[(2S)-2-methyl-3-sulfanylpropanoyl]pyrrolidine-2-carboxylic acid.

Chemical Structure

Uses:
- For the treatment of essential or renovascular hypertension (usually administered with other drugs, particularly thiazide diuretics).
- May be used to treat congestive heart failure in combination with other drugs (e.g. cardiac glycosides, diuretics, β-adrenergic blockers).
- May improve survival in patients with left ventricular dysfunction following myocardial infarction.
- May be used to treat nephropathy, including diabetic nephropathy.

Stability: Captopril solution prepared in water using tablets was stable for about 20 days when stored at 5°C.

Storage Condition:
- Captopril in powder papers is stable for at least 12 weeks when stored at room temperature under all three storage conditions.
- Store in a cool, dry place (room temperature; 15°C to 30°C (59°F to 86°F)), away from light.
- Liquid medicine: Store in the refrigerator.

Different types of Formulations: Tablet

Popular brand names: Topril, Aceril, Acenorm, Captolar, Angiopril.

Lisinopril

Classification: Angiotensin-Converting Enzyme (ACE) Inhibitors.

Chemical Name: (2*S*)-1-[(2*S*)-6-amino-2-[[(1*S*)-1-carboxy-3-phenylpropyl]amino] hexanoyl]pyrrolidine-2-carboxylic acid.

Chemical Structure

Uses:
- Lisinopril is indicated for the treatment of acute myocardial infarction, hypertension in patients, and as an adjunct therapy for heart failure.
- A combination product with hydrochlorothiazide is indicated for the treatment of hypertension.

Stability: Lisinopril can be prepared in either of 2 liquid dosage forms and stored for at least 13 weeks under refrigeration and 8 weeks at room temperature.

Storage Conditions
- Oral solution: Store at 20°C to 25°C (68°F to 77°F).
- Protect from freezing and excessive heat.
- Tablet: Store at 15°C to 30°C (59°F to 86°F).
- The suspension should be stored at or below 25°C (77°F).

Different types of Formulations: Tablet, Solution, Suspension.

Popular brand names: Lipril, Zestril, Biopril, Acinopril, Sopril, Sinopril, Dilace, Cipril, Hipril, Normopril.

Enalapril

Classification: Angiotensin-Converting Enzyme (ACE) Inhibitors.

Chemical Name: (2*S*)-1-[(2*S*)-2-[[(2*S*)-1-ethoxy-1-oxo-4-phenylbutan-2-yl]amino] propanoyl]pyrrolidine-2-carboxylic acid.

Chemical Structure

Uses

- Indicated for the management of essential or renovascular hypertension as monotherapy or in combination with other antihypertensive agents, such as thiazide diuretics, for an additive effect.
- Indicated for the treatment of symptomatic congestive heart failure, usually in combination with diuretics and digitalis.
- Indicated for the management of asymptomatic left ventricular dysfunction in patients with an ejection fraction of ≤35 percent to decrease the rate of development of overt heart failure and the incidence of hospitalization for heart failure.

Stability: Enalapril was found to be stable under oxidative stress. No decomposition was seen on exposure of solid drug powder to dry heat at 70 °C or 40 ± 2 °C/75 ± 5% RH for 27 days. The exposure of an aqueous solution of enalapril to UV and VIS radiation for 7 days resulted in a slight degradation to enalaprilat.

Storage Conditions

- Tablets should be stored at room temperature between 15°C - 30°C (59°F - 86°F).
- The injectable formulation should be stored at 20°C to 25°C (68°F to 77°F).

Different types of Formulations

- Tablet

Popular brand names: Enlarc, Dilvas, Enace, Enal, Oren, Lepril, Myoace, Nuril, Lapacrd, Envas

Benazepril Hydrochloride

Classification: Angiotensin-Converting Enzyme (ACE) Inhibitors.

Chemical Name: 6-chloro-1,1-dioxo-3,4-dihydro-$2H$-$1\lambda^6$,2,4-benzothiadiazine-7-sulfonamide.

Chemical Structure

Uses: Benazepril is indicated for the treatment of hypertension. It may be used alone or in combination with thiazide diuretics.

Stability: The drug degrades under the influence of direct light.

Storage Conditions
- Don't store benazepril at a temperature above 86°F (30°C).
- Don't freeze this drug.
- Keep this drug away from light.

Different types of Formulations: Tablet, film coated

Popular brand names: Benzil, Benace.

Quinapril Hydrochloride

Classification: Angiotensin-Converting Enzyme (ACE) Inhibitors.

Chemical Name: (3*S*)-2-[(2*S*)-2-[[(2*S*)-1-ethoxy-1-oxo-4-phenylbutan-2-yl]amino]propanoyl]-3,4-dihydro-1*H*-isoquinoline-3-carboxylic acid.

Chemical Structure

Uses:
- Quinapril is indicated for the treatment of hypertension and as an adjunct therapy in the treatment of heart failure.

- Quinapril in combination with hydrochlorothiazide is indicated for the treatment of hypertension.

Stability: Quinapril free base forms a stable salt with tris(hydroxymethyl)amino methane.

Storage Conditions

- Store quinapril at room temperature between 59°F and 86°F (15°C and 30°C).
- Keep it away from light.
- Don't freeze quinapril.
- Don't store this medication in moist or damp areas, such as bathrooms.

Different types of Formulations: Tablet, film coated

Popular brand names: Acupil, Q-Pril, Artisol.

Methyldopa Hydrochloride

Classification: Centrally Acting Cardiovascular Agents.

Chemical Name: ethyl (2*S*)-2-amino-3-(3,4-dihydroxyphenyl)-2-methylpropanoate.

Chemical Structure

Uses

- Methyldopa is indicated for the management of hypertension as monotherapy or in combination with hydrochlorothiazide.
- Methyldopa injection is used to manage hypertensive crises.

Stability

- Injectable dosage form is most stable at acid to neutral pH.
- Stability of parenteral admixture in D5W at room temperature (25°C) is 24 hours.
- Parenteral admixture is stable at room temperature for up to 125 hours

Storage Conditions

- Store in a well-closed container at controlled room temperature [15-30°C (59-86°F)].
- Oral suspension should be stored in tight, light-resistant containers at a temperature less than 26 °C and protected from freezing.

Different types of Formulations: Tablet, Liquid

Popular brand names: Alphadopa, Medop, Manodopa, Aldomet, Emdopa, Phynedopa, Medopres.

Clonidine Hydrochloride

Classification: Centrally Acting Alpha-Agonist.

Chemical Name: N-(2,6-dichlorophenyl)-4,5-dihydro-1H-imidazol-2-amine

Chemical Structure

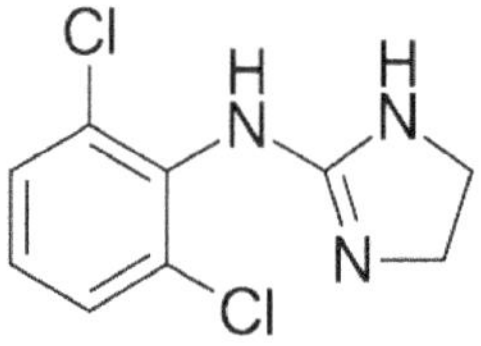

Uses

- Clonidine tablets and transdermal systems are indicated for the treatment of hypertension alone or in combination with other medications.
- A clonidine injection is indicated for use with opiates in the treatment of severe cancer pain where opiates alone are insufficient.
- An extended release tablet of clonidine is indicated for the treatment of ADHD either alone or in combination with other medications.
- Clonidine is also used for the diagnosis of pheochromocytoma, treatment of nicotine dependance, and opiate withdrawal.

Stability: This formulation is stable for at least 3 months at 5 °C +/− 3 °C in amber glass bottles and for one month when stored at room temperature.

Storage Conditions

- Clonidine should be stored at a temperature less than 30°C.
- Store at room temperature away from light and moisture.
- Do not store in the bathroom.
- Keep all medications away from children and pets.

Different types of Formulations: Tablet, Patch (extended release), Suspension.

Popular brand names: Clonilark, Arkamin, Clonomide, Clopresyn, Clonid, Nefropres, Elpres, Lonifa, Clodict, Arkadex

Reserpine

Classification: Centrally Acting Cardiovascular Agents.

Chemical Name: methyl(1R,15S,17R,18R,19S,20S)-6,18-dimethoxy-17-(3,4,5-trimethoxybenzoyl)oxy-1,3,11,12,14,15,16,17,18,19,20,21-dodecahydroyohimban-19-carboxylate.

Chemical Structure

Uses: It has been used as an antihypertensive and an antipsychotic as well as a research tool, but its adverse effects limit its clinical use.

Stability: Reserpine has a biocontamination factor of 72 and has a moderate potential for degradation.

Storage Conditions
- Store at room temperature between 68-77°F (20-25°C) away from light and moisture.
- Do not store in the bathroom.

Different types of Formulations: Tablet.

Popular brand names: Adelphane, Genophane, Sarpalzino, Serpasil, Serpalan.

Hydralazine

Classification: Vasodilators.

Chemical Name: phthalazin-1-ylhydrazine

Chemical Structure

Uses: It is used for the management of essential hypertension or severe hypertension associated with conditions requiring immediate action, heart failure, and pre-eclampsia or eclampsia.

Stability
- The pH profile indicates that hydralazine has maximum stability near pH 3.5.
- The drug decomposes to phthalazine and other products.

Storage Conditions

- Store at 20° to 25°C (68° to 77°F); excursions permitted to 15° to 30°C (59° to 86°F).
- Oral tablets: stored in light proof and air tight containers, between 15°C and 40°C (59°F to 104°F).
- Ampoules should be kept between the same temperatures described above and should not be frozen.
- Solutions containing glucose, fructose, lactose and maltose reduce the stability of the drug.

Different types of Formulations: Tablet, coated, Solution, Injections.

Popular brand names: Apresol, Aprezin, H-Zin, Naman, Bidil, Apresoline, Dralzine.

Nifedipine

Classification: Calcium Channel Blockers.

Chemical Name: dimethyl 2,6-dimethyl-4-(2-nitrophenyl)-1,4-dihydropyridine-3,5-dicarboxylate

Chemical Structure

Uses: It is indicated to treat vasospastic angina, chronic stable angina and hypertension.

Stability: Nifedipine 10 mg/mL was stable in an oral solution prepared from commercially available powder in a peppermint-flavored vehicle for at least 35 days when stored at 22-25 degrees C in amber glass bottles and for at least 14 days when stored in amber oral syringes wrapped in aluminum foil.

Storage Conditions

- Nifedipine is expected to be stable for at least two years when stored at 2-8°C.
- Store drug capsules at room temperature between 59°F - 77°F.
- The tablets should be protected from light and moisture and stored below 86°F.

Different types of Formulations: Tablet (film coated), Capsule

Popular brand names: Nicardia, Calcigard, Depin, Depicor, Cardules, Nifesta, Nifelat, Nifeditrix, Nicardiwyn, Cardif.

Isosorbide Dinitrate

Classification: Vasodilators.

Chemical Name: [(3S,3aS,6R,6aS)-3-nitrooxy-2,3,3a,5,6,6a-hexahydrofuro[3,2-b] furan-6-yl] nitrate.

Chemical Structure

Uses: For the prevention of angina pectoris due to coronary artery disease.

Stability: Solutions of isosorbide dinitrate 0.60 mg/mL in syringe of sodium chloride 0.9 % injection can be considered physically and chemically stable for 28 days when stored in syringes at 5°C ± 3°C with protection from light and may be prepared in advance by a centralized intravenous additive service.

Storage Conditions

- Isosorbide dinitra0074e should be stored at room temperature, 15°C - 30°C (59°F - 86°F).
- Store the medicine in a closed container at room temperature, away from heat, moisture, and direct light.
- Keep from freezing.

Different types of Formulations: Tablet (extended release), Capsule, extended release.

Popular brand names: Isonit, Nitra, Anzidin, Isolar, Sorbitrate, Sorbilarc, Vasodil, Sosodil, Angex, Sorbidine.

Amyl Nitrate

Classification: Vasodilators.

Chemical Name: Pentyl nitrate

Chemical Structure

Uses
- It is a fast acting vasodilator used for rapid relief of angina pectoris.
- Amyl Nitrite is an antihypertensive medicine and to treat heart diseases such as angina.
- Amyl nitrite is also used to treat cyanide poisoning.

Stability: Decomposes and has tendency to explode under heat and fire.

Storage Conditions
- The capsule contents are FLAMMABLE and should be protected from light.
- Storage should be in a cold place, $2°$-$8°C$ ($26°F$ - $46°F$).

Different types of Formulations: Tablet, Capsule

Popular brand names: Amyl, Amnitre

Multiple Choice Questions

1. Which of the following tissues has a conduction rate of 0.05 m/s?
   - (a) Ventricular muscle
   - (b) Bundle of His
   - (c) Atrial pathways
   - (d) AV node e. Purkinje system

2. All of the following increase cardiac output EXCEPT
   - (a) Eating
   - (b) Pregnancy
   - (c) Sleep
   - (d) High environmental temperature
   - (e) Exercise

3. Hydralazine
   - (a) Dilates veins but not arterioles
   - (b) Is contraindicated in the treatment of preeclampsia
   - (c) Can cause an SLE type syndrome in up to $10 - 20\%$ of patients
   - (d) Causes orthostatic hypotension in many cases

4. Which of the following drugs has the smallest volume of distribution?
   - (a) Chloroquine
   - (b) Verapamil
   - (c) Imipramine
   - (d) Warfarin
   - (e) Digoxin

5. Digoxin
    (a) Is poorly lipid soluble
    (b) Is extensively metabolized
    (c) Has a half life in the body of 40 hours
    (d) Has minimal GI toxicity e. Is 80% bound to plasma proteins
6. Contents of the normal gastric juice include all of the following EXCEPT
    (a) Intrinsic factor
    (b) Lipase
    (c) Pepsins
    (d) Sulphate
    (e) Calcium
7. The cause of fluid retention peripherally with congestive cardiac failure is
    (a) Increased renin
    (b) Increased GFR
    (c) Increased angiotensin II
    (d) Increased aldosterone
8. Angiotensinogen is liberated from
    (a) Lungs
    (b) Kidney
    (c) Stomach
    (d) Pancrease
9. Nitric oxide is
    (a) Vasodilator
    (b) Vasoconstrictor
    (c) Both
    (d) None
10. Renin is secreted from
    (a) Kidney
    (b) Lungs
    (c) Liver
    (d) Stomach

CHAPTER 8
Diuretics

Introduction

The chapter aims at providing the latest and pharmacopoeial information regarding some Diuretics (Acetazolamide, Furosemide, Bumetanide, Chlorthiazide, Benzthiazide, Xipmide, and Spironolactone) regarding their classification, chemical name, chemical structure, uses, stability, storage conditions, different types of formulations, and popular brand names.

Diuretics increase the rate of urine flow and sodium excretion, and are used to adjust the volume or composition of body fluids in a variety of clinical situations, including hypertension, heart failure, renal failure, nephritic syndrome, and cirrhosis. The normal fluid filtration in human body is 180 litres, and about 1.5 litres of urine is formed in 24 hrs.

The diuretics act primarily by inhibiting tubular reabsorption; just 1% decrease in tubular reabsorption would produce more than double urine output. The action depends upon the drug by acting on various symport and antiport present in the nephron. All the transports depend on the basolateral membrane porters, especially in tubular reabsorption, which is divided into four sites:

1. Proximal tubule (PT)
2. Ascending limb of loop of henle (AscLH)
3. Cortical diluting segment of loop of henle
4. Distal tubule (DT)
5. Collecting duct

Classification

Diuretics may be classified under the following two categories:

    I. **Mercurial diuretics:** Mersalyl, Mercurophyllin, Mercaptomerin, Chloromerodrin, Merethoxyline, Meralluride

II. Non mercurial diuretics: The nonmercurial diuretics may be classified on the basis of their chemical structure as follows:

(a) **Thiazide derivatives:** Chlorthiazide, Benzthiazide, Flumethiazide

(b) **Hydrothiazides:** Hydrochlorothiazide, Bendroflumethiazide, Cyclothi-azide, Hydro flumethiazide, Cyclopenthiazide, Trichloromethiazide, Buthi-azide, Methyclothiazide, Polythiazide

(c) **Carbonic anhydrase inhibitors:** Acetazolamide, Methazolamide, Ethoxozolamide, Dichlorophenamide, Disulfamide

(d) **Sulphonamide diuretics:** Quinethazone, Chlorothalidone, Metolazone, Indapamide, Clopamide, Xipamide, Clorexolone

(e) **Aldosterone inhibitors:** Spironolactone, canrenone, Amphenone B, Metyrapone, Eplerenone,

(f) **Pteridine derivatives and related compounds:** Triamterene, Amiloride

(g) **Sulphomoyl benzoic acid derivatives:** Furosemide, Bumetanide, Toresemide, Piretanide

(h) **Phenoxyacetic acid derivatives:** Ethacrynic acid,

(i) **Purine or Xanthine derivatives:** Caffeine, Theophylline, Theobromine

(j) **Osmotic diuretics:** Sodium and potassium salt, urea, sucrose, mannitol, trometamol, sodium acid phosphate, potassium acetate, and glycerine are the osmotic diuretics.

Urea, Isosorbide, Mannitol

(k) **Acidic diuretics:** Ammonium chloride is a acidic diuretic

(l) **Uricosuric diuretics:** Indacrinone

(m) **Miscellaneous:** Example: Muzolimine

Acetazolamide

Classification: Diuretics

Chemical Name: *N*-(5-sulfamoyl-1,3,4-thiadiazol-2-yl)acetamide

Chemical Structure

Uses

- Acetazolamide is a diuretic and carbonic anhydrase inhibitor medication that is used to treat several illnesses.
- Acetazolamide is used to prevent and reduce the symptoms of altitude sickness. This medication can decrease headache, tiredness, nausea, dizziness, and shortness of breath.

- Acetazolamide is used to lower intraocular pressure in the treatment of malignant (ciliary block) glaucoma, which may occur after inflammation surgery, trauma, or use of miotics.
- Acetazolamide has also been used with other medications to treat certain types of seizures (petit mal and unlocalized seizures).

Stability

- Insoluble in water.
- Reacts with Amides and Imides.
- A weak acid and a diazo derivative. Azo, diazo, azido compounds can detonate.

Storage Conditions: Store between 15 and 30 °C (59 and 86 °F), in a well-closed container, unless otherwise specified by manufacturer.

Different types of Formulations: Oral - Solid: 250 mg, Modified-release capsules

Popular brand names: Acetazolarc Tab, Actamid Tab, Avva SR Tab, Diamox Tab, Press Dt Tab, Iopar SR Tab, Cap SR 250mg Tab, Bell Zolamide Tab, Axytex 250mg Tab, Actex 250mg Tab.

Furosemide

Classification: Diuretics

Chemical Name: 4-chloro-2-(furan-2-ylmethylamino)-5-sulfamoylbenzoic acid

Chemical Structure

Uses

- Sodium Potassium Chloride Symporter Inhibitors (diuretic).
- Furosemide may be used in adults for the treatment of hypertension alone or in combination with other antihypertensive agents.
- Furosemide is indicated in adults and pediatric patients for the treatment of edema associated with congestive heart failure, cirrhosis of the liver, and renal disease, including the nephrotic syndrome.

Stability

- Stable under recommended storage conditions.
- Commercially available 40-mg furosemide tablets have an expiration date of 5 years and the commercially available injection has an expiration date

42 months following the date of manufacture. The 20-mg tablets do not have a specific expiration dating period.

- When heated to decomposition it emits very toxic fumes of /hydrogen chloride, nitrogen oxides and sulfur oxides.
- Melts between 203-205 ᵒC with decomposition.

Storage Conditions

- Keep container tightly closed in a dry and well-ventilated place.
- Furosemide injection should be stored at a temperature of 15-30 ᵒC and protected from light; injections having a yellow color should not be used. Exposure of furosemide tablets to light may cause discoloration; discolored tablets should not be dispensed.
- Furosemide tablets should be stored and dispensed in well-closed, light-resistant containers at a controlled room temperature of 15-30 ᵒC.

Different types of Formulations

- Furosemide Solution (Available from one or more manufacturer, distributor, and/or repackager by generic (nonproprietary) name).
- Furosemide Tablets (Available from one or more manufacturer, distributor, and/or repackager by generic (nonproprietary) name).
- Furosemide Injections (Available from one or more manufacturer, distributor, and/or repackager by generic (nonproprietary) name).

Popular brand names: Lasix, Tesix, Frusizex, Frusee, Frusenex, Frumide, Frumil, Lasiride, Amifru, Diucontin.

Bumetanide

Classification: Diuretics

Chemical Name: 3-(butylamino)-4-phenoxy-5-sulfamoylbenzoic acid

Chemical Structure

Uses: Bumetanide is used to reduce extra fluid in the body (edema) caused by conditions such as heart failure, liver disease, and kidney disease.

Stability: Protect from light; drug discolors when exposed to light and moisture.

Storage Conditions

- Store at 68 °C to 77°F (20 °C to 25 °C); excursions permitted between 59 °C to 86°F (15° to 30 °C).
- Dispense contents in a tight, light-resistant container as defined in the USP with a child-resistant closure, as required.
- Do not store in the bathroom.
- Keep all medications away from children and pets.
- Do not flush medications down the toilet or pour them into a drain unless instructed to do so.

Different types of Formulations: Tablet

Popular brand names: Bumex, Burinex

Chlorothiazide

Classification: Diuretics

Chemical Name: 6-chloro-1,1-dioxo-4H-1λ^6,2,4-benzothiadiazine-7-sulfonamide

Chemical Structure

Uses

- Thiazides are diuretics of choice for maintenance therapy in ambulatory patients with edema caused by chronic congestive heart failure but with normal renal function.
- Less common usages of thiazides includes treatment of diabetes insipidus and management of hypercalciuria in proximal tubule with recurrent urinary calculi composed of calcium.

Stability

- Insoluble in water.
- Reacts with Amines, Phosphines, and Pyridines.
- Alkaline aqueous solutions will decompose on standing or heating.

Storage Conditions

- Keep container tightly closed and store at room temperature, 15-30 °C (59-86°F).
- Protect from freezing, −20 °C (−4 °F)

Different types of Formulations: Oral Suspension, Tablet.

Popular brand names: Diuril, Chlotride, Microzide, Hydrodiuril

Benzthiazide

Classification: Diuretics

Chemical Name: 3-(benzylsulfanylmethyl)-6-chloro-1,1-dioxo-4*H*-1λ⁶,2,4-benzothi-adiazine-7-sulfonamide

Chemical Structure

Uses

- Thiazide drugs are usually first drug to be employed in treatment of hypertension. Since thiazides induce only limited (10%) reduction in blood pressure they are useful either in mild cases of hypertension or as adjunctive therapy to other drugs.
- They are effective as adjunctive therapy in edema assoc with congestive heart failure, hepatic cirrhosis, corticosteroid & estrogen therapy, as well as edema due to various forms of renal dysfunction & severe edema due to pregnancy.

Stability

- Stable in both light and air.
- When heated to decomposition it emits very toxic fumes of sulfoxides, nitroxides, and hydrogen chloride.

Storage Conditions

- It must be stored under room temperature (between 15°C to 25°C)

Different types of Formulations: Tablet, Solution, Solution.

Popular brand names: Aquatag, Dihydrex, Diucen, Edemax, Exna, Foven

Xipamide

Classification: Diuretics

Chemical Name: 4-chloro-*N*-(2,6-dimethylphenyl)-2-hydroxy-5-sulfamoylbenzamide

Chemical Structure

Uses

- Xipamide is used in Hypertension (high blood pressure). It treats edema (fluid overload) associated with heart, liver, kidney or lung disease.
- Xipamide is a thiazide diuretic. It lowers blood pressure and fluid retention in edema by removing the extra water and certain electrolytes from the body.

Stability: Degradation takes place under alkaline condition.

Storage Conditions

- Store in a cool, dry place, away from direct heat and light.
- Keep all medicines out of the reach and sight of children.

Different types of Formulations: Tablet, Capsule

Popular brand names: Aquaphor, Aquaphoril, Xipamid

Q. Write a detailed note on Spironolactone.

Classification: Diuretics

Chemical Name: S-[(7R,8R,9S,10R,13S,14S,17R)-10,13-dimethyl-3,5'-dioxospiro[2,6,7, 8,9,11,12,14,15,16-decahydro-1H-cyclopenta[a]phenanthrene-17,2'-oxolane]-7-yl] etha-nethioate

Chemical Structure

Uses

- Aldosterone Antagonists; Diuretics
- Spironolactone can be used with furosemide to control ascites.
- Spironolactone is used most frequently and is a competitive antagonist of aldosterone. Aldosterone is elevated in animals with congestive heart failure in which the renin-angiotensin system is activated in response to hyponatremia,

hyperkalemia, and reductions in blood pressure or cardiac output. Aldosterone is responsible for increasing sodium and chloride reabsorption and potassium and calcium excretion from renal tubules. Spironolactone competes with aldosterone at its receptor site, causing a mild diuresis and potassium retention.

Stability: Stable in Air

Storage Conditions

- Spironolactone tablets should be stored in tight, light-resistant containers at a temperature less than 40 °C, preferably between 15-30 °C.
- Oral suspensions of spironolactone prepared by pulverizing commercially available tablets of the drug and adding them to cherry syrup have been reported to be stable for one month at 2-8 °C.

Different types of Formulations

- Oral: Tablets, film-coated: 25 mg Aldactone (with povidone), (Pfizer) Spironolactone Tablets (Mutual), Spironolactone Tablets (Mylan), Spironolactone Tablets (Sandoz), Spironolactone Tablets (UDL), Spironolactone Tablets, (United Research); 50 mg Aldactone (with povidone; scored), (Pfizer), Spironolactone Tablets (Actavis), Spironolactone Tablets (Mutual), Spironolactone Tablets (Mylan), Spironolactone Tablets (United Research); 100 mg Aldactone (with povidone; scored), (Pfizer), Spironolactone Tablets (Actavis), Spironolactone Tablets (Mutual), Spironolactone Tablets (Mylan), Spironolactone Tablets (United Research).

Popular brand names: Vascoton, Spitone, Wellton, Silectone, Aldactone, Spirozone, Spilactone, Cglactone, Torlactone, Loopstar Plus

---

Multiple Choice Questions

---

1. Osmotic diuretics are contraindicated in..?
   (a) Increased intracranial tension
   (b) Increased intraocular tension
   (c) Established acute renal failure
   (d) Poisonings

2. Which of the following drug and their mechanism of action is not correct?
   (a) Acetazolamide: epithelial sodium channel blockers
   (b) Spironolactone: potassium-sparing diuretics
   (c) Hydrochlorothiazide: inhibit sodium chloride symporter
   (d) Bumetanide: inhibits NA+/K+/2Cl- cotransport

3. The following diuretic promotes calcium reabsorption:
   (a) Spironolactone   (b) Furosemide
   (c) Chlorothiazide   (d) Ethacrynic acid

4. Which of the following drugs is used for urinary incontinence?
    (a) Flavoxate   (b) Sodium citrate
    (c) Trimethoprim   (d) Phenazopyridine

5. Concurrent use of Spironolactone & ACE inhibitors should be avoided because of the danger of –
    (a) Hyperglycemia   (b) Hyperkalemia
    (c) Hypokalemia   (d) Hypoglycemia

6. Following are the uses of Amiloride, except?
    (a) Adjunct to K+ wasting diuretics
    (b) Lithium induced nephrogenic diabetes insipidus
    (c) Congestive heart failure
    (d) a and b
    (e) a, b and c

7. Which one of the following diuretics is effective in severe renal failure?
    (a) Loop diuretics   (b) K+ sparing diuretics
    (c) Thiazides   (d) Carbonic anhydrase inhibitors

8. The antidiuretic action of Desmopressin is due to activation of...................................?
    (a) V 1a receptor   (b) V 2 receptor
    (c) V 1b receptor   (d) V1 and V2 receptor

9. One among the following is not an osmotic diuretic
    (a) Ureanitrate   (b) Glycerol
    (c) Mannitol   (d) Isosorbide

10. One of the following diuretics acts on the llop of Henle
    (a) Spironolactone   (b) Ethacrynic acid
    (c) Clorexolone   (d) Dichlorphenamide

CHAPTER 9

Hypoglycemic Agents

Introduction

The chapter aims at providing the latest and pharmacopoeial information regarding some Hypoglycemic agents (Insulin & its preparations, Metformin, Tolbutamide, Glibenclamide, Glipizide, Glimepiride, Pioglitazone, and Ripaglinide) regarding their classification, chemical name, chemical structure, uses, stability, storage conditions, different types of formulations, and popular brand names.

Diabetes mellitus is a metabolic disorder characterized by hyperglycaemia, glycosuria, hyperlipidemia, negative nitrogen balance, and ketonaemia. Most patients can be classified, clinically, as having either type I diabetes mellitus (insulin dependent diabetes mellitus (IDDM) or type II noninsulin dependent diabetes mellitus (NIDDM). The incidence of each type of diabetes varies widely throughout the world. In the United States, about 5% to 10% of the diabetic patients have type I diabetes mellitus, with an incidence of 17 per 100,000 found in United Kingdom. The vast majority of diabetic patients have type II diabetes mellitus.

Type I diabetes is also called juvenile onset diabetes mellitus. There is β-cell destruction in the pancreatic islets of langerhans. Majority of the cases are due to autoimmune (type I A) antibodies that destroy β cells, are detectable in blood, but some are idiopathic (type I B) no β (beta) cell antibody is found. In all type I cases, circulating insulin levels are low or very low and ketosis may occur. Genetic predisposition is also a cause for this condition.

Type II diabetes is also called maturity onset diabetes mellitus. There is no loss or moderate reduction in the β cell mass, insulin in circulation levels is low and generally has a late onset of disease after middle age. This may be due to an abnormality in the glucoreceptors of β cells, therefore, they respond at higher glucose concentrations or at relative β cell defi ciency. The reduced sensitivity of peripheral tissues to insulin and reduction in the number of insulin receptors are a consequence for producing diabetes. When glucagons exceed a normal amount, it produces hypoglycaemia. The insulin is secreted by the β cells of langerhans, synthesized by a single chain precursor of 110 amino acid preproinsulin. After translocation through the membrane of rough endoplasmic reticulum, the 24 amino acid N-terminal peptide of preproinsulin is rapidly cleared off to form proinsulin. Here, the molecules folds and the disulphide bonds are formed. In the conversion of proinsulin to insulin in the Golgi complex, four basic amino acids and the remaining connector or C peptide are removed by proteolysis. This gives rise to two peptide chains (A and B) of insulin molecules, which contains one intrasubunit and two intersubunits disulphide bonds. The A chain consists of 21 amino acids and B with 30 amino acids and molecular mass is about 5734 daltons. The regulatory factors of insulin secretion are chemical, hormonal, and neural. Chemical regulation depends upon the glucose entry in to the β cells by glucose transport. Once, after the entry of glucose and its phosphorylation by glucokinase, glucoreceptor activation indirectly inhibits the adenosine triphosphate (ATP) sensitive potassium channels and increases intracellular calcium, which triggers the exocytic release of insulin. Hormonal change in corticosteroids modify the release of insulin. Insulin inhibits glucagon secretion and glucagons increase the insulin secretion.

Classification

I. **Sulphonylureas**

   (a) **First-generation drugs:** Carbutamide, Tolbutamide, Chloropropamide, Tolazamide, Acetohexamide

   (b) **Second-generation drugs:** Glibenclamide (Glyburide), Glipizide, Gliclazide, Glibornuride

II. **Biguanides:** Phenformin, Metformin, Buformin

III. **Substituted benzoic acid derivatives (Meglitinides):** Meglitinide, Repaglinide, Nateglinide

IV. **Thiazolidinediones (Glitazones):** Pioglitazone, Ciglitazone, Rosiglitazone

V. **α- Glucosidase inhibitors:** Acarbose, Miglitol

VI. **Aldose reductase inhibitors:** Sorbinil, Tolrestat

VII. **Miscellaneous:** Linogliride, Palmoxirate sodium, pirogliride

Metformin

Classification: Anti-diabetic Agents

Chemical Name: 3-(diaminomethylidene)-1,1-dimethylguanidine

Chemical Structure

Uses: Metformin is a biguanide drug used in conjunction with diet and exercise for glycemic control in type 2 diabetes mellitus and used off-label for insulin resistance in polycystic ovary syndrome (PCOS).

Stability: Incompatible materials: Strong oxidizing agents.

Storage Conditions
- Keep container tightly closed in a dry and well-ventilated place.
- Recommended storage temperature is 2 - 8 °C.

Different types of Formulations: Solutions, Tablets (extended-release), Tablets, film-coated

Popular brand names: Obimet, Okamet, Insuform, Metbay, Metform, Metchek, Metafort, Metatime, Melmet, Metaday.

Tolbutamide

Classification: Anti-diabetic Agents

Chemical Name: 1-butyl-3-(4-methylphenyl) sulfonylurea

Chemical Structure

Uses: Tolbutamide is an oral antihyperglycemic agent used for the treatment of non-insulin-dependent diabetes mellitus (NIDDM).

Stability
- It is insoluble in water.
- It reacts with Amides and Imides.
- It reacts with azo and diazo compounds to generate toxic gases

Storage Conditions: Store at room temperature (between 59 to 86 °F)

Different types of Formulations: Tablets

Popular brand names: Told, Rastinon, Orinase, Toltab

Glibenclamide

Classification: Anti-diabetic Agents

Chemical Name: 5-chloro-*N*-[2-[4-(cyclohexylcarbamoylsulfamoyl) phenyl] ethyl]-2-methoxybenzamide

Chemical Structure

Uses: Glibenclamide is a second-generation sulfonylurea used to treat patients with diabetes mellitus type II.

Stability: It forms water-soluble salts with alkali hydroxides.

Storage Conditions:
- Keep away from children.
- Keep in a cool, dry place, away from direct sunlight.

Different types of Formulations: Suspension, Tablets.

Popular brand names: Daonil, Glinil, Getrol, Glybovin, Diabetnil, Diaben, Gilly, Gimide, Glyboral, Gliconil.

Glipizide

Classification: Anti-diabetic Agents

Chemical Name: *N*-[2-[4-(cyclohexylcarbamoylsulfamoyl) phenyl] ethyl]-5-methylpyrazine-2-carboxamide

Chemical Structure

Uses: Glipizide is an oral hypoglycemic agent in the second-generation sulfonylurea drug class that is used to control blood sugar levels in patients with type 2 diabetes mellitus.

Stability: It forms water-soluble salts with alkali hydroxides.

Storage Conditions
- Store below 86°F (30°C).
- Recommended room temperature between 68°F and 77°F.

Different types of Formulations: Tablet (extended release)

Popular brand names: Glez, Glytop, Glynase, Zidetrix, Glicept, Sugarid, Metglib, Metglip, Glirum, Bionase.

Glimepiride

Classification: Anti-diabetic Agents

Chemical Name: 4-ethyl-3-methyl-*N*-[2-[4-[(4-methylcyclohexyl)carbamoyl-sulfamoyl]phenyl]ethyl]-5-oxo-2*H*-pyrrole-1-carboxamide

Chemical Structure

Uses: Glimepiride is a member of the second-generation sulfonylurea drug class used for the management of type 2 diabetes mellitus (T2DM) to improve glycemic control.

Stability: Glimepiride is stable to dry heat (50 °C for 31 days).

Storage Conditions
- Store glimepiride at room temperature.
- Keep it at a temperature between 68°F and 77°F (20°C and 25°C).
- Don't freeze glimepiride.

Different types of Formulations: Tablets

Popular brand names: Glador, Glimy, Glyree, Glimisave, Glimulin, Glycilarc, Glimiprex, Glimtide, Geniride, Glitaray

Pioglitazone

Classification: Anti-diabetic Agents

Chemical Name: 5-[[4-[2-(5-ethylpyridin-2-yl) ethoxy] phenyl] methyl]-1,3-thiazolidine-2,4-dione

Chemical Structure

Uses: Pioglitazone is an antihyperglycemic used as an adjunct to diet, exercise, and other antidiabetic medications to manage type 2 diabetes mellitus.

Stability: Hazardous decomposition products formed under fire conditions: Carbon oxides, Nitrogen oxides (NOx), Sulfur oxides, Hydrogen chloride gas.

Storage Conditions: Store at 20 °C to 25 °C (68 °F to 77 °F); excursions permitted to 15 °C to 30 °C (59 °F to 86 °F).

- Keep container tightly closed in a dry and well-ventilated place.

Different types of Formulations: Tablets

Popular brand names: Pizowyn, Arpie, Glitaris, Pioglar, Piogen, Pioglit, Piomed, Piopod, Piolon, Piosys.

Repaglinide

Classification: Anti-diabetic Agents

Chemical Name: 2-ethoxy-4-[2-[[(1S)-3-methyl-1-(2-piperidin-1-ylphenyl) butyl] amino]-2-oxoethyl] benzoic acid

Chemical Structure

Uses: Repaglinide is an oral antihyperglycemic agent used for the treatment of non-insulin-dependent diabetes mellitus (NIDDM).

Stability: Contact with alkalizing agents showed no degradation or spontaneous recrystallization in the formulation.

Storage Conditions

- Store at room temperature between 59-77 °F (15-25 °C) away from light and moisture.
- Do not store in the bathroom.

Different types of Formulations: Tablets

Popular brand names: Novonorm, Restrict, Repasafe, Reepag, Eurepa, Hirepa, Premeal, Repact, Regan, Repide

---

Multiple Choice Questions

1. Insulin Administer through the Route?
   - (a) Oral
   - (b) IV
   - (c) Sublingual
   - (d) Subcutaneous

2. Oral hypoglycemic agent most likely to be prescribed for patients with refractory obesity?
   - (a) Chlorpropamide
   - (b) Metformin
   - (c) Tolbutamide
   - (d) Glipizide

3. Fasting Glucose Level is?
   - (a) 80-120 mg/dl
   - (b) 50-80 mg/dl
   - (c) 100-140 mg/dl
   - (d) 150-200 mg/dl

4. Insulin Released from the Cells?
   - (a) Alpha Cells
   - (b) Beta Cells
   - (c) Delta Cells
   - (d) None

5. The pathogenesis of hyperglycemia in diabetic ketoacidosis includes all the following mechanisms except for:
   - (a) Increased glycogenolysis in the liver
   - (b) Increased gluconeogenesis in the kidneys
   - (c) Increased serum glucagon
   - (d) Increased gluconeogenesis in adipose tissue
   - (e) Decreased glucose uptake from the muscles

6. Which of the following confirmed values meet the diagnostic threshold for diabetes?
   - (a) fasting blood glucose ? 140 mg/dl
   - (b) random glucose > 160 mg/dl
   - (c) 2 hour post prandial glucose $\geq$ to 126 mg/dl
   - (d) Fasting blood glucose $\geq$ 126 mg/dl

7. Which of the following statements is correct?
   (a) Insulin suppresses the activity of glycogen synthase
   (b) Insulin mediates glucose uptake in the brain
   (c) "Prediabetes" is a condition characterized by an increased risk for the future development of type 2 diabetes
   (d) The rise in insulin concentration after meal ingestion is reduced in type 1 but not in type 2 diabetes

8. Insulin deficiency is associated with
   (a) Reduced lipolysis
   (b) Increased ketogenesis
   (c) Reduced gluconeogenesis
   (d) Reduced proteolysis

9. The risk factors for type 2 diabetes mellitus include:
   (a) Family history
   (b) Being overweight
   (c) High intake of dietary fat
   (d) All of the options listed are correct

10. What is the first-line drug for patients with type 2 diabetes and obesity?
    (a) Acarbose
    (b) Metformin
    (c) Sulphonylureas
    (d) Insulin

CHAPTER 10

Analgesic and Anti-Inflammatory Agents

Introduction

The chapter aims at providing the latest and pharmacopoeial information regarding some Analgesic and Anti-inflammatory agents (Morphine analogues, Narcotic antagonists, Aspirin, Diclofenac, Ibuprofen, Piroxicam, Celecoxib, Mefenamic Acid, and Paracetamol) regarding their classification, chemical name, chemical structure, uses, stability, storage conditions, different types of formulations, and popular brand names.

Nonsteroidal anti-inflammatory drugs (NSAIDs) are used primarily to treat inflammation, mild-to-moderate pain, and fever. Specific uses include the treatment of headache, arthritis, sports injuries, and menstrual cramps. Aspirin is used to inhibit the clotting of blood and prevent strokes and heart attacks in individuals at high risk. NSAIDs are also included in many cold and allergic preparations. NSAIDs are associated with a number of side effects. The frequency of side effects varies according to the drugs; the most common side effects are gastro intestinal tract (GIT) disturbances, such as nausea, diarrhoea, constipation, vomiting, decreased appetite, and peptic ulcer. NSAIDs may also cause fluid retention, leading to oedema; the most serious side effects are kidney failure, liver failure, ulcers, and prolonged bleeding after an injury of surgery. Some individuals are allergic to NSAIDs and may develop shortness of breath when NSAIDs are administered. People with asthma are at a higher risk for experiencing serious allergic reaction to NSAIDs. Use of aspirin in children and teenagers with chicken pox or influenza has been associated with the development of Reye's syndrome. Therefore, aspirin and salicylate should not be used in children and teenagers with suspected or confirmed chicken pox or influenza. Antipyretics are the drugs that reduce the elevated body temperature. Anti-inflammatory agents are used to cure or prevent inflammation caused by prostaglandin (PGE2). These drugs are widely utilized for the alleviation of minor aches, pains, fever, and symptomatic treatment of rheumatic fever, rheumatoid arthritis, and osteoarthritis.

NSAIDs are typically divided into groups based on their chemical structure and selectivity: acetylated salicylates (aspirin), non-acetylated salicylates (diflunisal, salsalate), propionic acids (naproxen, ibuprofen, acetic acids (diclofenac, indomethacin), enolic acids (meloxicam, piroxicam) anthranilic acids (meclofenamate, mefenamic acid), naphthylalanine (nabumetone), and selective COX-2 inhibitors (celecoxib, etoricoxib).

Classification

Salicylic acid derivatives

Acetylsalicyclic acid (Aspirin), Sodium Salicylate, Diflunisal, Salicylsalicyclic acid, Sulfasalazine, Olsalazine

Para-aminophenol derivatives

Acetaminophen

Indol and indene acetic acid

Indomethacin, Sulindac, Etodolac

Heteroaryl acetic acid

Ibuprofen, Neproxen, Flubiprofen, Ketoprofen, Fenoprofen, Oxaprozin

Anthranilic acid derivatives

Mefenamic acid, Meclofenamic acid

Enolic acid derivatives

Piroxicam, Tenoxicam, Meloxicam

Mechanism of Action

The main mechanism of action of NSAIDs is the inhibition of the enzyme cyclooxygenase (COX). Cyclooxygenase is required to convert arachidonic acid into thromboxanes, prostaglandins, and prostacyclins. The therapeutic effects of NSAIDs are attributed to the lack of these eicosanoids. Specifically, thromboxanes play a role in platelet adhesion, prostaglandins cause vasodilation, increase the temperature set-point in the hypothalamus, and play a role in anti-nociception.

There are two cyclooxygenase isoenzymes, COX-1 and COX-2. COX-1 gets constitutively expressed in the body, and it plays a role in maintaining gastrointestinal mucosa lining, kidney function, and platelet aggregation. COX-2 is not constitutively expressed in the body; and instead, it inducibly expresses during an inflammatory response. Most of the NSAIDs are nonselective and inhibit both COX-1 and COX-2. However, COX-2 selective NSAIDs (ex. celecoxib) only target COX-2 and therefore have a different side effect profile. Importantly, because COX-1 is the prime mediator for ensuring gastric mucosal integrity and COX-2 is mainly involved in inflammation, COX-2 selective NSAIDs should provide anti-inflammatory relief without compromising the gastric mucosa.

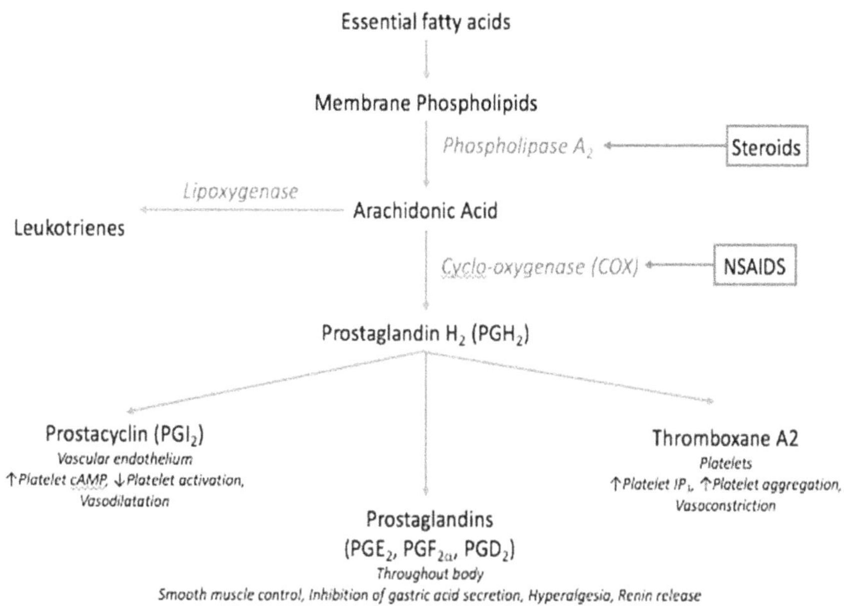

Fig. 1 Mechanism of action of NSAIDs in the inhibition of the enzyme cyclooxygenase (COX)

Analgesic and Anti-inflammatory Agents

Morphine Analogues

Narcotic agents are potent analgesics, which are effective for the relief of severe pain. They are selective central nervous system depressants used to relieve pain. In therapeutic doses, narcotic analgesics can cause respiratory depression, nausea, and drowsiness. Long-term administration of narcotics produces tolerance, psychic, and physical dependence called addiction.

Classification of Narcotic analgesic

Narcotic analgesics will be classified on the basis of their structural derivation from morphine. They may be classified into following categories:

1. **Natural alkaloids of opium:** Morphine and codeine.
2. **Semisynthetic analogs**. e.g.: Hydromorphone, oxymorphone, oxycodone.
3. **Synthetic agents** Ex: Meperidine, levorphanol, methadone, sufentanil, alfentanil, fentanyl, remifentanil, levomethadyl.

Morphine

The prototypic narcotic analgesic is (-)-morphine, the principal alkaloid obtained from the opium poppy (Papaver somniferum). Morphine was isolated as a pure alkaloid by a German pharmacist, Serturner in 1803.

Chemical name: (4R,4aR,7S,7aR,12bS)-3-methyl-2,4,4a,7,7a,13-hexahydro-1H-4,12-methanobenzofuro[3,2-e]isoquinoline-7,9-diol

Chemical Structure

Uses: This medication is used to help relieve moderate to severe pain. Morphine belongs to a class of drugs known as opioid analgesics. It works in the brain to change how your body feels and responds to pain.

Stability: The compatibility and stability studies were carried out at two different temperatures (25±0.5 °C and 37±0.5 °C), and all drug mixtures were protected from direct light exposure.

Storage conditions: Morphine solutions should preferably be stored at room temperature in order to avoid precipitation at low temperatures and water evaporation at higher temperatures causing increase in morphine concentration when stored in polymer reservoirs.

Different types of formulations with popular brand names: Kadian, MS Contin

Codeine

Conversion of the 3-OH to a 3-OCH$_3$, yields codeine, reduces activity to 15% of morphine. Codeine is available as a sulfate and phosphate salt and also as the free base and as tablets, elixir and solution for injection. The 3-methoxy group protects the 3-position from glucuronide as occurs with morphine. Codeine is used as an analgesic and antitussive.

Chemical name: Morphinan-6-ol,7,8-didehydro-4,5-epoxy-3-methoxy-17-methyl-(5α,6α)-, sulfate (2:1) (salt), trihydrate

Chemical Structure

Uses: This medication is used to help relieve mild to moderate pain. Codeine belongs to a class of drugs known as opioid analgesics. It works in the brain to change how your body feels and responds to pain.

Stability: codeine sulfate is predicted to have a room temperature shelf life of approximately 44 years between pH 1 and 10, significantly longer than the 1.1 year shelf life of codeine phosphate reported earlier.

Storage conditions: Mainly the drug should be kept at room temperature between 68°F and 77°F (20°C and 25°C).

Different types of formulations with popular brand names: Codeine Sulfate, Nalex, Pentazine, Ambophen, Phenergan.

Hydromorphone

The 7, 8-double bond of morphine also is not required for analgesic activity as indicated by the relative analgesic potency of dihydromorphine. Also, oxidation of the 6-OH of dihydromorphine to yield hydromorphone further increases activity. Substitution of a 14-OH group on the hydromorphone structure as in oxymorphone produces a further increase in analgesic activity (RP = 10). Oxidation of the 6-OH of morphine directly as in morphone (without reduction of the 7, 8-double bond) does not significantly alter analgesic activity. Hydromorphone is available as the HCl salt in tablets, liquid, suppository and injectable.

Chemical name: (4R,4aR,7aR,12bS)-9-hydroxy-3-methyl-1,2,4,4a,5,6,7a,13-octahydro-4,12-methanobenzofuro[3,2-e]isoquinolin-7-one

Uses: This medication is used to help relieve moderate to severe pain. Hydromorphone belongs to a class of drugs known as opioid analgesics. It works in the brain to change how your body feels and responds to pain.

Stability: Hydromorphone hydrochloride is affected by light; although hydromorphone hydrochloride injection may develop a slight yellowish discoloration, this change apparently does not indicate loss of potency.

Chemical Structure

Storage conditions: Store in airtight containers at a temperature of 25 °C, excursions permitted between 15 and 30 °C. Protect from light.

Different types of formulations with popular brand names: Dilaudid, Exalgo, Hydrostat, Vicoprofen.

Oxymorphone

Oxymorphone is a semisynthetic narcotic analgesic related to hydromorphone and other opiates, Oxymorphone, hydroxy-dihydromorphinone, affects the central nervous system and smooth muscles by activation of specific opiate receptors. Similar to morphine, but more potent and without cough suppressant activity, it is used in treatment of moderate to severe pain, including obstetrical pain, or as an adjunct to anaesthesia.

Chemical name: (4R,4aS,7aR,12bS)-4a,9-dihydroxy-3-methyl-2,4,5,6,7a,13-hexahydro-1H-4,12-methanobenzofuro[3,2-e]isoquinolin-7-one

Chemical Structure

Uses: oxymorphone is used to relieve moderate to severe pain in people whose pain is not controlled with other medications. Oxymorphone is in a class of medications called opiate (narcotic) analgesics. It works by changing the way the body responds to pain.

Stability: oxycodone and its metabolites are stable in human plasma for up to 24 h at room temperature, for 460 days at −20°C and after three freeze–thaw cycles.

Storage conditions: Store it at room temperature (20°-25° C), and in an airtight container. Keep away from children.

Different types of formulations with popular brand names: Numorphan HCl, Opana, Opana ER

Meperidine

Meperidine (Pethidine). Meperidine is the most common substitute for morphine and is 10 times less potent than morphine. Meperidine belongs to phenylpiperidine group of synthetic opoids. Chemically it is 1-methyl-4-phenyl-4-piperidine carboxylate.

Meperidine is a synthetic piperidine ester with opioid analgesic activity. Meperidine mimics the actions of endogenous neuropeptides via opioid receptors, thereby producing the characteristic morphine-like effects on the mu-opioid receptor, including analgesia, euphoria, sedation, respiratory depression, miosis, bradycardia and physical dependence.

Chemical name: ethyl 1-methyl-4-phenylpiperidine-4-carboxylate

Chemical Structure

Uses: Meperidine is used to help relieve moderate to severe pain. It belongs to a class of drugs known as opioid analgesics and is similar to morphine. It works in the brain to change how your body feels and responds to pain. Meperidine should not be used to treat long-term or ongoing pain. It should only be used to treat sudden episodes of moderate to severe pain. See also Precautions section.This drug is not recommended for use in newborns due to an increased risk of serious side effects. Ask the doctor or pharmacist for details.

Stability: Pethidine hydrochloride injection 100 mg/mL was stable for at least 24 hours at room temperature when diluted to a concentration of 300 mg/L in glucose 5% and 4% and in sodium chloride injection (0.9%) and sodium chloride injection (0.9%) diluted 1 in 5.

Storage conditions: Meperidine hydrochloride preparations should be protected from light and stored at a temperature less than 40 °C; meperidine hydrochloride tablets should be stored at 15-30 °C and meperidine hydrochloride injections should be stored at 15-25 °C. Freezing of meperidine hydrochloride oral solutions or injections should be avoided. Meperidine hydrochloride oral solutions or tablets should be stored in tight or well-closed containers, respectively.

Different types of formulations with popular brand names: Demerol, Meperitab

Levorphanol

Levorphanol is a synthetic derivative of morphine with analgesic activities. Levorphanol mimics the actions of morphine, however, it is about 8 times more potent than morphine. This agent binds to opioid mu receptors, thereby producing analgesia, euphoria, sedation, respiratory depression, miosis, bradycardia, and physical dependence.

Chemical name: (1R,9R,10R)-17-methyl-17-azatetracyclo[7.5.3.01,10.02,7]heptadeca-2(7),3,5-trien-4-ol

Chemical Structure

Uses: Levorphanol Tartrate Tablets USP are indicated for the management of moderate to severe pain where an opioid analgesic is appropriate.

Stability: Stable under recommended storage conditions.

Storage conditions: Keep container tightly closed in a dry and well-ventilated place. Light sensitive. Keep in a dry place. Store at 20 deg to 25 °C (68 deg to 77 °F).

Different types of formulations with popular brand names: Levo-Dromoran

Methadone

Methadone is a synthetic opioid with analgesic activity. Methadone mimics the actions of endogenous peptides at CNS opioid receptors, primarily on the mu-receptor and has actions similar to those of morphine and morphine-like agents. The characteristic morphine-like effects include analgesia, euphoria, sedation, respiratory depression, miosis, bradycardia and physical dependence. However, the detoxification symptoms between morphine-like agents and methadone differ in that the onset of methadone's withdrawal symptoms is slower, the course is more prolonged and the symptoms are less severe.

Chemical name: (1R,9R,10R)-17-methyl-17-azatetracyclo[7.5.3.01,10.02,7]heptadeca-2(7),3,5-trien-4-ol

Chemical Structure

Uses: Levorphanol Tartrate Tablets USP are indicated for the management of moderate to severe pain where an opioid analgesic is appropriate.

Stability: Stable under recommended storage conditions.

Storage conditions: Keep container tightly closed in a dry and well-ventilated place. Light sensitive. Keep in a dry place. Store at 20 deg to 25 °C (68 deg to 77 °F).

Different types of formulations with popular brand names: Dolophine, Methadose, Methadose Sugar-Free, Diskets

Narcotic Antagonists

- **Nalmefene (Revex)** – Reverses the effects of narcotics; manages known or suspected narcotic overdose
- **Naloxone (Narcan)** – Reverses adverse effects of narcotics; diagnoses suspected acute narcotic overdose
- **Naltrexone (ReVia)** – Used orally in the management of alcohol or narcotic dependence

Nalmefene

Nalmefene is an opiate receptor antagonist which is used to treat acute opioid overdose and to help in the management of alcohol dependence and addictive behaviors. Nalmefene has not been linked to serum enzyme elevations during therapy or to clinically apparent liver injury.

Chemical name: (4R,4aS,7aS,12bS)-3-(cyclopropylmethyl)-7-methylidene-2,4,5,6,7a, 13-hexahydro-1H-4,12-methanobenzofuro[3,2-e]isoquinoline-4a,9-diol

Chemical Structure

Uses: Nalmefene is an opiate receptor antagonist which is used to treat acute opioid overdose and to help in the management of alcohol dependence and addictive behaviors.

Stability: Parenteral drug products should be inspected visually for particulate matter and discoloration prior to administration, whenever solution and container permit.

Storage conditions: Keep container tightly closed in a dry and well-ventilated place.

Different types of formulations with popular brand names: Revex, Selincro.

Naloxone

Naloxone is a thebaine derivate with competitive opioid antagonistic properties. Naloxone reverses the effects of opioid analgesics by binding to the opioid receptors in the CNS, and inhibiting the typical actions of opioid analgesics, including analgesia, euphoria, sedation, respiratory depression, miosis, bradycardia, and physical dependence. Naloxone binds to mu-opioid receptors with a high affinity, and a lesser degree to kappa- and gamma-opioid receptors in the CNS.

Chemical name: (4R,4aS,7aR,12bS)-4a,9-dihydroxy-3-prop-2-enyl-2,4,5,6,7a,13-hexahydro-1H-4,12-methanobenzofuro[3,2-e]isoquinolin-7-one

Chemical Structure

Uses: Naloxone is an opioid antagonist medication used to block or reverse the effects of opioid drugs, particularly within the setting of drug overdoses which are rapidly becoming a leading cause of death worldwide. More specifically, naloxone has a high affinity for μ-opioid receptors, where it acts as an inverse agonist, causing the rapid removal of any other drugs bound to these receptors. When taken in large quantities, opioid medications such as morphine, hydromorphone, methadone, heroin, or fentanyl are capable of causing life-threatening symptoms such as respiratory depression, reduced heart rate, slurred speech, drowsiness, and constricted pupils

Stability: Parenteral drug products should be inspected visually for particulate matter and discoloration prior to administration, whenever solution and container permit.

Storage conditions: Keep container tightly closed in a dry and well-ventilated place.

Different types of formulations with popular brand names: Bunavail, Evzio, Kloxxado, Narcan, Suboxone, Targin, Targiniq, Zubsolv.

Naltrexone

Naltrexone is a noroxymorphone derivative with competitive opioid antagonistic property. Naltrexone reverses the effects of opioid analgesics by binding to the various opioid receptors in the central nervous system, including the mu-, kappa- and gamma-opioid receptors. This leads to an inhibition of the typical actions of opioid analgesics, including analgesia, euphoria, sedation, respiratory depression, miosis, bradycardia, and physical dependence. Naltrexone is longer-acting and more potent compared to naloxone.

Chemical name: (4*R*,4*aS*,7*aR*,12*bS*)-3-(cyclopropylmethyl)-4*a*,9-dihydroxy-2,4,5,6,7*a*, 13-hexahydro-1*H*-4,12-methanobenzofuro[3,2-e]isoquinolin-7-one

Chemical Structure

Uses: Naltrexone blocks the effects of opioid medication, including pain relief or feelings of well-being that can lead to opioid abuse. An opioid is sometimes called a narcotic. Vivitrol is used as part of a treatment program for drug or alcohol dependence.

Stability: Stable under recommended storage conditions.

Storage conditions: Keep container tightly closed in a dry and well-ventilated place. Recommended storage temperature 2 - 8 °C. Light sensitive. Keep in a dry place.

Different types of formulations with popular brand names: Contrave, Embeda, Vivitrol

Aspirin*

Aspirin is an orally administered non-steroidal antiinflammatory agent. Acetylsalicylic acid binds to and acetylates serine residues in cyclooxygenases, resulting in decreased synthesis of prostaglandin, platelet aggregation, and inflammation. This agent exhibits analgesic, antipyretic, and anticoagulant properties.

Acetylsalicylic acid is an acetyl derivative of salicylic acid. It was introduced into medicine by Dreser in 1899. Acetyl salicylic acid (aspirin) can be prepared by the reaction between salicylic acid and acetic anhydride. In this reaction, the hydroxyl group on the benzene ring in salicylic acid reacts with acetic anhydride to form an ester funtional group. Thus, the formation of acetyl salicylic acid is referred to as an esterification reaction.

Chemical name: 2-Acetoxybenzoic acid,

Chemical Structure

Properties: Aspirin occurs as colorless crystals or powder. It is slightly soluble in water and soluble in alcohol, chloroform, ether and glycerin.

Uses: Aspirin is used to reduce fever and relieve mild to moderate pain from conditions such as muscle aches, toothaches, common cold, and headaches. It may also be used to reduce pain and swelling in conditions such as arthritis. Aspirin is known as a salicylate and a nonsteroidal anti-inflammatory drug (NSAID)

Stability: Slowly hydrolyzes in moist air. Has been involved in dust cloud explosions. Water insoluble. Solution in water is acid to methyl red indicator.

Storage conditions: Chewable aspirin tablets containing 81 mg of the drug should be stored in child-resistant containers holding not more than 36 tablets each in order to limit the potential toxicity associated with accidental ingestion in children. Aspirin suppositories should be stored at 2-15 °C.

Different types of formulations with popular brand names: Cotaspirin, Covasa, Aspitec, Delisprin, Loprin, Sprin, Zosprin, Ecoswyn, Ecosprin, Aspeeday

Diclofenac

Chemical name: 2-[2-(2,6-dichloroanilino)phenyl]acetic acid

Chemical Structure

Properties

Property	Value	Source
Melting point (°C)	283-285 °C	Not Available
Water solubility	2.37 mg/L (at 25 °C)	FINI,A ET AL. (1986)
logP	4.51	AVDEEF,A (1997)
pKa	4.15	SANGSTER (1994)

Uses: Diclofenac is a medicine that reduces swelling (inflammation) and pain. It's used to treat aches and pains, as well as problems with joints, muscles and bones. These include: rheumatoid arthritis and osteoarthritis.

Stability: Stored in a well closed container

Storage conditions: Diclofenac sodium delayed-release (enteric-coated) tablets, diclofenac sodium extended-release tablets, and diclofenac potassium tablets should be protected from moisture and stored in tight containers at a temperature not exceeding 30 °C. Commercially available diclofenac sodium and misoprostol tablets should be stored in a dry area at a temperature not exceeding 25 °C.

Diclofenac sodium 1% gel and diclofenac epolamine transdermal system should be stored at 25 °C but may be exposed to temperatures ranging from 15-30 °C. Diclofenac gel should not be frozen.

Different types of formulations with popular brand names: Zobid, Fenac, Eldofen, Diclonac, Dicloran, Voveran, Jonac, Diclohil, Dicloflam, Densaid

Ibuprofen*

Ibuprofen is a propionic acid derivate and nonsteroidal anti-inflammatory drug (NSAID) with anti-inflammatory, analgesic, and antipyretic effects. Ibuprofen inhibits the activity of cyclo-oxygenase I and II, resulting in a decreased formation of precursors of prostaglandins and thromboxanes. This leads to decreased prostaglandin synthesis, by prostaglandin synthase, the main physiologic effect of ibuprofen. Ibuprofen also causes a decrease in the formation of thromboxane A2 synthesis, by thromboxane synthase, thereby inhibiting platelet aggregation. (NCI05).

Chemical name: 2-[4-(2-methylpropyl)phenyl]propanoic acid

Chemical Structure

Uses: Ibuprofen is an everyday painkiller for a range of aches and pains, including back pain, period pain, toothache. It also treats inflammation such as strains and sprains, and pain from arthritis. It's available as tablets and capsules, and as a syrup that you swallow.

Stability: Undiluted ibuprofen (5 mg/mL) stored in glass vials and ibuprofen diluted to 2.5 mg/mL with either NS or D5W and stored in polypropylene syringes will retain more than 92% of its initial concentration with storage for up to 14 days at 4°C.

Storage conditions: Keep out of reach and sight of children.

Store ibuprofen at room temperature away from heat, sunlight, and moisture.

Do not store in the bathroom or toilets.

Keep refrigerated after opening (Suspension).

Different types of formulations with popular brand names: Brufen, Alfam, Ibuwin, Dolocyl, Myofen, Bruriff, Fenlong, Norswel, Icparil, Ibutas

Piroxicam

Piroxicam is a nonsteroidal oxicam derivative with anti-inflammatory, antipyretic and analgesic properties. As a non-selective, nonsteroidal anti-inflammatory drug (NSAID), piroxicam binds and chelates both isoforms of cyclooxygenases (COX1 and COX2), thereby stalling phospholipase A2 activity and conversion of arachidonic acid into prostaglandin precursors at the rate limiting cyclooxygenase enzyme step. This results in inhibition of prostaglandin biosynthesis. As a second, independent effect, piroxicam inhibits the activation of neutrophils thereby contributing to its overall anti-inflammatory effects.

Chemical name: 4-hydroxy-2-methyl-1,1-dioxo-N-pyridin-2-yl-1λ6,2-benzothiazine-3-carboxamide

Chemical Structure

Uses: Piroxicam is used to relieve pain, tenderness, swelling, and stiffness caused by osteoarthritis (arthritis caused by a breakdown of the lining of the joints) and rheumatoid arthritis (arthritis caused by swelling of the lining of the joints). Piroxicam is in a class of medications called NSAIDs.

Stability: Photochemical degradation of piroxicam solution at pH 2.0 (maximum degradation) showed absorption maxima at 242 and 356 nm.

Storage conditions:
- Store below 25°C in a dry place.
- Protect from light.
- Store this drug at a temperature between 59°F and 86°F (15°C and 30°C).

Different types of formulations with popular brand names: Doloforce, Piricam, Pirox, Doloxicam, Greatin, Feloxigen, Inflavan, Pinij, Dolcare, Pironat

Celecoxib

- Celecoxib is a nonsteroidal anti-inflammatory drug (NSAID) with a diaryl-substituted pyrazole structure. Celecoxib selectively inhibits cyclo-oxygenase-2 activity (COX-2); COX-2 inhibition may result in apoptosis and a reduction in tumor angiogenesis and metastasis.
- **Chemical name:** 4-[5-(4-methylphenyl)-3-(trifluoromethyl)pyrazol-1-yl]benzene-sulfonamide

Chemical Structure

Uses: Celecoxib is used to relieve pain, tenderness, swelling and stiffness caused by osteoarthritis (arthritis caused by a breakdown of the lining of the joints), rheumatoid arthritis (arthritis caused by swelling of the lining of the joints), and ankylosing spondylitis (arthritis that mainly affects the spine).

Stability:

- Store at room temperature away from light and moisture.
- Do not store in the bathroom.
- Keep all medications away from children and pet.

Storage conditions: Keep container tightly closed in a dry and well-ventilated place. Store at room temperature 20 °C to 25 °C (68 °F to 77 °F); excursions permitted between 15 °C to 30 °C (59 °F to 86 °F).

Different types of formulations with popular brand names: Sionara, Revibra, Coxigen, Zycel, Celeheal, Cobix, Celebrex, Colcibra, Cril, Celcib

Mefenamic Acid

Mefenamic acid is an NSAID used to treat mild to moderate pain for no more than a week, and primary dysmenorrhea. Mefenamic acid binds the prostaglandin synthetase receptors COX-1 and COX-2, inhibiting the action of prostaglandin synthetase. As these receptors have a role as a major mediator of inflammation and/or a role for prostanoid signaling in activity-dependent plasticity, the symptoms of pain are temporarily reduced.

Chemical name: 2-(2,3-dimethylanilino)benzoic acid

Chemical Structure

Uses: Mefenamic acid is a fenamate nonsteroidal anti-inflammatory (NSAI) drug, which is used for several years for pain management. However, it has been rarely reported that, mefenamic acid can induce central nervous system toxicity both in toxic doses and therapeutic usage.

Stability: Darkens on prolonged exposure to light, It is stable at 25 °C, 37 °C and 45 °C.

Storage conditions: Store mefenamic acid at room temperature between 68°F and 77°F (20°C and 25°C).

Don't store this medication in moist or damp areas, such as bathrooms.

Different types of formulations with popular brand names: Meftal, Mictal, Lymef, Mefnir, Geftal, Mefalgin, Mefzen, Nefmic, Mefdol Forte, Azispas

Paracetamol*

Acetaminophen is a p-aminophenol derivative with analgesic and antipyretic activities. Although the exact mechanism through which acetaminophen exert its effects has yet to be fully determined, acetaminophen may inhibit the nitric oxide (NO) pathway mediated by a variety of neurotransmitter receptors including N-methyl-D-aspartate (NMDA) and substance P, resulting in elevation of the pain threshold. The antipyretic activity may result from inhibition of prostaglandin synthesis and release in the central nervous system (CNS) and prostaglandin-mediated effects on the heat-regulating center in the anterior hypothalamus.

Chemical name: N-(4-hydroxyphenyl)acetamide

Chemical Structure

Uses: Paracetamol is a common painkiller used to treat aches and pain. It can also be used to reduce a high temperature. It's available combined with other painkillers and anti-sickness medicines. It's also an ingredient in a wide range of cold and flu remedies.

Stability: Stable under recommended storage conditions.

Storage conditions: Store in well closed air tight light resistant container.

Different types of formulations with popular brand names: Dolopar, Metamol, Macfast, Malidens, Calpol, Fepanil, Febrex, Munpal, Crocin, Algina

Aceclofenac

Aceclofenac is a monocarboxylic acid that is the carboxymethyl ester of diclofenac. A non-steroidal anti-inflammatory drug related to diclofenac, it is used in the management of osteoarthritis, rheumatoid arthritis, and ankylosing spondylitis. It has a role as an EC 1.14.99.1 (prostaglandin-endoperoxide synthase) inhibitor, a non-steroidal anti-inflammatory drug and a non-narcotic analgesic. It is a monocarboxylic acid, a carboxylic ester, a secondary amino compound, an amino acid and a dichlorobenzene. It derives from a diclofenac.

Chemical name: 2-[2-[2-(2,6-dichloroanilino)phenyl]acetyl]oxyacetic acid

Chemical Structure

Uses: Paracetamol is a common painkiller used to treat aches and pain. It can also be used to reduce a high temperature. It's available combined with other painkillers and anti-sickness medicines. It's also an ingredient in a wide range of cold and flu remedies.

Stability: Stable under recommended storage conditions.

Storage conditions: Store in well closed air tight light resistant container.

Different types of formulations with popular brand names: Acebloc tab, Aceclofenac, Aceclofenac.

Multiple Choice Questions

1. Agents that often cause vasoconstriction include all of the following except
   (a) Angiotensin II
   (b) Methysergide
   (c) PGF2a
   (d) Prostacyclin
   (e) Thromboxane

2. Which of the following is a reversible inhibitor of platelet cyclooxygenase?
   (a) Alprostadil
   (b) Aspirin
   (c) Ibuprofen
   (d) LTC4
   (e) Misoprostol

3. Vasodilation by prostaglandins involves
   (a) Arterioles
   (b) Precapillary sphincters
   (c) Postcapillary venules
   (d) All of the above

4. Fentanyl transdermal patches have been used postoperatively to provide transdermal analgesia. The most dangerous adverse effect of this mode of administration is
   (a) Cutaneous reactions
   (b) Diarrhea
   (c) Hypertension
   (d) Relaxation of skeletal muscle
   (e) Respiratory depression

5. Following is an example of paraaminophenol NSAID
   (a) Diclofenac
   (b) Acetaminophen
   (c) Piroxicam
   (d) Celecoxib

6. Which one of the following effects does not occur in salicylate intoxication ?
   (a) Hyperventilation
   (b) Hypothemia
   (c) Metabolic acidosis
   (d) Respiratory alkalosis
   (e) Tinnitus

7. Which one of the following drugs is not useful in dysmenorrhea?
   (a) Aspirin
   (b) Colchicine
   (c) Ibuprofen
   (d) Rofecoxib
   (e) Naproxen

8. Following is an example of preformed and not lipid derived mast cell mediator of inflammatory process
   (a) LTC4
   (b) PGD2
   (c) PAF
   (d) Histamine

9. A drug that decreases blood pressure and has analgesic and spasmolytic effects when given intrathecally is
   - (a) Atenolol
   - (b) Clonidine
   - (c) Morphine
   - (d) Nitroprusside
   - (e) Prazosin

10. Diamprit is an agonist of _______ receptors, except
    - (a) H1
    - (b) H2
    - (c) H3
    - (d) All of the above

CHAPTER 11

Anti-Infective Agents

Introduction

The chapter aims at providing the latest and pharmacopoeial information regarding some Anti-infective agents (Amphotericin-B and Griseofulvin, Econoazole nitrate, Miconazole, Ketoconazole, Itraconazole, Fluconazole, Naftifine hydrochloride, Tolnaftate, Nalidixic Acid, Cinoxacin, Norfloxacin, Ciprofloxacin, Ofloxacin, Lomefloxacin, Sparfloxacin, Isoniazid, Ethionamide, ethambutol, Pyrazinamide, Para amino salicylic acid, Rifampicin, Amantadine hydrochloride, Idoxuridine, Acyclovir, Gancyclovir, Foscarnet, Zidovudine, Lamivudine, Ribavirin, Quinine sulphate, Chloroquine phosphate, Primaquine phosphate, Quinacrine hydrochloride, Mefloquine, Cycloguanil, Proguanil, Pyrimethamine, Sulfanilamide, Sulfadiazine, Sulfamethoxazole, Sulfacetamide, Mefenide acetate and Cotrimoxazole) regarding their classification, chemical name, chemical structure, uses, stability, storage conditions, different types of formulations, and popular brand names.

Antifungal Agents

Human-fungi-parasitic relationship result in mycotic illnesses. Most fungal infections (mycoses) involve superficial invasion of the skin or mucous membrane of the body orifices. These diseases can usually be controlled by local application of the antifungal agents. Fungi have different shapes and sizes. Some are large while others are minute, parasitic, and saprophytic cells. They differ from the following organisms in some important aspects:

- Algae by lack of photosynthetic ability.
- Protozoa by the lack of motility, possession of chitinuous cell wall, and ease of culture on simple media.
- Bacteria by greater size and having certain intracellular structure such as mitochondria and nuclear membrane

Classification

The antifungal agents can be divided into the following classes, based on their chemical structure, mechanism of action, and source:

I. **Antibiotics:** Amphotericin B, Nystatin, Griseofulvin

II. **Azoles** (imidazole, triazole derivates)

   Triazoles - Fluconazole, Itraconzole, Terconazole

   Imidazoles - Clotrimazole, Ketoconazole, Miconazole, Bifonazole, Butoconazole, and Zinoconazole

III. **Fluorinated pyrimidines:** Flucytosine

IV. **Chitin synthetase inhibitors:** Nikomycin Z

V. **Peptides/proteins:** Cispentacin

VI. **Miscellaneous:** Ciclopirox, Tolnaftate, Naftifine, and Terbinafine

Amphotericin-B

Classification: Antifungal antibiotic

Chemical Name: (1R,3S,5R,6R,9R,11R,15S,16R,17R,18S,19E,21E,23E,25E,27E,29E, 31E,33R,35S,36R,37S)-33-[(2R,3S,4S,5S,6R)-4-amino-3,5-dihydroxy-6-methyloxan-2-yl]oxy-1,3,5,6,9,11,17,37-octahydroxy-15,16,18-trimethyl-13-oxo-14,39-dioxabicyclo[33.3.1]nonatriaconta-19,21,23,25,27,29,31-heptaene-36-carboxylic acid

Chemical Structure:

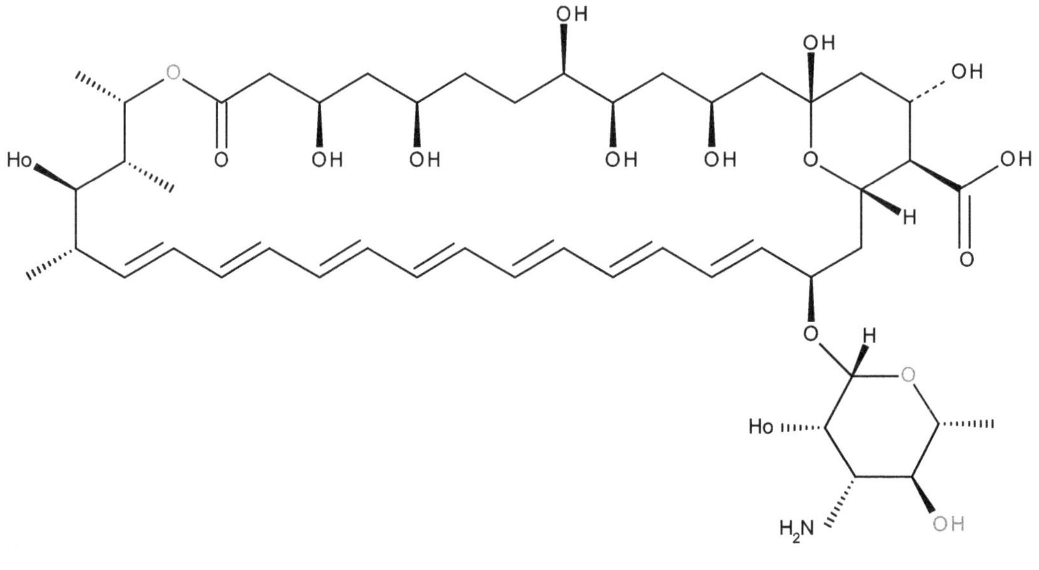

Uses

- Used to treat potentially life threatening fungal infections.

Stability

- Prior to reconstitution Amphotericin B Intravenous should be stored in the refrigerator, protected against exposure to light.
- The reconstituted solution may be stored in the dark, at room temperature for 24 hours, or at refrigerator temperatures for 1 week with minimal loss of potency and clarity.

Storage Conditions

- Keep the container tightly closed under an inert atmosphere, and store under refrigerated temperatures.
- Protect this chemical from exposure to light.

Different types of Formulations:

- Powder for solution
- Powder for suspension
- Lyophilized
- Injection
- Powder

Popular brand names: Ambisone, Amfocare, Amphotin, Abhope, Fungizone, Amphocrit, Amphogard, Amphomul, Amphoject, Mycoflu

Griseofulvin

Classification: Antifungal

Chemical Name: (2*S*,5'*R*)-7-chloro-3',4,6-trimethoxy-5'-methylspiro[1-benzofuran-2,4'-cyclohex-2-ene]-1',3-dione

Chemical Structure

Uses

- For the treatment of ringworm infections of the skin, hair, and nails, namely: tinea corporis, tinea pedis, tinea cruris, tinea barbae, cradle cap or other conditions caused by *Trichophyton* or *Microsporum* fungi.

Stability
- Keep away from oxidizing materials.

Storage Conditions
- Store this drug under ambient temperatures.
- Griseofulvin preparation should generally be stored at a temperature less than 40°C, preferably between 15-30°C.
- Microsize griseofulvin oral suspension should be protected from freezing and stored in light-resistant containers.

Different types of Formulations
- Tablet, film coated
- Suspension

Popular brand names: Rimask, Grisofit, Grisomed, Grisof, Grisonus, Grisure, Cytofulvin, Grisken, Fulvinem, Amigris

Econazole Nitrate

Classification: Topical antifungal

Chemical Name: 1-[2-[(4-chlorophenyl)methoxy]-2-(2,4-dichlorophenyl)ethyl]imidazole

Chemical Structure

Uses
- For topical application in the treatment of tinea pedis, tinea cruris, and tinea corporis caused by Trichophyton rubrum, Trichophyton mentagrophytes, Trichophyton tonsurans, Microsporum canis, Microsporum audouini, Microsporum gypseum, and Epidermophyton floccosum, in the treatment of cutaneous candidiasis, and in the treatment of tinea versicolor.

Stability
- Econazole topical foam is flammable. Avoid heat, flame, and smoking during and immediately following application.

- Do not expose containers to heat and/or store at temperatures above 120°F (49°C) even when empty.

Storage Conditions

- Store at controlled room temperature 20°C to 25°C (68°F to 77°F) with excursions permitted between 15°C and 30°C (59°F and 86°F).
- Do not store in direct sunlight.
- Do not refrigerate or freeze.

Different types of Formulations

- Tablet, film coated
- Suspension

Popular brand names: Spectazole, Ecanol, Aurozole, Cucon G

Miconazole

Classification: Antifungal

Chemical Name: 1-[2-(2,4-dichlorophenyl)-2-[(2,4-dichlorophenyl)methoxy]ethyl] imidazole

Chemical Structure

Uses

- Miconazole is indicated for the local treatment of oropharyngeal candidiasis in adult patients and for the adjunctive treatment of diaper dermatitis complicated by candidiasis in immunocompetent patients aged four weeks and older.
- Miconazole is available as both a suppository and cream for the treatment of vaginal yeast infections and the relief of associated vulvar itching and irritation. Lastly, miconazole cream is effective in treating athlete's foot (tinea pedis), jock itch (tinea cruris), ringworm infections (tinea corporis), pityriasis (formerly tinea) versicolor, and cutaneous candidiasis.

Stability

- Protect the tablets from moisture.

Storage Conditions

- Store miconazole tablets at room temperature, 68°F to 77°F (20°C to 25°C).
- Store miconazole vaginal suppositories at 59°F to 86°F (15°C to 30°C).
- Store it in room temperature and keep away from children.

Different types of Formulations

- Tablet
- Cream
- Suppository

Popular brand names: Condiderm, Hitrimazole, Micowyn, Fungitop, Fungirex, Conzole, Fungiguard, Clobital, Micasulf, Micogel

Ketoconazole

Classification: Azole antifungals

Chemical Name: 1-[4-[4-[[(2*R*,4*S*)-2-(2,4-dichlorophenyl)-2-(imidazol-1-ylmethyl)-1,3-dioxolan-4-yl]methoxy]phenyl]piperazin-1-yl]ethanone

Chemical Structure

Uses

- Ketoconazole is used in the treatment or prevention of fungal infections including blastomycosis, candidiasis, coccidioidomycosis, histoplasmosis, chromomycosis, and paracoccidioidomycosis.
- In Europe, it is also used in the treatment of endogenous Cushing's syndrome.

Stability

- Provision to contain effluent from fire extinguishing. Well closed. Separated from food and feedstuffs. Store in an area without drain or sewer access.

Storage Conditions

- Store at controlled room temperature 15°C - 25 °C (59°F - 77°F).
- Protect from moisture.
- Ketoconazole topical cream should be stored at a temperature less than 25°C and should not be frozen. The cream should not be stored at high temperatures (e.g., warmer than 37 °C), since creams generally separate at these temperatures.
- Ketoconazole 2% shampoo should be stored at temperatures not exceeding 25°C and should be protected from light; the 1% shampoo should be stored between 2°C-30°C and should be protected from light and freezing.

Different types of Formulations

- Tablet
- Aerosol
- Cream
- Shampoo

Popular brand names: Nizral, Ketomac, Kevon, Ketafung, Exizol, Soluken, Ketocip, Belzole, Sebandro, Arcolane

Itraconazole

Classification: Azole antifungals

Chemical Name: 2-butan-2-yl-4-[4-[4-[4-[[(2R,4S)-2-(2,4-dichlorophenyl)-2-(1,2,4-triazol-1-ylmethyl)-1,3-dioxolan-4-yl]methoxy]phenyl]piperazin-1-yl]phenyl]-1,2,4-triazol-3-one

Chemical Structure

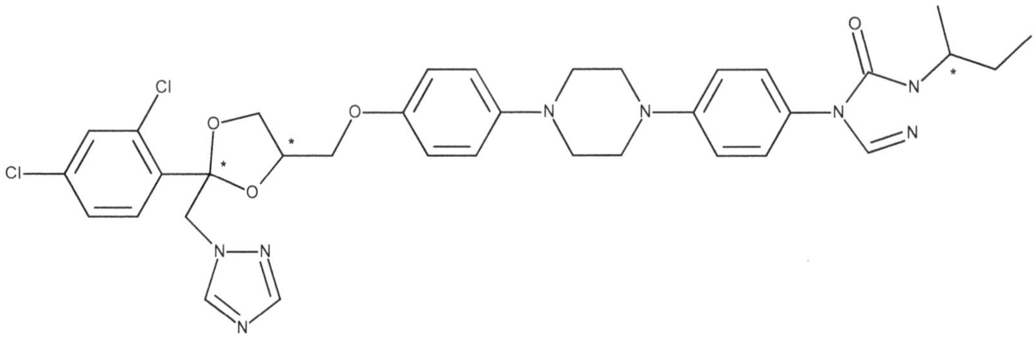

Uses
- For the treatment of the following fungal infections in immunocompromised and non-immunocompromised patients: pulmonary and extrapulmonary blastomycosis, histoplasmosis, aspergillosis, and onychomycosis.

Stability
- The injection should be protected from light during storage, but may be exposed to normal room light during administration.

Storage Conditions
- Itraconazole capsules should be stored at a controlled room temperature of 15-25°C and protected from light and moisture.
- Itraconazole oral solution should be stored at 25°C or lower and should not be frozen.
- Commercially available itraconazole injection should be stored at 25°C or lower and protected from light; freezing should be avoided. Following dilution of itraconazole injection in the 0.9% sodium chloride injection diluent supplied by the manufacturer, itraconazole injections may be stored at 2-8 deg or 15-25 °C for up to 48 hours.

Different types of Formulations
- Tablet
- Capsule
- Solution
- Coated pellets

Popular brand names: Itrawyn, Eukarit, Clobitra, Ceastra, Canzap, Apexitra, Itapro, Itracoe, Itratuf, Itrazole

Fluconazole

Classification: Triazole antifungals

Chemical Name: 2-(2,4-difluorophenyl)-1,3-bis(1,2,4-triazol-1-yl)propan-2-ol

Chemical Structure

Uses: Fluconazole can be administered in the treatment of the following fungal infections:

1. Vaginal yeast infections caused by Candida
2. Systemic Candida infections
3. Both esophageal and oropharyngeal candidiasis
4. Cryptococcal meningitis
5. UTI (urinary tract infection) by Candida
6. Peritonitis (inflammation of the peritoneum) caused by Candida

Fungal Infection Prophylaxis

Patients receiving bone marrow transplantation who are treated with cytotoxic chemotherapy and/or radiation therapy may be predisposed to candida infections, and may receive fluconazole as prophylactic therapy.

Stability

- Fluconazole 2 mg/mL is stable in potassium chloride plus 5% dextrose injection and in theophylline plus 5% dextrose injection for 72 hours.
- Fluconazole is stable in the other injectable solutions for 24 hours.

Storage Conditions

- Fluconazole tablets should be stored in tight containers at a temperature less than 30°C.

- Fluconazole powder for oral suspension should be stored at a temperature less than 30°C.

Different types of Formulations

- Tablet
- Powder for suspension
- Solution

Popular brand names: Nixican, Nuforce, Fumycin, Conflu, Fusys, Gocan, Fluconex, Flutican, Flutas, Fluclox

Naftifine Hydrochloride

Classification: Allylamine Antifungal

Chemical Name: (*E*)-*N*-methyl-*N*-(naphthalen-1-ylmethyl)-3-phenylprop-2-en-1-amine

Chemical Structure

Uses:

- For the topical treatment of tinea pedis, tinea cruris, and tinea corporis caused by the organisms *Trichophyton rubrum, Trichophyton mentagrophytes, Trichophyton tonsurans* and *Epidermophyton floccosum*.

Stability

- Cream is stable for 24 months after the date of manufacture.

Storage Conditions

- Store Cream / Gel at 25°C (77°F); excursions permitted to 15-30°C (59-86°F).

Different types of Formulations

- Cream
- Gel

Popular brand names

- Sporofine

Tolnaftate

Classification: Antifungal

Chemical Name: *O*-naphthalen-2-yl *N*-methyl-*N*-(3-methylphenyl)carbamothioate

Chemical Structure

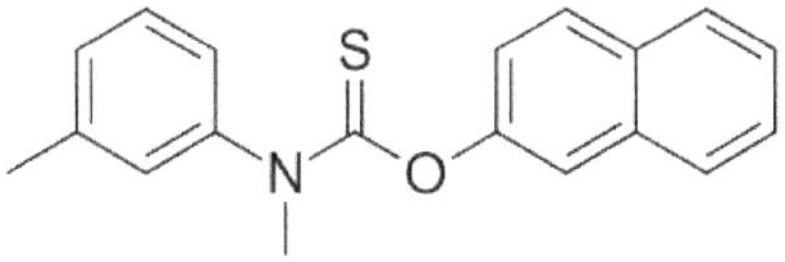

Uses

- Tolnaftate topical is used to treat skin infections such as athlete's foot, jock itch, and ringworm infections.
- Tolnaftate is also used, along with other antifungals, to treat infections of the nails, scalp, palms, and soles of the feet.
- The powder and powder aerosol may be used to prevent athlete's foot.

Stability

- Reconstituted solutions are stable at room temperature for 12 hours (6 to 12 hours in 5% dextrose in water).

Storage Conditions

- Keep container tightly closed in a dry and well-ventilated place at recommended temperature at 2-8°C.
- Avoid freezing.

Different types of Formulations: Powder, Liquid, Cream, Solution, Spray, Tincture, Aerosol, Soap, Oil, Cream, Injection

Popular brand names: Naftate, Tinaderm, Tinavate, Tinaderm, Tigboderm, Mycopar, Begent, Quiss, Novaderm, Dermitop

Urinary Tract Anti-infective Agents

Urinary anti-infectives are drugs that are used to prevent or treat urinary tract infections. There are several classes of antibacterial agents in this category and they have different mechanisms of action. However, majority of these drugs tend to have high concentration in the urine and therefore are ideal to treat urinary tract infections, or used as prophylaxis for urinary tract infections.

Classification

1. **Quinolones:** Nalidixic acid, Norfloxacin, Enoxacin, Ciprofloxacin, Ofloxacin, Lomefloxacin, Sparfloxacin, Gatifloxacin, Moxifloxacin.
2. **Nitrofurans:** Furazolidine, Nitrofurantoin
3. **Methanamine and its salts:** methanamine, Methenamine mandelate and hippurate

Nalidixic Acid

Classification: Anti-Bacterial Agents

Chemical Name: 1-ethyl-7-methyl-4-oxo-1,8-naphthyridine-3-carboxylic acid

Chemical Structure

Uses
- For the treatment of urinary tract infections caused by susceptible gram-negative microorganisms, including the majority of *E. coli*, *Enterobacter* species, *Klebsiella* species, and *Proteus* species.

Stability
- Nalidixic acid is stable enough to withstand boiling or autoclaving.

Storage Conditions
- Nalidixic acid tablets and oral suspension should be stored in tight containers at a temperature less than 40°C, preferably between 15°C-30°C.
- Freezing of the suspension should be avoided.

Different types of Formulations
- Tablet

Popular brand names: Negadix, Gramoneg, Ordixic

Cinoxacin

Classification: Topoisomerase II Inhibitors

Chemical Name: 1-ethyl-4-oxo-[1,3]dioxolo[4,5-g]cinnoline-3-carboxylic acid

Chemical Structure

Uses

- For the treatment of initial and recurrent urinary tract infections in adults caused by the following susceptible microorganisms: *Escherichia coli*, *Proteus mirabilis*, *Proteus vulgaris*, *Klebsiella* species (including *K. pneumoniae*), and *Enterobacter* species.

Stability

- Degradation results from light. Prevent it from direct sunlight.

Storage Conditions

- Store at controlled room temperature, 59° to 86° F (15°C to 30°C).
- Store in a well closed container, below 40°C.
- Protect from Sunlight and Moisture.

Different types of Formulations: Tablet, Capsule

Popular brand names: Cinobac

Norfloxacin

Classification: Topoisomerase II Inhibitors

Chemical Name: 1-ethyl-6-fluoro-4-oxo-7-piperazin-1-ylquinoline-3-carboxylic acid

Chemical Structure

Uses

- Norfloxacin is a broad-spectrum fluoroquinolone antibiotic with variable activity against gram-positive and gram-negative bacteria.
- Typically reserved for the treatment of UTIs due to accumulation in the urine.

Stability: Norfloxacin is most stable at acidic and basic pH, in darkness, in the absence of oxygen and at low temperature.

Storage Conditions: Store norfloxacin tablets between temperatures of 15°C - 30°C (59°F - 86°F), in a tightly closed container.

Different types of Formulations

- Tablet, film coated
- Solution

Popular brand names: Norflox, Biofloxin, Norbid, Floxnor, Norflokem, Emnorcin, Enflox, Bruflox, Embenor, Norilet

Ciprofloxacin

Classification: Topoisomerase II Inhibitors

Chemical Name: 1-cyclopropyl-6-fluoro-4-oxo-7-piperazin-1-ylquinoline-3-carboxylic acid

Chemical Structure

Uses

- Ciprofloxacin is only indicated in infections caused by susceptible bacteria.
- Ciprofloxacin immediate release tablets, oral suspensions, and intravenous injections are indicated for the treatment of skin and skin structure infections, bone and joint infections, complicated intra-abdominal infections, nosocomial pneumonia, febrile neutropenia, adults who have inhaled anthrax, plague, chronic bacterial prostatitis, lower respiratory tract infections including acute exacerbations of chronic bronchitis, urinary tract infections, complicated urinary tract infections in pediatrics, complicated pyelonephritis in pediatrics, and acute sinusitis.

- A ciprofloxacin otic solution and otic suspension with hydrocortisone are indicated for acute otitis externa.
- Ciprofloxacin suspension with dexamethasone is indicated for acute otitis media in pediatric patients with tympanostomy tubes or acute otitis externa.
- A ciprofloxacin eye drop is indicated for bacterial corneal ulcers and conjunctivitis.

Stability: Stable at concentration of 0.5-2 mg/mL in distilled water or normal saline for 14 days at room temperature.

Storage Conditions

- Store the tablets and extended-release tablets at room temperature and away from excess heat and moisture (not in the bathroom).
- Store the suspension in the refrigerator or at room temperature, closed tightly, for up to 14 days.
- Do not freeze ciprofloxacin suspension.

Different types of Formulations: Tablet (film coated), Solution, Ointment, Drops, Kit, Liquid, Suspension

Popular brand names: Baycip, Cebran, Cifran, Ciplox, Zoxan, Alquin, Alcipro, Floxip, Ciprobid, Ciprolet

Ofloxacin

Classification: Anti-Bacterial Agents

Chemical Name: 7-fluoro-2-methyl-6-(4-methylpiperazin-1-yl)-10-oxo-4-oxa-1-azatricyclo $[7.3.1.0^{5,13}]$trideca-5(13),6,8,11-tetraene-11-carboxylic acid

Chemical Structure

Uses: For the treatment of infections (respiratory tract, kidney, skin, soft tissue, UTI), urethral and cervical gonorrhoea.

Stability: An injectable formulation of ofloxacin was stable for at least 3 days at 24°C, 14 days at 5°C, and 26 weeks at -20°C.

Storage Conditions

- Store the medicine in a closed container at room temperature, away from heat, moisture, and direct light.
- Store at room temperature between 59-77°F (15-25°C) away from light and moisture.
- Do not store in the bathroom.

Different types of Formulations

- Tablet, coated
- Solution
- Drops

Popular brand names: Oflorite, Oflin, Ofler, Oxanic, Oflox, Flodal, Ojen, Flith, Tarivid, Ronflox

Lomefloxacin

Classification: Topoisomerase II Inhibitors

Chemical Name: 1-ethyl-6,8-difluoro-7-(3-methylpiperazin-1-yl)-4-oxoquinoline-3-carboxylic acid

Chemical Structure

Uses

- For the treatment of bacterial infections of the respiratory tract (chronic bronchitis) and urinary tract, and as a pre-operative prophylactic to prevent urinary tract infection caused by: *S.pneumoniae, H.influenzae, S.aureus, P.aeruginosa, E. cloacae, P. mirabilis, C. civersus, S. asprphyticus, E.coli,* and *K.pneumoniae.*

Stability: Lomefloxacin has a shelf-life of 60 months.

Storage Conditions
- Keep this medication in the container it came in, tightly closed, and out of reach of children.
- Store at 59° to 77°F (15° to 25°C), protect from sunlight and heat.

Different types of Formulations: Tablet, film coated

Popular brand names: Lomitas, Maxalom, Hilome, Soloflox, Lomaday, Qumax, Vivo, Floxaday, Lom Eye

Sparfloxacin

Classification: Topoisomerase II Inhibitors

Chemical Name: 5-amino-1-cyclopropyl-7-[(3*R*,5*S*)-3,5-dimethylpiperazin-1-yl]-6,8-difluoro-4-oxoquinoline-3-carboxylic acid

Chemical Structure

Uses
- For the treatment of adults with the following infections caused by susceptible strains microorganisms: community-acquired pneumonia (caused by *Chlamydia pneumoniae, Haemophilus influenzae, Haemophilus parainfluenzae, Moraxella catarrhalis, Mycoplasma pneumoniae,* or *Streptococcus pneumoniae*) and acute bacterial exacerbations of chronic bronchitis (caused by *Chlamydia pneumoniae, Enterobacter cloacae, Haemophilus influenzae, Haemophilus parainfluenzae, Klebsiella pneumoniae, Moraxella catarrhalis, Staphylococcus aureus,* or *Streptococcus pneumoniae*).

Stability: Degradation results from light. Prevent it from direct sunlight.

Storage Conditions
- Store it at controlled room temperature (20 to 25°C).
- Store the medicine in a closed container at room temperature, away from heat and direct sunlight.

Different types of Formulations: Tablet, Capsule, Cream, Ointment, Gel, Cream, Liquid, Injection

Popular brand names: Zospar, Bluspar, Sparit, Floxy, Novospar, Alaska, Rexpar, Sparta, Sparnole, Sparit

Anti-tubercular Agents

Tuberculosis is the most prevalent infectious disease worldwide and a leading killer caused by a single infectious agent, that is, Mycobacterium tuberculosis. According to World Health Organization (WHO) report, M. tuberculosis, currently infects over 2 billion people worldwide, with 30 million new cases reported every year. This intracellular infection accounts for at least 3 million deaths annually. Common infection sites of the tuberculosis are lungs (primary site), brain, bone, liver, and kidney. The main symptoms are cough, tachycardia, cyanosis, and respiratory failure. Depending upon the site of infection, the disease can be categorized as follows:

- Pulmonary tuberculosis (respiratory tract).
- Genitourinary tuberculosis (genitourinary tract).
- Tuberculous meningitis (nervous system).
- Miliary tuberculosis (a widespread infection).

Drugs used in the treatment of tuberculosis can be divided into two major categories:

1. **First-line drugs:** Isoniazid, streptomycin, rifampicin, ethambutol, and pyrazinamide.
2. **Second-line drugs:** Ethionamide, p-amino salicylic acid, ofloxacin, ciprofloxacin, cycloserine, amikacin, kanamycin, viomycin, and capreomycin.

Isoniazid

Classification: Antitubercular Agents

Chemical Name: pyridine-4-carbohydrazide

Chemical Structure

Uses

- Isoniazid is an antibiotic used to treat mycobacterial infections; most commonly use in combination with other antimycobacterial agents for the treatment of active or latent tuberculosis.

Stability

- Isoniazid is generally considered to be a relatively stable compound.
- Isoniazid injection is less stable in 5% dextrose injection, especially at a concentration of 0.5 mg/mL at room temperature.

Storage Conditions

- Store isoniazid oral solution at room temperature, 68°F to 77°F (20°C to 25°C).
- Store isoniazid tablets at 68°F to 77°F (20°C to 25°C) and protect them from moisture and light.
- Keep isoniazid in the container that it came in and keep the container tightly closed.

Different types of Formulations

- Tablet
- Powder
- Syrup

Popular brand names: Docina, Macox, Mycocox, Rinizide, Binex, Arzade, Rifadin, Monto, Acrifa, Antex

Ethionamide

Classification: Antitubercular Agents

Chemical Name: 2-ethylpyridine-4-carbothioamide

Chemical Structure

Uses

- For use in the treatment of pulmonary and extrapulmonary tuberculosis when other antitubercular drugs have failed.

Stability

- It is quite stable at all ordinary temperatures and levels of humidity.

Storage Conditions

- Store at room temperature between 68-77°F (20-25°C) away from light and moisture.
- Do not store in the bathroom. Keep all medicines away from children and pets.

- Do not flush medications down the toilet or pour them into a drain unless instructed to do so.

Different types of Formulations
- Tablet, film coated

Popular brand names: Ethide, Thiomid, Ethimax, Zonamide, Ethio, Ethiobin, Mycotuf, Etamid, Ethiocid, Sitromide

Ethambutol

Classification: Antitubercular Agents

Chemical Name: (2S)-2-[2-[[(2S)-1-hydroxybutan-2-yl]amino]ethylamino]butan-1-ol

Chemical Structure

Uses
- Ethambutol is indicated in combination with other anti-tuberculosis drugs in the treatment of pulmonary tuberculosis.
- Ethambutol is commonly used in combination with isoniazid, rifampin, and pyrazinamide.

Stability
- It is hygroscopic when exposed to high relative humidity.

Storage Conditions
- Ethambutol hydrochloride should be preserved in a well-closed container, and it is stable in both light and heat.
- Store at room temperature between 68-77°F (20-25°C) away from light and moisture. Do not store in the bathroom.
- Keep all medicines away from children and pets.
- Do not flush medications down the toilet or pour them into a drain unless instructed to do so.

Different types of Formulations
- Tablet, film coated

Popular brand names: Mycobutol, Ecox, Tabutol, Beethom, Actol, Mycostat, Hitol, Tolbin, Resicox, Cavibutol

Pyrazinamide

Classification: Antitubercular Agents

Chemical Name: pyrazine-2-carboxamide

Chemical Structure

Uses

- For the initial treatment of active tuberculosis in adults and children when combined with other antituberculous agents.

Stability

- It is stable for at least 90 days at room temperature.

Storage Conditions

- Store in a well-closed container at controlled room temperature, 15°C to 30°C (59°F to 86°F).
- Dispense in a well-closed container with a child-resistant closure.

Different types of Formulations

- Tablet

Popular brand names: Macrozide, Pyzina, Cavizide, Isomide, Montozin, Kemide, Zypyra, Hituber, Mzide, Pyratis

Para Aminosalicylic Acid

Classification: Antitubercular Agents

Chemical Name: 4-amino-2-hydroxybenzoic acid

Chemical Structure

Uses

- Aminosalicylic acid is an aminosalicylate drug used to induce remission in ulcerative colitis.

Stability
- Para aminosalicylic acid decomposes most rapidly under conditions promoting oxidation and is most stable under conditions tending to inhibit oxidation.

Storage Conditions
- Store below 59°F (15°C) (in a refrigerator or freezer).
- Patients are urged to store product (aminosalicylic acid) in a refrigerator or freezer.
- The packets may be stored at room temperature for short periods of time.
- Avoid excessive heat.

Different types of Formulations
- Granule, delayed release
- Tablet

Popular brand names: Paser, Granupas, Cosacol, Elmes, Salofalk

Rifampicin

Classification: Antibiotics, Antitubercular

Chemical Name: [(7S,9E,11S,12R,13S,14R,15R,16R,17S,18S,19E,21Z)-2,15,17,27, 29-pentahydroxy-11-methoxy-3,7,12,14,16,18,22-heptamethyl-26-[(E)-(4-methylpi perazin-1-yl)iminomethyl]-6,23-dioxo-8,30-dioxa-24-azatetracyclo[23.3.1.14,7.05,28] triaconta-1(29),2,4,9,19,21,25,27-octaen-13-yl] acetate

Chemical Structure

Uses

- Rifampicin is an antibiotic used to treat several types of mycobacterial infections including *Mycobacterium avium* complex, leprosy, and in combination with other antibacterials to treat latent or active tuberculosis.

Stability

- It is susceptible to degradation where under acidic condition, rifampicin forms 3-formyl rifamycin.

Storage Conditions

- Rifampin was found to be chemically stable in each suspension for 56 days at room temperature.
- Suspensions prepared from the capsules may be non-homogeneous and lead to unsatisfactory dosing.

Different types of Formulations

- Capsule
- Injection, powder, lyophilized, for solution

Popular brand names: Rcin, Ticin, Hifam, Exact Kid, Rifampila, Macox, Monocin, Tricin, Serom, Rifacure

Antiviral Agents

Antiviral agents are substances used in the treatment and prophylaxis of diseases caused by viruses. Viral diseases include influenza, rabies, yellow fever, poliomyelitis, ornithosis, mumps, measles, ebola, human immuno deficiency virus (HIV), herpes, warts, and small pox. Viruses are not proper living things, but consists of a genome; they are smaller in size with simple chemical composition, sometimes a few enzymes stored in a capsule made up of protein and rarely covered with a lipid layer. The viruses only replicate within the host cell and the viral replication depends primarily on the metabolic processes of the invaded cell. Viruses does not possess cell wall, but they have RNA or DNA enclosed in a shell of protein known as capsid. The capsid is composed of several subunits known as capsomers. In certain cases, capsid may be surrounded by an outer protein or lipoprotein envelope. One group of RNA virus that deserves special mention are reteroviruses. They are responsible for acquired immuno deficiency syndrome (AIDS) and T-leukaemias. Reteroviruses contain reverse transcriptase (RT) enzyme activity that makes a DNA copy of the viral RNA template. Then, the DNA copy is integrated into the host genome, at which it is referred to as provirus and is transcribed into both the genomic RNA and mRNA for translocation into the viral proteins, giving generation to new virus particles.

Life cycle of virus

- **Adsorption:** Attachment of the virus to the host cell.
- **Penetration:** Penetration of virus into the cell.
- **Uncoating:** The genetic material or viral genome (DNA or RNA) passes into the host cell leaving the capsid covering outside the host cell.
- **Transcription:** Production of the viral mRNA from the viral genome.
- **Translation:** The viral genome enters the cytoplasm or the nucleoplasma and directs or utilizes the host nucleic acid machinery for the synthesis of the new viral protein and for the production of more viral genome. The viral protein modifies the host cell and allows the viral genome to replicate by using host and viral enzyme. This is often the stage at which the cell is irreversibly modified and eventually killed.
- **Assembly of the viral particle:** New viral coat protein assembles into capsid and viral genomes.
- **Release of the mature virus** from the cell and the budding process or rupture of the cell and repeat of the process, in a fresh host cell

Classification According to its Mechanism of Action

Antiviral drugs may be classified on the basis of its mechanism of action as follows:

I. Nucleoside RT inhibitors
   (a) Purine nucleosides and nucleotides: Aciclovir, Ganciclovir, Valaciclovir, Vidarabine, Penciclovir, Famciclovir, Abacavir
   (b) Pyrimidine nucleosides and nucleotides: Iodoxuridine, Trifluridine, Cidofovir
   (c) Thiosemicarbazones: Methisazone
   (d) Adamantane amines: Amantadine, Rimantadine, Somantadine, Tromantadine

II. Non-nucleoside RT inhibitors: Nevirapine, Delavirdine, Efavirenz, Emivirine, Loviride, Trovidine

III. HIV protease inhibitors: Saquinavir, Indinavir, Ritonavir, Nelfinavir

IV. Miscellaneous: Foscarnet sodium, Ribavirin

Amantadine Hydrochloride

Classification: Antiviral Agents

Chemical Name: Adamantan-1-amine

Chemical Structure

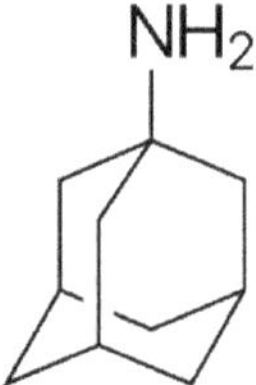

Uses

- For the chemoprophylaxis, prophylaxis, and treatment of signs and symptoms of infection caused by various strains of influenza A virus.
- Also for the treatment of parkinsonism and drug-induced extrapyramidal reactions.

Stability

- Both compounds were quite stable after storage for at least 25 years at ambient temperature; they both retained full antiviral activity after long-term storage or after boiling and holding at 65-85°C for several days.

Storage Conditions

- Store amantadine at room temperature between 68°F and 77°F (20°C and 25°C).
- It can be temporarily stored in temperatures from 59°F to 86°F (15°C to 30°C).
- Don't store this medication in moist or damp areas, such as bathrooms.

Different types of Formulations

- Capsule, coated pellets
- Tablet, extended release
- Solution
- Syrup

Popular brand names: Ensorex, Extadin, Manotrel, Amantex, Amantrel, Amantalarc, Comantrel, Parkitidin

Idoxuridine

Classification: Antiviral Agents

Chemical Name: 1-[(2R,4S,5R)-4-hydroxy-5-(hydroxymethyl)oxolan-2-yl]-5-iodopy-rimidine-2,4-dione

Chemical Structure

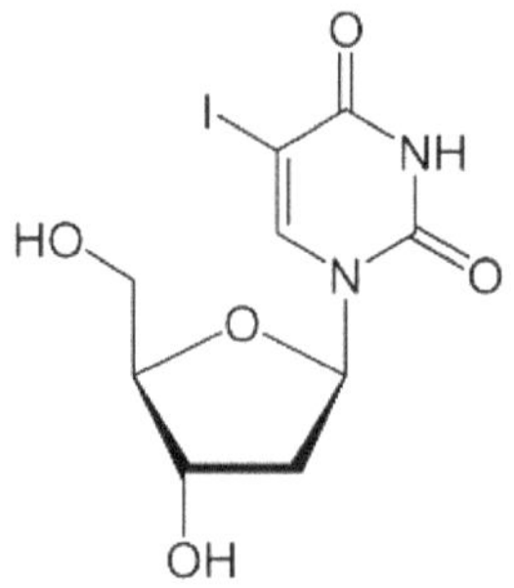

Uses

- Idoxuridine is a pyrimidine analog antiviral used for the treatment of viral eye infections, including herpes simplex keratitis.

Stability

- Idoxuridine is rapidly inactivated by deaminases or nucleotidases.
- To ensure stability, the ophthalmic solution should not be mixed with other medications. Burning after application or failure to respond to treatment may suggest deterioration of the ophthalmic solution; replace with fresh solution.

Storage Conditions

- Store between 2 °C and 8 °C (36 and 46 °F). Store in a tight, light-resistant container.
- Store between 8 and 15 °C (46 and 59 °F). Store in a collapsible ophthalmic ointment tube.

Formulations

- Solution
- Drops
- Liquid

Popular brand names: Ridinox, Toxil, Idurin, Xurin, Ifex, Herplex, Dendrid

Acyclovir

Classification: Antiviral Agents

Chemical Name: 2-amino-9-(2-hydroxyethoxymethyl)-1*H*-purin-6-one

Chemical Structure

Uses

- An acyclovir topical cream is indicated to treat recurrent herpes labialis in immunocompetent patients 12 years and older.
- Acyclovir oral tablets, capsules, and suspensions are indicated to treat herpes zoster, genital herpes, and chickenpox.

Stability

- Acyclovir 5 mg/mL in 100 mL of NaCl 0.9% infusion remains stable at least for 21 days at 5°C with or without freezing at -20°C during the three previous months.

Storage Conditions

- Keep container tightly closed in a dry and well-ventilated place.
- Store acyclovir tablets at 59°F to 77°F (15°C to 25°C) and protect them from moisture and light.
- Store acyclovir suspension at 59°F to 77°F (15°C to 25°C) and protect it from light.
- Store acyclovir capsules at room temperature, 68°F to 77°F (20°C to 25°C), and protect them from moisture.

Different types of Formulations

- Tablet, delayed release
- Capsule
- Powder for solution
- Solution
- Ointment
- Cream
- Suspension
- Injection, powder, lyophilized, for solution

Popular brand names: Acivir, Alovir, Zovirax, Ocuvir, Biovir, Autic, Aviral, Zovir, Zovistar, Herpikind

Ganciclovir

Classification: Antiviral Agents

Chemical Name: 2-amino-9-(1,3-dihydroxypropan-2-yloxymethyl)-1*H*-purin-6-one

Chemical Structure

Uses

- For induction and maintenance in the treatment of cytomegalovirus (CMV) retinitis in immunocompromised patients, including patients with acquired immunodeficiency syndrome (AIDS). Also used in the treatment of severe cytomegalovirus (CMV) disease, including CMV pneumonia, CMV gastrointestinal disease, and disseminated CMV infections, in immune-compromised patients.

Stability

- The drug is stable at room temperature for 12 hours in vial.
- When further diluted with normal saline or distilled water, the final solution should be refrigerated until ready for use.

Storage Conditions

- The diluted ganciclovir intravenous solution should be kept in the refrigerator (2 - 8°C).
- It is recommended that the solution be used within 24 hours of dilution.
- Keep well out of the reach of children.

Different types of Formulations

- Powder, for solution
- Capsule
- Injection, powder, lyophilized, for solution
- Gel
- Solution
- Implant

Popular brand names: Ganguard, Gavir, Natclovir, Cymevene, Cytogan, Gancicel, Dendrigel, Ganpyar Eye, Grevir, Ganov

Foscarnet

Classification: Antiviral Agents

Chemical Name: phosphonoformic acid

Chemical Structure

Uses

- For the treatment of CMV retinitis in patients with acquired immunodeficiency syndrome (AIDS) and for treatment of acyclovir-resistant mucocutaneous HSV infections in immunocompromised patients.

Stability

- Foscarnet sodium 12 mg/mL in 0.9% sodium chloride injection was stable for up to 30 days when stored at 25°C and exposed to light, 25°C and protected from light, or 5°C and protected from light.

Storage Conditions

- Store at room temperature between 59-86°F (15-30°C) away from light and heat. Keep below 104 degrees F (40°C).
- The diluted solutions should be used as soon as possible after preparation but can be stored for up to 24 hours if kept refrigerated.

Different types of Formulations

- Injection
- Solution

Popular brand names: Foscavir, Triapten

Zidovudine

Classification: Anti-HIV Agents

Chemical Name: 1-[(2R,4S,5S)-4-azido-5-(hydroxymethyl)oxolan-2-yl]-5-methylpyrimidine-2,4-dione

Chemical Structure

Uses

- Used in combination with other antiretroviral agents for the treatment of human immunovirus (HIV) infections.

Stability

- Zidovudine 4 mg/mL in admixtures with 5% dextrose injection or 0.9% sodium chloride injection stored in polyvinyl chloride infusion bags was stable for up to 192 hours (eight days) at room temperature and under refrigeration.

Storage Conditions

- Store zidovudine tablets at room temperature, 68°F to 77°F (20°C to 25°C).
- Store zidovudine capsules and oral solution between 59°F and 77°F (15°C to 25°C).

Different types of Formulations

- Tablet, film coated
- Injection
- Solution
- Capsule
- Syrup

Popular brand names: Zidovir, Retrovir, Viro Z, Ziv, Zidohope, Zyvud, Zido, Zidine, Zidovex, Zidolam

Lamivudine

Classification: Anti-HIV Agents

Chemical Name: 4-amino-1-[(2*R*,5*S*)-2-(hydroxymethyl)-1,3-oxathiolan-5-yl]pyrimidin-2-one

Chemical Structure

Uses

- For the treatment of HIV infection and chronic hepatitis B (HBV).

Stability
- It also degraded extensively under oxidative environment.
- It remained stable to light and thermal stress.

Storage Conditions
- Keep lamivudine tablets at room temperature between 68°F and 77°F (20°C and 25°C).
- The tablets can occasionally be in temperatures between 59°F and 86°F (15°C and 30°C).
- Keep bottles of tablets tightly closed to keep them fresh and potent.

Different types of Formulations
- Tablet, film coated
- Solution

Popular brand names: Lamivir, Heptavir, Hepitec, Hivir, Shanvudin, Cytocom, Virocomb, Lazid, Duovir, Trezav

Ribavirin

Classification: Antiviral Agents

Chemical Name: 1-[(2R,3R,4S,5R)-3,4-dihydroxy-5-(hydroxymethyl)oxolan-2-yl]-1,2,4-triazole-3-carboxamide

Uses
- Indicated for the treatment of chronic Hepatitis C virus (HCV) infection in combination with other antiviral agents with the intent to cure or achieve a sustained virologic response (SVR). Typically added to improve SVR and reduce relapse rates.
- The addition of ribavirin in Technivie therapy indicated for treating HCV genotype 1a and 4 infections is recommended in patients with or without cirrhosis.

Chemical Structure

Stability

- Ribavirin for inhalation solution is physically and chemically stable for at least 45 days when frozen, refrigerated, or kept at room temperature after reconstitution to a concentration of approximately 67 mg/mL and placed in syringes or glass vials.

Storage Conditions

- Store ribavirin tablets and capsules at room temperature, between 68°F and 77°F (20°C to 25°C).
- Store ribavirin oral solution at room temperature, between 68°F and 77°F (20°C to 25°C), or in the refrigerator, between 36°F and 46°F (2°C to 8°C).
- Keep ribavirin in the container that it came in and keep the container tightly closed.

Different types of Formulations

- Tablet, film coated
- Capsule
- Powder, for solution

Popular brand names: Ribavin, Ribahep, Heptos, Gatorib, Ribocare, Rebetol, Ribapro, Heplovir, Rinhib, Ribanol

Antimalarials

Antimalarial agents are drugs used for the treatment or prophylaxis of malaria. Malaria is caused by four species of Plasmodium, such as Plasmodium falciparum, P. malariae, P. ovale, and P. vivax. Three of which produces the mild forms of malaria by destroying red blood cells in peripheral capillaries and thus, causing anaemia. The bouts of fever correspond to the reproductive cycle of the parasite. However, the most dangerous is the P. falciparum. In this case, the infected red blood cells become sticky and form lumps in the capillaries of the deep organs of the body and cause microcirculatory arrest. This disease still affects about 200 millions people and causes at least 2 million deaths per year.

The different stages of the reproductive cycle of the malarial parasite and the drugs acting at different stages of this cycle are given below:

- Stage-I: No drug is effective in this stage.
- Stage-II: Primaquine and pyrimethamine can block at this stage.
- Stage-III: Primaquine can only prevent because fever occurs at this stage.
- Stage-IV: Chloroquine, amodiaquine, santoquine, proguanil.
- Stage-V: Primaquine only.

Two important phases of the parasite life cycle are the following:

1. Asexual cycle—occurs in the infected host.
2. Sexual cycle—occurs in the mosquito.

After the insect bite, the parasite forms rapidly. They leave the circulation and localize in the hepatocytes whereby they transform, multiply, and develop into tissue schizonts. The primary asymptomatic tissue stage lasts for 15 days and the tissue schizonts rupture, each releasing thousands of merozites. The released merozites invade more erythrocytes to continue the cycle's synchronous rupture of erythrocytes to continue the cycle. Synchronous rupture of erythrocytes and release of merozytes into the circulation lead febrile pattern attacks on day 1 and 3; hence, the designation is 'tertian malaria'. Some erythrocyte parasites differentiate into several forms known as gametophytes. After infecting human blood, female mosquito ingests them. Then the exflagellation of male gametocyte is followed by the male gametogenesis and the fertilization of the female gametocytes in the insect's guts. The resulting zygote, which develops as an oocyte in the gut wall, eventually gives rise to infective sporozoite, which invades the salivary glands of the mosquito. The insect then can infect another human by taking a blood meal.

Classification

I. **Cinchona alkaloids:** Quinine, Quinidine, Cinchonine, Cinchonidine

II. **7-Chloro-4-Amino Quinolines:** Cholorquine, Amodiaquine, Hydroxychloroquine, Sontoquine, Amopyroquine

III. **8-Amino Quinolines:** Primaquine, Pamaquine, Pentaquine phosphate, Isopentaquine, Quinocide HCl

IV. **Acridine derivatives (9-amino acridine derivatives):** Quinacrine, Acriquine

V. **Antifolates:**
   (a) **Biguanids:** Proguanil, Chloro proguanil, Bromoguanil, Nitroguanil
   (b) **Diamino pyrimidines:** Pyrimethamine (Daraprim), Trimethoprim

VI. **Sulphonamides and Sulphones:** Sulphadoxine, Sulphadiazine, Sulphamethoxazole

VII. **Phenanthrine methanol:** Halofentamine

VIII. **Miscellaneous drugs:** Halofantrine (Hafan), Mefloquine, Dapsone, Artemether, Artemotil, Artesunate

Quinine Sulphate

Classification: Antimalarials

Chemical Name: (*R*)-[(2*S*,4*S*,5*R*)-5-ethenyl-1-azabicyclo[2.2.2]octan-2-yl]-(6-methoxy-quinolin-4-yl)methanol

Chemical Structure

Uses

- It is used to treat uncomplicated Plasmodium falciparum malaria and leg cramps.

Stability

- Quinine was stable for at least 24 hr in all of the infusion fluids studied and did not require protection from light during 24 hr. However, some decrease in concentration was observed on storage. Therefore, quinine admixtures should still be used as soon after preparation as possible.

Storage Conditions

- Store at room temperature away from light and moisture.
- Do not store in the bathroom.
- Keep all medicines away from children and pets.

Different types of Formulations

- Capsule

Popular brand names: Cinkona, Qinarsol, Swiquin, Rubiquin, Safequin, Lequin, Nofalsi, Quininga, Quinarsol, Osquin

Chloroquine Phosphate

Classification: Antimalarials

Chemical Name: 4-*N*-(7-chloroquinolin-4-yl)-1-*N*,1-*N*-diethylpentane-1,4-diamine

Chemical Structure

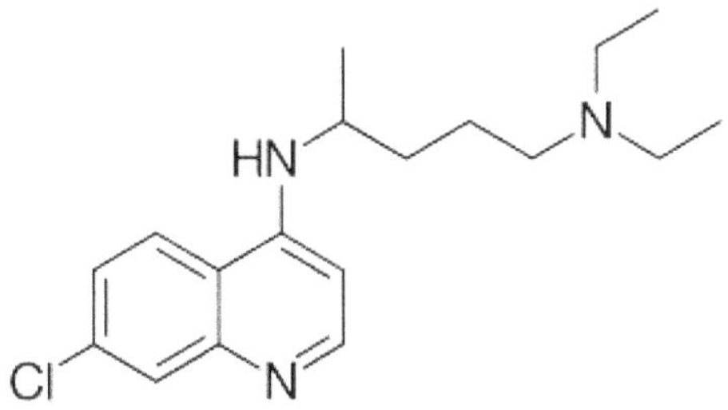

Uses

- Chloroquine is indicated to treat infections of *P. vivax*, *P. malariae*, *P. ovale*, and susceptible strains of *P. falciparum*.
- It is also used to treat extraintestinal amebiasis.
- Chloroquine is also used off label for the treatment of rheumatic diseases, as well as treatment and prophylaxis of Zika virus.
- Chloroquine is currently undergoing clinical trials for the treatment of COVID-19.

Stability

- In lyophilized form, the chemical is stable for 24 months.
- Once in solution, use within 3 months to prevent loss of potency.
- Aliquot to avoid multiple freeze/thaw cycles.
- Product in powder form is stable for 6 months at room temperature when properly stored.

Storage Conditions

- Chloroquine is shipped at room temperature.
- Store at room temperature (15-25 °C).
- Protect from light.

Different types of Formulations

- Tablet, film coated

Popular brand names: Lariago, Resochin, Anaquin, Falcin, Cloquin, Loroquin, Mahaquin, Malacure, Malarbin, Nivaquine

Primaquine Phosphate

Classification: Antimalarials

Chemical Name: 4-*N*-(6-methoxyquinolin-8-yl)pentane-1,4-diamine

Chemical Structure

Uses
- It is an antimalarial indicated to prevent relapse of vivax malaria.

Stability
- Photochemical degradation of primaquine takes place in an aqueous-medium.

Storage Conditions
- Primaquine tablets should be stored in well-closed, light-resistant containers at a temperature less than 40°C.

Different types of Formulations
- Tablet, film coated

Popular brand names: Malirid, Primaline, Evaquin, Primal, Vexaprim, Primacip, Primarid, Prematin, Premadiff, Primelife

Quinacrine Hydrochloride

Classification: Antimalarials

Chemical Name: 4-*N*-(6-chloro-2-methoxyacridin-9-yl)-1-*N*,1-*N*-diethylpentane-1,4-diamine

Chemical Structure

Uses
- For the treatment of giardiasis and cutaneous leishmaniasis and the management of malignant effusions.

Stability
- Stable in solid forms under ordinary storage conditions.
- Degradation may happen in aqueous solutions.

Storage Conditions
- Store below 40 °C (104 °F), preferably between 15 and 30 °C (59 and 86 °F) in a light-resistant container.

Different types of Formulations
- Tablet
- Injection
- Capsule
- Suppositories

Popular brand names: Mepalex, Maladin

Mefloquine

Classification: Antimalarials

Chemical Name: [2,8-bis(trifluoromethyl)quinolin-4-yl]-piperidin-2-ylmethanol

Chemical Structure

Uses
- Mefloquine is indicated for the treatment of mild to moderate cases of malaria caused by Plasmodium falciparum and Plasmodium vivax.
- It is effective against chloroquine-resistant forms of Plasmodium falciparum. Mefloquine is also indicated for the prophylaxis of malaria caused by Plasmodium falciparum and Plasmodium vivax, including chloroquine-resistant forms of Plasmodium falciparum.

Stability
- Photochemical decomposition of mefloquine occurs in water.

Storage Conditions
- It should be stored at 25°C but may be exposed to 15-30°C.
- Keep away from children.
- Keep in a cool, dry place, away from direct sunlight.

Different types of Formulations
- Tablet

Popular brand names: Meflotas, Mefloc, Altimef, Mefax, Meflife, Falcimef, Devexquin, Larium, Maxquin, Meflosain

Cycloguanil

Classification: Antimalarials

Chemical Name: 1-(4-chlorophenyl)-6,6-dimethyl-1,3,5-triazine-2,4-diamine

Chemical Structure

Uses
- Cycloguanil is a dihydrofolate reductase inhibitor, and is a metabolite of the antimalarial drug proguanil; its formation in vivo has been thought to be primarily responsible for the antimalarial activity of proguanil.
- However, more recent work has indicated that, while proguanil is synergistic with the drug atovaquone (as in the combination Malarone), cycloguanil is in fact antagonistic to the effects of atovaquone, suggesting that, unlike cycloguanil, proguanil may have an alternative mechanism of antimalarial action besides dihydrofolate reductase inhibition.

Stability
- Strong oxidizing agents degrade the drug material.

Storage Conditions
- Store at -20°C temperature.

Different types of Formulations
- Tablet
- Capsule

Popular brand names: Malarone

Pyrimethamine

Classification: Antimalarials

Chemical Name: 5-(4-chlorophenyl)-6-ethylpyrimidine-2,4-diamine

Chemical Structure

Uses
- For the treatment of toxoplasmosis and acute malaria; For the prevention of malaria in areas non-resistant to pyrimethamine

Stability
- Stable, but light sensitive.

Storage Conditions
- Store at 15 °C to 25 °C (59 °F to 77 °F) in a dry place in a closed container and protect from light.

Different types of Formulations
- Tablet

Popular brand names: Laridox, Pyralfin, Amalar, Reziz, Metafin, Rimodkar, Malin, Malocide, Malcidal, Croydoxin

Sulfonamides

Sulfonamides are synthetic antibacterial compounds and are generally wide-spectrum drugs active against a range of bacterial species, both Gram-positive and Gram-negative. Most sulfonamide formulations are supplied as combination products having two main components, a sulfonamide and the synthetic diaminopyrimidines, trimethoprim or ormethoprim. These combinations are believed to act synergistically on specific targets in bacterial DNA synthesis.

Classification

(a) **Short acting:** Sulfadiazine, Sulfadimidine, Sulfacetamide

(b) **Intermediate acting:** Sulfamethoxazole

(c) **Long acting:** Sulfadoxine, Sulfamethoxypyrazine, Sulfadimethoxine

(d) Topically used: Mafenide, Silver sulfadiazine and Sulfacetamide

(e) Ulcerative colitis: Sulfasalzine

Sulfanilamide

Classification: Anti-Bacterial Agents

Chemical Name: 4-aminobenzenesulfonamide

Chemical Structure

Uses
- For the treatment of vulvovaginitis caused by Candida albicans.

Stability
- Sulfanilamide is a stable substance under normal temperature and pressure conditions.
- It is sensitive to light and incompatible with strong oxidizing agents.

Storage Conditions
- Store the medicine in a closed container at room temperature, away from heat, moisture, and direct light.

Different types of Formulations
- Cream

Popular brand names: Sulphakream-N, Avc, Albexan, Albosal, Ambeside, Antistrept, Astreptine, Astrocid, Bacteramid, Bactesid

Sulfadiazine

Classification: Anti-Bacterial Agents

Chemical Name

4-amino-*N*-pyrimidin-2-ylbenzenesulfonamide

Chemical Structure

Uses

- Sulfadiazine is a sulfonamide antibiotic used in a variety of infections, such as urinary tract infections, trachoma, and chancroid.

Stability

- The solution prepared from powder remains stable for 3 days under refrigerated condition.
- The sulfadiazine suspension remains stable for 14 days at room temperature.

Storage Conditions

- Store sulfadiazine tablets at room temperature, 68°F to 77°F (20°C to 25°C).
- Protect sulfadiazine tablets from light.
- Keep sulfadiazine in the container that it came in and keep the container tightly closed.

Different types of Formulations

- Tablet

Popular brand names: Burnosaf, Safoderm, Burnhit, Burnomed, Burncare, Silva, Silvolar, Silverine, Silverdina, Silzine

Sulfamethoxazole

Classification: Anti-Infective Agents

Chemical Name: 4-amino-*N*-(5-methyl-1,2-oxazol-3-yl)benzenesulfonamide

Chemical Structure

Uses

- Sulfamethoxazole is indicated in combination with trimethoprim, in various formulations, for the following infections caused by bacteria with documented susceptibility: urinary tract infections, acute otitis media in pediatric patients (when clinically indicated), acute exacerbations of chronic bronchitis in adults, enteritis caused by susceptible *Shigella*, prophylaxis and treatment of *Pneumocystis jiroveci* pneumonia, and travelers' diarrhea caused by enterotoxigenic *E. coli*.

Stability

- Sulfamethoxazole is stable for 48 hours in 5% dextrose injection and 0.9% sodium chloride injection.

Storage Conditions

- Store sulfamethoxazole tablets at room temperature, 68°F to 77°F (20°C to 25°C).
- Do not refrigerate the injection solution.
- Commercially available sulfamethoxazole tablets and oral suspension should be protected from light and stored at a temperature less than 40°C.
- Keep all medications away from children and pets.

Different types of Formulations

- Tablet

Popular brand names: Septra, Bactrim-Iv, Sulfatrim

Sulfacetamide

Classification: Anti-Bacterial Agents

Chemical Name: *N*-(4-aminophenyl)sulfonylacetamide

Chemical Structure

Uses

- For the treatment of bacterial vaginitis, keratitis, acute conjunctivitis, and blepharitis.

Stability

- Research proved that it is more toxic in the presence of light than in the dark. Sulfacetamide is slightly irritant when UV-A light is present. In the presence of light sulfacetamide gets sensitized and degraded which might cause irritation which will lead to toxicity when it is used continuously. In the dark only slight irritation has been shown. Therefore it should be stored in the dark.

Storage Conditions

- Store at room temperature between 68-77°F (20-25°C).

Different types of Formulations: Solution, Liquid, Drops, Ointment, Lotion, Cream, Shampoo, Aerosol, Swab

Popular brand names: Klaron, Clenia, Rosac, Vasocidin, Sulfatol-C, Blephamide, Rosanil, Plexion, Isopto, Fml-S

Mafenide Acetate

Classification: Anti-Bacterial Agents

Chemical Name: 4-(aminomethyl)benzenesulfonamide

Chemical Structure

Uses

- Indicated for use as an adjunctive topical antimicrobial agent to control bacterial infection when used under moist dressings over meshed autografts on excised burn wounds.

Stability

- The drug should be used within 48 hours after mixing.
- Stable up to 28 days in unopened containers.

Storage Conditions

- The 5% topical solution is to be stored at room temperature, 25°C - 30°C (77°F-86°F) in a dry place.

Different types of Formulations

- Powder, for solution
- Cream

Popular brand names: Sulfamylon

Cotrimoxazole

Classification: Anti-Bacterial Agents

Chemical Name: 4-amino-*N*-(5-methyl-1,2-oxazol-3-yl)benzenesulfonamide;

5-[(3,4,5-trimethoxyphenyl)methyl]pyrimidine-2,4-diamine

Chemical Structure

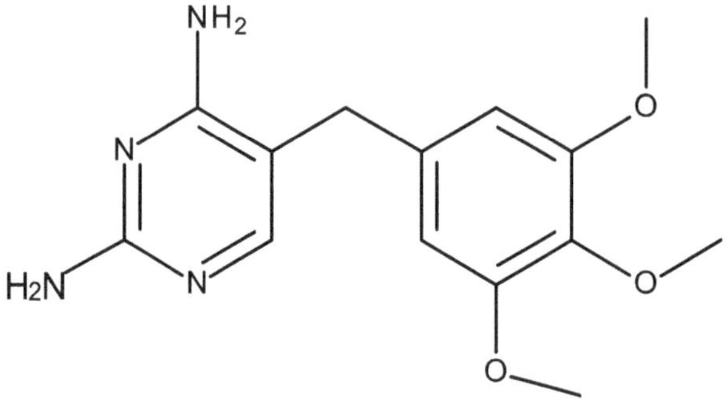

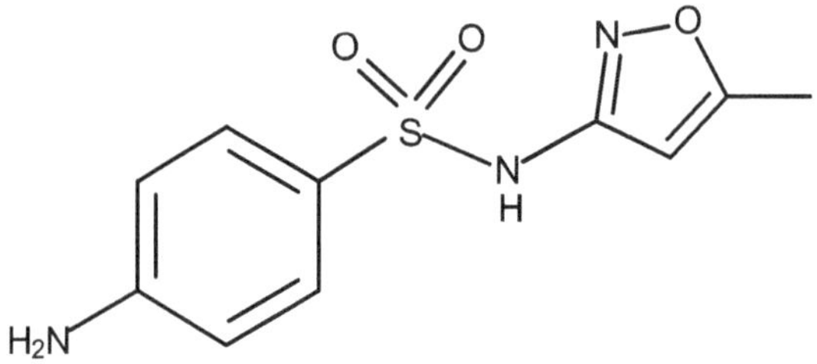

Uses

- Co-trimoxazole is used to treat certain bacterial infections, such as pneumonia (a lung infection), bronchitis (infection of the tubes leading to the lungs), and infections of the urinary tract, ears, and intestines.
- It also is used to treat 'travelers' diarrhea.

Stability

- Cotrimoxazole in peritoneal dialysis fluid stored in polyvinyl chloride bags and glass ampoules at room temperature for up to nine days.

Storage Conditions

- Store below 25°C in a dry place.
- Protect from light.

Different types of Formulations

- Tablet

Popular brand names: Cotrimox, Larprim, Wypal, Tabrol, Alcorim-F, Cosulf, Kombina, Antrima, Colizole, Otrim.

Multiple Choice Questions

1. Which of the following combination is correct?
   (a) Penicillin: inhibition of cell wall synthesis
   (b) Cephalosporin: inhibition of protein synthesis
   (c) Aminoglycoside: inhibition of cell wall synthesis
   (d) Fluoroquinolones: inhibition of cell wall synthesis

2. Amoxycillin is similar to Ampicillin in different respects except in ....
   (a) Antibacterial spectrum   (b) Penicillinase resistance
   (c) Hypersensitivity reaction   (d) Oral absorption

3. Which of the following group of antibiotics show bacteriostatic action?
   (a) Fluoroquinolones   (b) Aminoglycosides
   (c) Macrolides   (d) Monobactams

4. Which of the following group of antibiotics in accordance with the structure and mode of action of penicillin?
   (a) Chloramphenicol   (b) Polymyxins
   (c) Cycloserines   (d) Cephalosporins

5. Gray baby syndrome in neonates can be caused by
   (a) Penicillin   (b) Chloramphenicol
   (c) Quinolones   (d) Sulphonamides

6. Followings are the penicillinase-resistant penicillin, except:
   (a) Carbenicillin   (b) Methicillin
   (c) Nafcillin   (d) Cloxacillin

7. Which of the following antibiotics acts as a protein synthesis inhibitor?
   (a) Erythromycin, Chloramphenicol (b) Vancomycin, Cephamycin
   (c) Gentamicin, Tetracycline   (d) Options a and c
   (e) Options b and c

8. All of the followings are the adverse effects of tetracycline, except:
   (a) Ototoxicity   (b) Phototoxicity
   (c) Fatal hepatotoxicity   (d) Yellow discoloration of teeth

9. The following cephalosporin is associated with bleeding complications
   (a) Cefotaxime   (b) Cefuroxime
   (c) Cefotetan   (d) Cefazolin

10. Redman syndrome is toxicity associated with
    (a) Amoxicillin   (b) Daptomycin
    (c) Linezolid   (d) Vancomycin

11. One cycle of liver invasion and multiplication:
    (a) P vivax
    (b) P falciparum
    (c) P. malariae
    (d) P ovale

12. Factors which determine antimalarial agent efficacy:
    (a) Species
    (b) Life-cycle stage-dependencies
    (c) Both
    (d) Neither

13. Asserting a malarial diagnosis:
    (a) Fever/flu-like symptoms in individual returning from travel (or native to) a malarious geographical region
    (b) Disease ruled out the patient has taken prophylactic drugs during travel
    (c) Both
    (d) Neither

14. Treatment of malaria caused by chloroquine (Aralen)-resistant P falciparum: oral: quinine sulfate and clindamycin (Cleocin):
    (a) True
    (b) False

15. Which of the following antiviral drug is used to treat influenza A?
    (a) Dextran sulfate
    (b) Amantadine
    (c) Ganciclovir
    (d) Cidofovir

16. Which of the following is used to treat eye infection?
    (a) Rimantadine
    (b) Ganciclovir
    (c) TFT
    (d) ACV

17. Which of the following is used to treat CMV infections?
    (a) Foscarnet
    (b) Saquinavir
    (c) Ritonavir
    (d) Nelfinavir

18. Which of the following is used to treat genital herpes infections?
    (a) Penciclovir
    (b) Pleconaril
    (c) Oseltamivir
    (d) Efavirenz

19. Why antiviral drugs cannot cure HIV?
    (a) They do not block viral replication
    (b) They cannot block viral translation
    (c) They cannot block viral transcription
    (d) They do not penetrate the cells

20. Which of the following cannot be treated by antiviral drugs?
    (a) Tuberculosis
    (b) Smallpox
    (c) Hepatitis
    (d) Wartsw

CHAPTER 12

Antibiotics

Introduction

The chapter aims at providing the latest and pharmacopoeial information regarding some Antibiotics (Penicillin G, Ampicillin, Amoxicillin, Cloxacillin, Clavulenic acid, Cephalosporins, Streptomycin, Neomycin, Tetracycline, Doxycycline, Minocycline, Erythromycin, Azithromycin, Chloramphenicol, and Clindamycin) regarding their classification, chemical name, chemical structure, uses, stability, storage conditions, different types of formulations, and popular brand names.

The term antibiotic has its origin in the word antibiosis (i.e. against life). Antibiotics are chemical substances obtained from various species of microorganisms (bacteria, fungi, actinomycetes) that suppress the growth of other microorganisms and eventually may destroy them. The probable points of difference amongst the antibiotics may be physical, chemical, pharmacological properties, antibacterial spectra, and mechanism of action. They have made it possible to cure diseases caused by bacteria, such as pneumonia, tuberculosis, and meningitis, and they save the lives of millions of people around the world.

Antibiotics came into worldwide prominence with the introduction of penicillin in 1941. Since then they have revolutionized the treatment of bacterial infections in humans and other animals. They are, however, ineffective against viruses.

Classification of Antibiotics

Aminoglycosides (inhibit protein synthesis): gentamicin, tobramycin

Cephalosporins (inhibit cell wall synthesis): cefaclor, cefamandole, cefazolin, ceftriaxone, cefuroxime, cephalexin

Chloramphenicols (inhibit protein synthesis): chloramphenicol

Fluoroquinolones (interfere with DNA synthesis): ciprofloxacin, norfloxacin

Lincosamides (inhibit protein synthesis): clindamycin

Macrolides (inhibit protein synthesis): azithromycin, clarithromycin, erythromycin

Nitrofurans (inactivate essential cell components): nitrofurantoin

Penicillins (inhibit cell wall synthesis): amoxicillin, ampicillin, penicillin G, piperacillin, ticarcillin

Tetracyclines (inhibit protein synthesis): tetracycline

Miscellaneous antibiotics: aztreonam, imipenem-cilastatin, isoniazid, metronidazole, rifampin, trimethoprim-sulfamethoxazole, vancomycin

Penicillin G

Classification: Anti-Bacterial Agents

Chemical Name: (2S,5R,6R)-3,3-dimethyl-7-oxo-6-[(2-phenylacetyl)amino]-4-thia-1-azabicyclo[3.2.0]heptane-2-carboxylic acid

Chemical Structure

Uses

- For use in the treatment of severe infections caused by penicillin G-susceptible microorganisms when rapid and high penicillin levels are required such as in the treatment of septicemia, meningitis, pericarditis, endocarditis and severe pneumonia.

Stability

- When refrigerated, penicillin solutions may be stored for seven days without loss of potency.

Storage Conditions

- Store product in a refrigerator, 2° to 8°C (36° to 46°F).
- Keep from freezing.
- Store dry powder at 20º to 25ºC (68º to 77ºF).

Different types of Formulations: Injection suspension, Powder for solution, Suspension

Popular brand names: Pentids, Pentas, Bistrepen, Benzathine, Sodicillin, Bpg, Pentab, Fpp

Ampicillin

Classification: Anti-Bacterial Agents

Chemical Name: (2*S*,5*R*,6*R*)-6-[[(2*R*)-2-amino-2-phenylacetyl]amino]-3,3-dimethyl-7-oxo-4-thia-1-azabicyclo[3.2.0]heptane-2-carboxylic acid

Chemical Structure

Uses

- For treatment of infection (Respiratory, GI, UTI and meningitis) due to E. coli, P. mirabilis, enterococci, Shigella, S. typhosa and other Salmonella, nonpenicillinase-producing N. gononhoeae, H. influenzae, staphylococci, streptococci, etc.

Stability

- Ampicillin rapidly loses activity when stored above a pH of 7.0. 4,5,11.

Storage Conditions

- Ampicillin capsules and powder for oral suspension should be stored in tight containers at 15-30°C.
- Ampicillin can be prepared and stored in a refrigerator for up to 72 hours prior to continuously infusing at room temperature over 24 hours.

Different types of Formulations: Powder for solution, Injection powder for solution, Capsule

Popular brand names: Biocilin, Ampilon, Ampilin, Neocillin, Synthocilin, Roscillin, Synpen, Sultacin, Ampiace, Sulboxa

Amoxicillin

Classification: Anti-Bacterial Agents

Chemical Name: (2*S*,5*R*,6*R*)-6-[[(2*R*)-2-amino-2-(4-hydroxyphenyl)acetyl]amino]-3,3-dimethyl-7-oxo-4-thia-1-azabicyclo[3.2.0]heptane-2-carboxylic acid

Chemical Structure

Uses

- Amoxicillin alone is indicated to treat susceptible bacterial infections of the ear, nose, throat, genitourinary tract, skin, skin structure, and lower respiratory tract.
- Amoxicillin is given with calvulanic acid to treat acute bacterial sinusitis, community acquired pneumonia, lower respiratory tract infections, acute bacterial otitis media, skin and skin structure infections, and urinary tract infections.
- Amoxicillin is given with omeprazole in the treatment of *H. pylori*.

Stability

- Amoxicillin sodium is unstable in aqueous solutions stored between 0°C and -20°C.

Storage Conditions

- Store the capsules and tablets at room temperature and away from excess heat and moisture (not in the bathroom). The liquid medication preferably should be kept in the refrigerator, but it may be stored at room temperature. Do not freeze.

Different types of Formulations: - Capsule, Suspension, Tablet film coated, Granule for suspension, Powder for suspension, Tablet chewable, Tablet film coated extended release

Popular brand names: Amoxyrite, Blumox, Novamox, Gatmox, Wymox, Evoxil, Cipmox, Elmox, Amoxil, Almox

Clavulanic Acid

Classification: beta-Lactamase Inhibitors

Chemical Name: (2*R*,3*Z*,5*R*)-3-(2-hydroxyethylidene)-7-oxo-4-oxa-1-azabicyclo[3.2.0] heptane-2-carboxylic acid

Chemical Structure

Uses

- Clavulanic acid combined with other antibiotics is indicated to prevent the development of drug-resistant strains of bacteria and promotes their therapeutic antibacterial effects.

The following conditions, when they produced beta-lactamases, have been treated with a combination of amoxicillin and clavulanic acid or ticarcillin and clavulanic acid:

- Acute otitis media caused by H. influenzae and M. catarrhalis
- Sinusitis due to H. influenzae and M. catarrhalis
- Lower respiratory tract infections due to Haemophilus influenzae, S.aureus, Klebsiella species, and Moraxella catarrhalis
- Skin and skin structure infections caused by Staphylococcus aureus, Escherichia coli, and Klebsiella species
- Urinary Tract Infections due to E. coli, Klebsiella species of bacteria, and Enterobacter species of bacteria, S. marcescens, or S. aureus
- Gynecologic infections due to a variety of bacteria, including P. melaninogenicus, Enterobacter species, E. coli species, Klebsiella species, S. aureus, S.epidermidis
- Septicemia due to a variety of bacteria, including Klebsiella species, E. coli species, S. aureus, or Pseudomonas species
- Bone and joint infections due to S.aureus
- Intraabdominal infections due to E.Coli, K.pnemoniae, or B.fragilis group.

A note on susceptibility: It should be noted that it is only to be administered in infections that are confirmed or highly likely to be caused by susceptible bacteria. Culture and susceptibility tests should be performed if possible and used in selecting whether this antibiotic is prescribed. When beta-lactamase enzyme production is not detected during microbiological testing, clavulanic acid should not be used.

Stability

- The stability of clavulanic acid in aqueous solutions has been investigated over a pH range of 3.15 to 10.10 at 35°C and at an ionic strength of 0.5.

Storage Conditions

- Store the tablets at room temperature and away from excess heat and moisture (not in the bathroom).
- Keep liquid medication in the refrigerator, tightly closed, and dispose of any unused medication after 10 days.

Different types of Formulations: Tablet coated, Injection, Powder for suspension

Popular brand names: Valirol, Ticarvib, Clatiplus, Timentin, Yestic, Timcyn, Ticarset, Ticarnic, Ticarset, Clatiplus

Cephalosporins

Classification: Anti-Bacterial Agents

Chemical Name: (2R)-2-[(R)-[[(6R)-6-amino-6-carboxyhexanoyl]amino]-carboxy-methyl]-5-methylidene-2H-1,3-thiazine-4-carboxylic acid

Chemical Structure

Uses: Healthcare providers use cephalosporins to treat a variety of bacterial infections, especially for people who are allergic to penicillin, another common antibiotic. Some examples of infections that cephalosporins can treat include: - Skin or soft tissue infections, urinary tract infections (UTIs), strep throat, ear infections, pneumonia, sinus infections, meningitis, gonorrhea

Stability

- At room temperature, losses were much more rapid.
- Cefazolin sodium and ceftriaxone sodium retained at least 90% of their initial concentrations through 7 days and 5 days, respectively, when stored at 23°C.
- Ceftazidime remained stable for only 1 day at 23°C.

Storage Conditions

- Store tablets at controlled room temperature 68° to 77°F. (20°C to 25°C).
- Store the capsules at room temperature between 59-86°F.
- The tablets and powder for oral suspension should be stored at for oral suspension should be stored at controlled room temperature 15°C - 30°C.
- Suspension should be stored in a cool place, preferably a refrigerator.
- Solutions prior to reconstitution should be stored below 40°C.

Different types of Formulations

Tablet, Capsule, Solution, Suspension, Ointment, Injection

Popular brand names: Ancef, Kefazol, Ceclor, Cefaclor, Cefdinir, Ceftin, Zinacef, Duricef, Keflex, Keftabs

Streptomycin

Classification: Anti-Bacterial Agents

Chemical Name: 2-[(1R,2R,3S,4R,5R,6S)-3-(diaminomethylideneamino)-4-[(2R,3R,4R,5S)-3-[(2S,3S,4S,5R,6S)-4,5-dihydroxy-6-(hydroxymethyl)-3-(methylamino)oxan-2-yl]oxy-4-formyl-4-hydroxy-5-methyloxolan-2-yl]oxy-2,5,6-trihydroxycyclohexyl]guanidine

Chemical Structure

Uses

- Although streptomycin was the first antibiotic available for the treatment of mycobacterium tuberculosis, it is now largely a second line option due to resistance and toxicity.
- Streptomycin may also be used to treat a variety of other infections caused by susceptible strains of aerobic bacteria where other less toxic agents are ineffective.

Stability

- Streptomycin is stable at pH 6.0, 7.0, and 8.0 for a period of three months.

Storage Conditions

- Streptomycin can be stored under controlled room temperature. 15 mg/kg/day (max 1 gram), 5-7 days per week; 15 mg/kg/dose, 2-3 times per week after initial period of daily administration.

Different types of Formulations: Powder for solution, Liquid, Injection powder lyophilized for solution, Injection solution

Popular brand names: Ambistryn, Merstrep, Streptomac

Neomycin

Classification: Anti-Bacterial Agents

Chemical Name: (2R,3S,4R,5R,6R)-5-amino-2-(aminomethyl)-6-[(1R,2R,3S,4R,6S)-4,6-diamino-2-[(2S,3R,4S,5R)-4-[(2R,3R,4R,5S,6S)-3-amino-6-(aminomethyl)-4,5-dihydroxyoxan-2-yl]oxy-3-hydroxy-5-(hydroxymethyl)oxolan-2-yl]oxy-3-hydroxycyclohexyl]oxyoxane-3,4-diol

Uses

- Oral neomycin sulfate is indicated as an adjunctive therapy in hepatic coma (portal-system encephalopathy) by reducing ammonia-forming bacteria in the intestinal tract.

- It is strongly recommended that oral neomycin is only used in infections that are proven or strongly suspected to be caused by susceptible bacteria to reduce the risk of the development of drug-resistant bacteria.
- Neomycin, in combination with polymyxin B sulfates and hydrocortisone in otic suspensions, is used in the treatment of superficial bacterial infections of the external auditory canal caused by organisms susceptible to the antibiotics.

Chemical Structure

Neomycin	R^1	R^2
B	CH_2NH_2	H
C	H	CH_2NH_2

Stability
- Neomycin is a water-soluble polybasic antibiotic relatively stable in solution over a range of pH 2.0 to 9.0.

Storage Conditions
- Store neomycin at room temperature between 68°F and 77°F (20°C and 25°C). Keep this drug in a tightly closed container. Store it away from light.

Different types of Formulations: Solution, Gel, Cream, Ointment, Tablet

Popular brand names: Nyocin, Neos, Neozen, Neostar, Cortilate, Nebal, Sofrazen, Sofracare, Ledercort-N

Tetracycline

Classification: Anti-Bacterial Agents

Chemical Name: (4*S*,4a*S*,5a*S*,6*S*,12a*R*)-4-(dimethylamino)-1,6,10,11,12a-pentahydroxy-6-methyl-3,12-dioxo-4,4a,5,5a-tetrahydrotetracene-2-carboxamide

Chemical Structure

Uses

- Used to treat bacterial infections such as Rocky Mountain spotted fever, typhus fever, tick fevers, Q fever, rickettsialpox and Brill-Zinsser disease. May be used to treat infections caused by Chlamydiae spp., B. burgdorferi (Lyme disease), and upper respiratory infections caused by typical (S. pneumoniae, H. influenzae, and M. catarrhalis) and atypical organisms (C. pneumoniae, M. pneumoniae, L. pneumophila). May also be used to treat acne. Tetracycline may be an alternative drug for people who are allergic to penicillin.

Stability

- Tetracycline is stable in water for three days.

Storage Conditions

- Store in a cool, dry place, away from direct heat and light.
- Storage at body temperature (37°C) resulted in no activity loss.

Different types of Formulations: Tablet, film coated, Capsule, Ointment, Liquid, Syrup, Spray

Popular brand names: Resteclin, elwintra, rancycline, teravin, arcycline, cadicycline, tetrapex, tetracon, tetralab, tetlin

Doxycycline

Classification: Anti-Bacterial Agents

Chemical Name: (4S,4aR,5S,5aR,6R,12aR)-4-(dimethylamino)-1,5,10,11,12a-pentahydroxy-6-methyl-3,12-dioxo-4a,5,5a,6-tetrahydro-4H-tetracene-2-carboxamide

Chemical Structure

Uses

- Doxycycline is indicated for the treatment of various infections by gram-positive and gram-negative bacteria, aerobes and anaerobes, as well other types of bacteria. A complete list of organisms is available in the FDA label and in the "indications" section of this drug entry.
- The following are some of the major infections that may be treated with doxycycline.
- Rocky mountain spotted fever, typhus fever and the typhus group, Q fever, rickettsialpox, and tick fevers caused by Rickettsiae
- Respiratory tract infections caused by Mycoplasma pneumoniae
- Lymphogranuloma venereum caused by Chlamydia trachomatis
- Psittacosis (ornithosis) caused by Chlamydia psittaci
- Trachoma caused by Chlamydia trachomatis, although the infectious agent is not always eliminated as judged by immunofluorescence
- Inclusion conjunctivitis caused by Chlamydia trachomatis
- Uncomplicated urethral, endocervical or rectal infections in adults caused by Chlamydia trachomatis
- Nongonococcal urethritis caused by Ureaplasma urealyticum
- Relapsing fever due to Borrelia recurrentis

A note regarding anti-microbial resistance:

- It is important to note that doxycycline is not the drug of choice in the treatment of any type of staphylococcal infection. Up to 44 percent of strains of Streptococcus pyogenes and 74 percent of Streptococcus faecalis have been found to be resistant to tetracyclines. Therefore, tetracyclines such as doxycycline should not be used to treat streptococcal infections unless the microorganism has been demonstrated to be susceptible.

Stability

- Doxycycline hyclate for injection will retain potency for 12 hours at room temperature or 72 hours refrigerated after reconstitution at concentrations up to 1 mg/mL.

Storage Conditions

- Tablets, capsules, and syrup should be kept at room temperature 15°C to 30°C (59°F to 86°F) in tight, light resistant containers.
- Powder for injection should be stored at or below 25°C (77 F) and protected from light.

Different types **of Formulations:** Tablet, film coated, Tablet, delayed release, Kit, Powder, for suspension, Powder, Syrup, Capsule, delayed release pellets

Popular brand names: Befadox, Doxberry, Doxicip, Ceedox, Codox, Doxypal, Detab, Doxytop, Doxilak, Doxil

Minocycline

Classification: - Anti-Bacterial Agents

Chemical Name: - (4*S*,4*aS*,5*aR*,12*aR*)-4,7-bis(dimethylamino)-1,10,11,12*a*-tetrahydroxy-3,12-dioxo-4*a*,5,5*a*,6-tetrahydro-4*H*-tetracene-2-carboxamide

Chemical Structure

Uses

- Oral and topical minocycline are indicated to treat inflammatory lesions of acne vulgaris. Subgingival microspheres are indicated as an adjunct treatment in the reduction of pocket depth in adults with periodontitis.
- Oral and intravenous formulations are indicated to treat infections of susceptible microorganisms. These include *rickettsiae*, *Mycoplasma pneumoniae*, *Chlamydia trachomatis*, *Chlamydophila psittaci etc.*

Stability

- Minocycline hydrochloride remained stable for at least seven days at 24°C and 4°C.

Storage Conditions

- Store below 25°C in a dry place.
- Protect from light.
- Do not store in the bathroom.
- Keep all medications away from children and pets.

Different types of Formulations: Powder, Capsule, coated pellets, Aerosol, Injection, Kit, Tablet extended release, Tablet film coated

Popular brand names: Minoz, Minolox, Climin, Minima, Divaine, Megacyclin, Minotag, Minocyn, Minopride, Mynomin

Erythromycin

Classification: - Anti-Bacterial Agents

Chemical Name

(3*R*,4*S*,5*S*,6*R*,7*R*,9*R*,11*R*,12*R*,13*S*,14*R*)-6-[(2*S*,3*R*,4*S*,6*R*)-4-(dimethylamino)-3-hydroxy-6-methyloxan-2-yl]oxy-14-ethyl-7,12,13-trihydroxy-4-[(2*R*,4*R*,5*S*,6*S*)-5-hydroxy-4-

methoxy-4,6-dimethyloxan-2-yl]oxy-3,5,7,9,11,13-hexamethyl-oxacyclotetradecane-2,10-dione

Chemical Structure

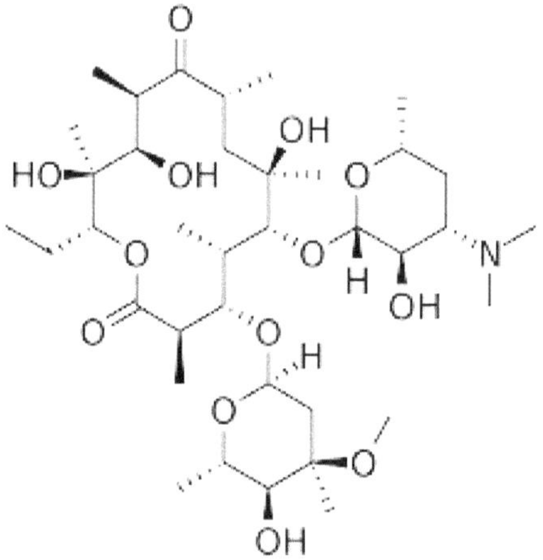

Uses

- Erythromycin is indicated in the treatment of infections caused by susceptible strains of various bacteria. The indications for erythromycin have been summarized by body system below:

Respiratory infections

- Mild to moderate upper respiratory tract infections caused by Streptococcus pyogenes, Streptococcus pneumoniae, or Haemophilus influenzae (when used concomitantly with appropriate doses of sulfonamides) can be treated with erythromycin.
- Mild to moderate lower-respiratory tract infections due to susceptible strains of Streptococcus pneumoniae or Streptococcus pyogenes may also be treated. Listeriosis caused by Listeria monocytogenes may also be treated with erythromycin. Erythromycin is indicated to treat pertussis (whooping cough) caused by Bordetella pertussis.
- It is effective in eliminating the causative organism from the nasopharynx of infected individuals, rendering them noninfectious.

Skin infections

- Mild to moderate skin or skin structure infections caused by Streptococcus pyogenes or Staphylococcus aureus may be treated with erythromycin, however, resistant staphylococcal organisms may emerge.
- Erythromycin can also be used to treat erythrasma, an infectious condition caused by Corynebacterium minutissimum.

Gastrointestinal infections

- Intestinal amebiasis caused by Entamoeba histolytica can be treated with oral erythromycin. Extraenteric amebiasis warrants treatment with other antimicrobial drugs.

Genital infections/STIs

- Erythromycin can be used as an alternative drug in treating acute pelvic inflammatory disease caused by N. gonorrheae in female patients who have demonstrated hypersensitivity or intolerance to penicillin. Syphilis, caused by Treponema pallidum, can be treated with erythromycin. It serves as an alternative treatment for primary syphilis in patients who have demonstrated penicillin hypersensitivity.
- Erythromycin can also be used in the primary stage of primary syphilis. Another approved indication of erythromycin is to treat chlamydial infections that cause conjunctivitis of the newborn, pneumonia of infancy, and urogenital infections occurring in pregnancy.
- It is indicated as an alternative option to tetracyclines for the treatment of uncomplicated rectal, urethral and endocervical infections in adults caused by Chlamydia trachomatis. Erythromycin can be used in nongonococcal urethritis can be used when tetracyclines cannot be administered.
- Finally, erythromycin is indicated to treat nongonococcal urethritis due to Ureaplasma urealyticum.

Stability

- The stability is influenced by the pH and by the presence of water.
- The influence of the pH on the stability of erythromycin was investigated even with the use of dimethyi isosorbide as co-solvent instead of water.

Storage Conditions

- Erythromycin should be stored at temperatures below 86°F (30°C).
- It is important to protect tablets from moisture and excessive heat.

Different types of Formulations: Granule, for suspension, Ointment, Tablet, film coated, Suspension, Capsule delayed release

Popular brand names: Althrocin, Eltocin, Etomin, Erycin, Eryster, Erythro, Elwicin, Elocin, Rekcin, Rethrocin

Azithromycin

Classification: Anti-Bacterial Agents

Chemical Name: (2R,3S,4R,5R,8R,10R,11R,12S,13S,14R)-11-[(2S,3R,4S,6R)-4-(dime-thylamino)-3-hydroxy-6-methyloxan-2-yl]oxy-2-ethyl-3,4,10-trihydroxy-13-[(2R,4R,5S, 6S)-5-hydroxy-4-methoxy-4,6-dimethyloxan-2-yl]oxy-3,5,6,8,10,12,14-heptamethyl-1-oxa-6-azacyclopentadecan-15-one

Uses
- Azithromycin should be used only to treat or prevent infections that are proven or strongly suspected to be caused by susceptible bacteria in order to prevent the development antimicrobial resistance and maintain the efficacy of azithromycin.

Chemical Structure

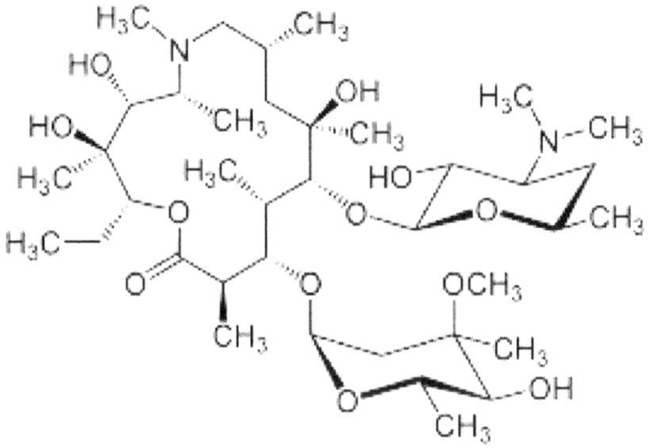

Adults
- Acute bacterial exacerbations of chronic obstructive pulmonary disease due to *Haemophilus influenzae, Moraxella catarrhalis* or *Streptococcus pneumoniae*
- Acute bacterial sinusitis due to *Haemophilus influenzae, Moraxella catarrhalis* or *Streptococcus pneumoniae*
- Community-acquired pneumonia due to *Chlamydophila pneumoniae, Haemophilus influenzae, Mycoplasma pneumoniae* or *Streptococcus pneumoniae* in patients appropriate for oral therapy
- Pharyngitis/tonsillitis caused by *Streptococcus pyogenes* as an alternative to first-line therapy in individuals who cannot use first-line therapy. Uncomplicated skin and skin structure infections due to *Staphylococcus aureus, Streptococcus pyogenes,* or *Streptococcus agalactiae.* Abscesses usually require surgical drainage.
- Urethritis and cervicitis due to *Chlamydia trachomatis* or *Neisseria gonorrhoeae.*
- Genital ulcer disease in men due to *Haemophilus ducreyi* (chancroid). Due to the small number of women included in clinical trials, the efficacy of azithromycin in the treatment of chancroid in women has not been established.

Pediatric Patients
- Acute otitis media caused by Haemophilus influenzae, Moraxella catarrhalis or Streptococcus pneumoniae
- Community-acquired pneumonia due to Chlamydophila pneumoniae, Haemophilus influenzae, Mycoplasma pneumoniae or Streptococcus pneumoniae in patients appropriate for oral therapy.

- Pharyngitis/tonsillitis caused by Streptococcus pyogenes as an alternative to first-line therapy in individuals who cannot use first-line therapy.

Stability

- Azithromycin decomposition occurs primarily via acid-catalyzed hydrolysis of the ether bond to the neutral cladinose sugar.
- Solution stability profile was generated for azithromycin over the pH range of 1.0 to 4.1 at 30°C.
- Stability was found to improve ten-fold for each unit increase in pH.

Storage Conditions

- Store azithromycin tablets, suspension, and extended-release suspension at room temperature and away from excess heat and moisture (not in the bathroom).
- Do not refrigerate or freeze the extended-release suspension.
- Discard any azithromycin suspension that is left over after 10 days or no longer needed.

Different types of Formulations: Tablet film coated, Solution, Drops, Powder for solution, Powder for suspension, Injection, Granule, for suspension, extended release

Popular brand names: Azibact, Azibest, Azicip, Azilide, Azeelarc, Azifast, Aziwok, Azitus, Azisafe, Azipro

Chloramphenicol

Classification: Anti-Bacterial Agents

Chemical Name: 2,2-dichloro-N-[(1R,2R)-1,3-dihydroxy-1-(4-nitrophenyl)propan-2-yl]acetamide

Chemical Structure

Uses

- Used in treatment of cholera, as it destroys the vibrios and decreases the diarrhea.
- It is effective against tetracycline-resistant vibrios.
- It is also used in eye drops or ointment to treat bacterial conjunctivitis.

Stability

- Degradation of chloramphenicol in aqueous solution is catalyzed by general acids and bases.
- The drug solution should be stored refrigerated and used within 30 days.

Storage Conditions

- Chloramphenicol eye drops (including single-use units) must be kept in a fridge (2°C to 8°C).
- Keep out of the sight and reach of children.
- Do not store the tube above 25 °C.
- Protect from light.

Different types of Formulations: Liquid, Solution, Ointment, Drops, Capsule

Popular brand names: Paraxin, Labchlor, Nicophenicol, Larmycetin, Dachlor, Denicol, Klorum, Elphenicol, Colonil, Biophenicol

Clindamycin

Classification: Anti-Bacterial Agents

Chemical Name: (2*S*,4*R*)-*N*-[(1*S*,2*S*)-2-chloro-1-[(2*R*,3*R*,4*S*,5*R*,6*R*)-3,4,5-trihydroxy-6-methylsulfanyloxan-2-yl]propyl]-1-methyl-4-propylpyrrolidine-2-carboxamide

Chemical Structure

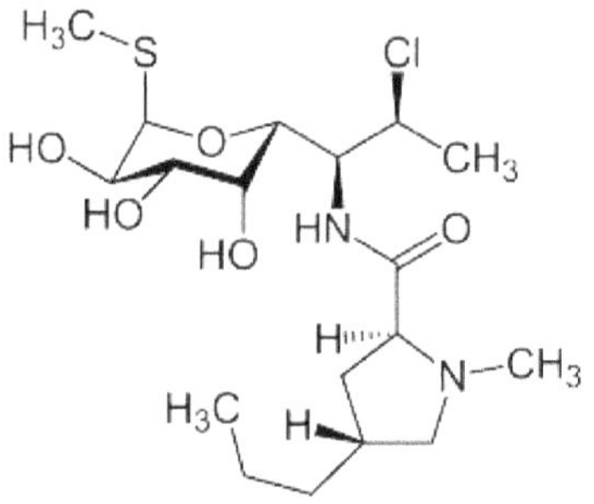

Uses

- In oral and parenteral formulations, clindamycin is indicated for the treatment of serious infections caused by susceptible anaerobic bacteria, as well as susceptible staphylococci, streptococci, and pneumococci.
- Used topically, it is indicated for the treatment of acne vulgaris and is available in combination with benzoyl peroxide or tretinoin for this purpose.
- Clindamycin is also indicated as a vaginal cream or suppository for the treatment of bacterial vaginosis in non-pregnant females.

Stability

- Clindamycin showed maximum stability at pH 3-5; however, high temperature studies indicated that not more than 10% degradation will occur in the pH range 1-6.5 after two years at 25°C.

Storage Conditions

- Keep this medication in the container it came in, tightly closed, and out of reach of children.
- Store it at room temperature and away from excess heat and moisture (not in the bathroom).
- Do not refrigerate clindamycin liquid because it may thicken and become hard to pour.

Different types of Formulations: Cream, Suppository, Injection, Solution, Capsule, Gel, Lotion.

Popular brand names: Dalacin, Camyda, Cliford, Clindatec, Clinox, Clintal, Clindamark, Clindak, Clynex, Maileed.

Multiple Choice Questions

1. The Crystalline Sodium or Potassium Salts are Slightly Soluble in:
   - (a) Ether
   - (b) Dioxane
   - (c) Water
   - (d) Chloroform

2. Streptomyces Orientalis Produces Which of the Following Antibiotics?
   - (a) Cephalosporins
   - (b) Cycloserine
   - (c) Bacitracin
   - (d) Vancomycin

3. Which of the Following Interferes with the Regeneration of the Monophosphate Form of Bactoprenol from the Pyrophosphate Form?
   - (a) Vancomycin
   - (b) Ampicillin
   - (c) Bacitracin
   - (d) Cephalosporins

4. Which of the Following Antibiotics is Effective in treating oral Candidiasis:
   - (a) Nystatin
   - (b) Bacitracin
   - (c) Tetracycline
   - (d) Griseofulvin

5. In Which of the Following Substances is Chlortetracycline Soluble:
   - (a) Water
   - (b) Ether
   - (c) Organic solvents
   - (d) All of the above

6. Which of the Following Fermentation Processes is Used in the Production of Penicillin?
   - (a) Aerobic fermentation followed by anaerobic fermentation
   - (b) Anaerobic fermentation
   - (c) Aerobic fermentation
   - (d) Anaerobic fermentation followed by aerobic fermentation

7. Streptomycin is Produced by Which of the Following Organisms?
   (a) Streptomyces noursei   (b) Streptomyces nodosus
   (c) Streptomyces fradiae   (d) Streptomyces griseus

8. Which of the Following Penicillin has Bes Gram-Negative Spectrum:
   (a) Nafcillin   (b) Ampicillin
   (c) Methicillin   (d) Penicillin V

9. Cell-wall Biosynthesis is Inhibited by Antibiotics by Inhibiting the Biosynthesis of Which of the following?
   (a) Lipopolysaccharide   (b) Cellulose
   (c) Peptidoglycan   (d) Proteins

10. What is the Typical Drug of Choice for Most Orofacial Infection?
    (a) Penicillin   (b) Tetracycline
    (c) Trimethoprim   (d) Ciprofloxacin

CHAPTER 13
Anti-Neoplastic Agents

Introduction

The chapter aims at providing the latest and pharmacopoeial information regarding some Anti-neoplastic agents (Mechlorethamine, Cyclophosphamide, Busulfan, Thiotepa, Mercaptopurine, Fluorouracil, Floxuridine, Cytarabine, Methotrexate, Azathioprine, Dactinomycin, Daunorubicin hydrochloride, Doxorubicin hydro-chloride, Etoposide, Vinblastine sulphate, Vincristine sulphate, Cisplatin, Mitotane, and Dromostanolone propionate) regarding their classification, chemical name, chemical structure, uses, stability, storage conditions, different types of formulations, and popular brand names.

Antineoplastic agents are drugs used for the treatment of cancer, malignancy, tumour, carcinoma, sarcoma, leukaemia, or neoplasm (Greek neo = new, Plasm = formation). Neoplasm refers to a group of diseases caused by several agents, namely, chemical compounds and radiant energy. Cancer is characterized by an abnormal and uncontrolled, division of cells, which produces tumours and invades adjacent normal tissues. Often, cancer cells separate themselves from the primary tumour, and are carried by the lymphatic system to reach distant sites of the organs, where they divide and form secondary tumours (metastasis).

Cell Cycle Kinetics

Two key aspects of cellular life are the following:

1. DNA synthesis and mitosis to produce new cells.
2. Cell differentiation that produces specialized cells.

Antineoplastic agents are classified as follows:

I. Alkylating agents
   (a) Nitrogen mustards: Mechlorethamine, Ifosamide, Cyclophosphamide, Melphalan, Uracil mustard, Chlorambucil, Estramustine
   (b) Alkyl Sulphonate: Busulfan
   (c) Nitrosoureas: Carmustine, Lomustine, Semustine, Chlorozotocin
   (d) Aziridines
   (e) Altretamine: Triethylene melamine, 4 (1-aziridinyl)-2,6-dimethoxy triazine
   (f) Methylhydrazines: Procarbazine, Dacarbazine

II. Antimetabolites
   (a) Pyrimdine analogues: 5-Flurouracil (5-FU), Capectitabine, Floxuridine, Cytarabine
   (b) Purine Analogues: 6-Mercaptopurine, 6-Thioguanine, Fludarabine
   (c) Folic acid analogues: Aminopterin, Methotrexate

III. Antibiotics
   (a) Anthracyclines: Daunorubicin, Doxorubicin, Carminomycin, Idarubicin, Epirubicin, Valrubicin
   (b) Bleomycin
   (c) Mitomycin C
   (d) Dactinomycin C or Actinomycin D
   (e) Plicamycin or Mithramycin

IV. Plant products
   (a) Vinca alkaloids: Vinorelbine, Vincristine, Vinblastine
   (b) Camptothecin Derivatives: Camptothecin, Irinotecan, Topotecan
   (c) Epipodophyllo toxins: Etoposide, Teniposide
   (d) Taxol derivatives: Paclitaxel, Docetaxel

V. Enzymes: L-asparaginase, Pegaspargase

VI. Hormones
   (a) Estorgenic derivatives: 17-β-Estradiol, Ethinyl estradiol, Diethylstilbosterol
   (b) Progestine derivatives: Progesterone, Progestins
   (c) Testosterone derivatives: Testosterone, Testosterone propionate, Testolactone
   (d) Steroidal anti-inflammatory agents: Prednisone, Flutamide (Nonsteroidal antiandrogen)
   (e) Miscellaneous agents: Mitotane, Tamoxifen, Letrozole, Dromostanolone, Pipobroman, Aminoglutethimide

VII. Immunotherapy: Interferon α-2a; Interferon-2b; Interferon α-n3; Aldesleukin, Diftitox, Denileukin; and Bucillus calmette-Guerin (BCG)

VIII. Monoclonal Antibodies: Rituximab, Gemtuzumab, Ozogamicin
 IX. Radio-therapeutic agents: Chromic phosphate P-32; Sodium phosphate P-32; Sodium iodide I-131; Strontium-89 chloride; Samarium, Sm 153 lexidronam
  X. Cytoprotective agents: Mesna, Amifostine, Dexrazoxane
 XI. Miscellaneous: Cisplastin, Carboplastin, Hydroxy urea, Gallium nitrate Mitoxantrone

Mechlorethamine

Classification: Alkylating Agents

Chemical Name: 2-chloro-*N*-(2-chloroethyl)-*N*-methylethanamine

Chemical Structure

Uses
- For the palliative treatment of Hodgkin's disease (Stages III and IV), lymphosarcoma, chronic myelocytic or chronic lymphocytic leukemia, polycythemia vera, mycosis fungoides, and bronchogenic carcinoma.
- Also, for the palliative treatment of metastatic carcinoma resulting in effusion.

Stability
- Drug is highly reactive and has a short stability and biologic half-life.
- Approximately 10% drug degradation takes place by 8 months.

Storage Conditions
- Store mechlorethamine gel in the refrigerator away from any food.
- Dispose of any mechlorethamine gel that is not used after 60 days.

Different types of Formulations: Powder, for solution, Gel

Popular brand names: Ledaga, Mustargen, Valchlor

Cyclophosphamide

Classification: Alkylating Agents

Chemical Name: N, N-bis(2-chloroethyl)-2-oxo-1,3,2λ^5-oxazaphosphinan-2-amine

Chemical Structure

Uses

- Cyclophosphamide is indicated for the treatment of malignant lymphomas, multiple myeloma, leukemias, mycosis fungoides (advanced disease), neuroblastoma (disseminated disease), adenocarcinoma of the ovary, retinoblastoma, and carcinoma of the breast.
- It is also indicated for the treatment of biopsy-proven minimal change nephrotic syndrome in pediatric patients.

Stability

- Cyclophosphamide is chemically and physically stable for 24 hours at room temperature or for six days in the refrigerator.

Storage Conditions

- It should be stored under refrigeration in glass containers and used within 14 days.
- Store vials at or below 25°C (77°F).

Different types of Formulations: Injection powder lyophilized for solution, Capsule, Injection, solution, Powder, for solution, Tablet

Popular brand names: Endoxan, Cycloxan, Cyclocel, Oncomide, Oncophos, Phosmid, Cysmide, Cyphos, Chophos

Busulfan

Classification: Alkylating Agents

Chemical Name: 4-methylsulfonyloxybutyl methanesulfonate

Chemical Structure

Uses

- For use in combination with cyclophosphamide as a conditioning regimen prior to allogeneic hematopoietic progenitor cell transplantation for chronic

myelogenous (myeloid, myelocytic, granulocytic) leukemia (FDA has designated busulfan as an orphan drug for this use).
- It is also used as a component of pretransplant conditioning regimens in patients undergoing bone marrow transplantation for acute myeloid leukemia and nonmalignant diseases.

Stability
- Solution is stable for 12 hours under refrigeration (2–8°C) or 3 hours at room temperature.

Storage Conditions
- Busulfan must be stored under refrigerated conditions between 2°C to 8°C (36°F to 46°F).

Different types of Formulations
- Injection solution, Injection powder solution, Solution, Tablet film coated

Popular brand names: Busulfex, Myleran

Thiotepa

Classification: Alkylating Agents

Chemical Name: tris(aziridin-1-yl)-sulfanylidene-λ^5-phosphane

Chemical Structure

Uses
- ThioTEPA is used a as conditioning treatment prior to allogeneic or autologous hematopoietic progenitor cell transplantation (HPCT) in hematological diseases in adult and pediatric patients.
- Also, when high dose chemotherapy with HPCT support it is appropriate for the treatment of solid tumors in adult and pediatric patients.

Stability
- When reconstituted with sterile water for injection, solutions of thiotepa should be stored in a refrigerator and used within 8 hours.

Storage Conditions
- Store intact vials under refrigeration (2-8°C).

Different types of Formulations: Injection powder for solution, Powder for solution

Popular brand names: Thioplan

Mercaptopurine

Classification: Antimetabolites

Chemical Name: 3,7-dihydropurine-6-thione

Chemical Structure

Uses
- For remission induction and maintenance therapy of acute lymphatic leukemia.

Stability
- The drug is susceptible to oxidative degradation which is increased by contact with water, exposure to light and alkaline pH.

Storage Conditions
- Store it at room temperature and away from excess heat and moisture (not in the bathroom).
- Mercaptopurine suspension can be kept at room temperature for up to 6 weeks after the bottle is opened for the first time.

Different types of Formulations: Tablet, Suspension

Popular brand names: Purinetone, Purinethol, Mercapto, Empurine, Puri-Nethol, 6-Mp

Fluorouracil

Classification: Antimetabolites

Chemical Name: 5-fluoro-1*H*-pyrimidine-2,4-dione

Chemical Structure

Uses
- For the topical treatment of multiple actinic or solar keratoses.

- In the 5% strength it is also useful in the treatment of superficial basal cell carcinomas when conventional methods are impractical, such as with multiple lesions or difficult treatment sites.
- Fluorouracil injection is indicated in the palliative management of some types of cancer, including colon, esophageal, gastric, rectum, breast, biliary tract, stomach, head and neck, cervical, pancreas, renal cell, and carcinoid.

Stability

- The stability of 5-fluorouracil has been tested in several solutions and containers and at various temperatures ranging from 4°C to 35°C.
- 5-Fluorouracil was stable when prepared in NS and stored in polyolefin bags at 5°C for 28 days.

Storage Conditions

- Store below 25°C.
- Do not refrigerate or freeze.
- Keep vial in the outer carton in order to protect from light.
- Store unopened vials of Fluorouracil Injection USP (50 mg/mL) between 15°C and 25°C.

Different types of Formulations: Solution, Liquid, Cream, Injection solution

Popular brand names: Fivocil, Fivoflu, Flocil, Flonida, Florac, Flucel, Flucil, Fludin, Fluonco, Flutas

Floxuridine

Classification: Antimetabolites

Chemical Name: 5-fluoro-1-[(2R,4S,5R)-4-hydroxy-5-(hydroxymethyl)oxolan-2-yl]pyrimidine-2,4-dione

Chemical Structure

Uses

- For palliative management of gastrointestinal adenocarcinoma metastatic to the liver, when given by continuous regional intra-arterial infusion in carefully selected patients who are considered incurable by surgery or other means.
- Also for the palliative management of liver cancer (usually administered by hepatic intra-arterial infusion).

Stability

- Floxuridine showed a decomposition product after 7 weeks of storage under room temperature.

Storage Conditions

- The sterile powder should be stored at 20° to 25°C (68° to 77°F)
- Reconstituted vials should be stored under refrigeration 2° to 8°C (36° to 46°F) for not more than 2 weeks.

Different types of Formulations

- Injection, powder, lyophilized, for solution

Popular brand names: Fudr, Fudf

Cytarabine

Classification: Antimetabolites

Chemical Name: 4-amino-1-[(2R,3S,4S,5R)-3,4-dihydroxy-5-(hydroxymethyl)oxolan-2-yl]pyrimidin-2-one

Chemical Structure

Uses

- For the treatment of acute non-lymphocytic leukemia, acute lymphocytic leukemia and blast phase of chronic myelocytic leukemia.
- Cytarabine is indicated in combination with daunorubicin for the treatment of newly-diagnosed therapy-related acute myeloid leukemia (t-AML) or AML with myelodysplasia-related changes (AML-MRC) in adults and pediatric patients 1 year and older.

Stability

- Solutions reconstituted with Bacteriostatic Water for Injection USP with benzyl alcohol may be stored at controlled room temperature, 15° to 30°C (59° to 86°F), for 48 hours.

Storage Conditions
- Cytarabine should not be stored at refrigerated temperatures (2-8°C).
- Protect from light. Retain in carton until time of use. Store at 20°C to 25°C (68°F to 77°F).
- Protect this material from exposure to light, and store it in a refrigerator.

Different types of Formulations: Injection suspension, Powder for solution, Injection lipid complex, Liquid

Popular brand names: Arasid, Biobin, Cybin-Pf, Cytalon, Cytabin, Cytostar, Cytaraside, Cytarine, Remcyta, Oncotar

Methotrexate

Classification: Antimetabolites

Chemical Name: (2S)-2-[[4-[(2,4-diaminopteridin-6-yl)methyl-methylamino]benzoyl]amino]pentanedioic acid

Chemical Structure

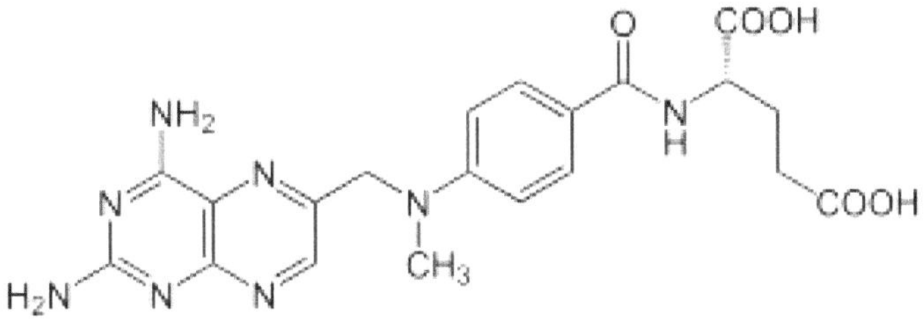

Uses
- Methotrexate oral solution is indicated for pediatric acute lymphoblastic leukemia and pediatric polyarticular juvenile idiopathic arthritis.4 Methotrexate injections for subcutaneous use are indicated for severe active rheumatoid arthritis, polyarticular juvenile idiopathic arthritis and severe, recalcitrant, disabling psoriasis.
- It is also used in the maintenance of acute lymphocytic leukemia.
- Methotrexate is also given before treatment with leucovorin to prolong relapse-free survival following surgical removal of a tumour in non-metastatic osteosarcoma.

Stability
- At concentrations of 0.2 and 20 mg/mL, methotrexate in 0.9% sodium chloride injection was found to be stable for 28 days when stored at 25 °C and protected from light.

Storage Conditions
- Store multi-dose vials between 15°C and 25°C.
- After the vials are punctured, the vials should be stored between 2°C and 8°C for a maximum of four weeks (30 days).
- Protect from light and freezing.

Different types of Formulations: Tablet, Solution, Injection, solution, Powder for solution, Liquid

Popular brand names: Mevotrex, Folitrax, Melcyl, Imotrax, Auratrex, Biotrexate, Mexate, Dermotrex, Meditrex, Nidtrex

Azathioprine

Classification: Antimetabolites

Chemical Name: 6-(3-methyl-5-nitroimidazol-4-yl)sulfanyl-7*H*-purine

Chemical Structure

Uses
- Azathioprine is an immunosuppressant used to prevent renal transplant rejection, treat rheumatoid arthritis, Crohn's disease, and ulcerative colitis.

Stability
- Azathioprine is stable in solution at neutral or acid pH but hydrolysis to mercaptopurine occurs in excess sodium hydroxide (0.1 N), especially on warming. Conversion to mercaptopurine also occurs in the presence of sulfhydryl compounds such as cysteine, glutathione, and hydrogen sulfide.

Storage Conditions
- Azathioprine tablets should be protected from light and stored at a temperature that does not exceed 35°C.
- Keep away from children. Keep in a cool, dry place, away from direct sunlight. Store at room temperature.

Different types of Formulations: Tablet, Powder for solution, Injection powder lyophilized for solution

Popular brand names: Azoran, Azr, Imuran, Azotrim, Aretha, Azarid, Imoprine, Innomune, Azofit, Azasis

Dactinomycin

Classification: Antibiotics, Antineoplastic

Chemical Name: 2-amino-4,6-dimethyl-3-oxo-1-*N*,9-*N*-bis[(3*R*,6*S*,7*R*,10*S*,16*S*)-7,11,14-trimethyl-2,5,9,12,15-pentaoxo-3,10-di(propan-2-yl)-8-oxa-1,4,11,14-tetrazabicyclo[14.3.0]nonadecan-6-yl]phenoxazine-1,9-dicarboxamide

Chemical Structure

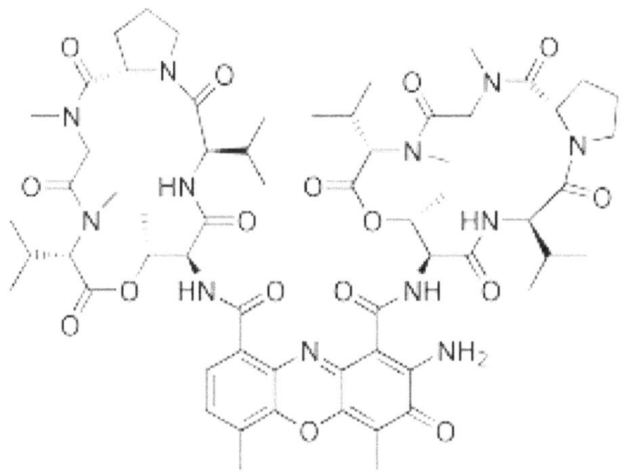

Uses
- For the treatment of Wilms' tumor, childhood rhabdomyosarcoma, Ewing's sarcoma and metastatic, nonseminomatous testicular cancer as part of a combination chemotherapy and/or multi-modality treatment regimen.

Stability
- Recommended final concentrations (>10 mcg/mL) in dextrose 5% in distilled water or normal saline should be stored for no more than 4 hours from reconstitution to completion of infusion.
- The most stable storage pH range is in buffer solution 5 to 7. Drug in distilled water and stored 5°C (refrigeration) preserved its stability for at least 150 days.

Storage Conditions
- Store at 20-25°C (68-77°F).
- Store intact vials at 20°C to 25°C (68°F to 77°F).
- Protect from light and humidity.

Different types of Formulations: Injection powder lyophilized for solution, Powder for solution

Popular brand names: Dacilon, Actinocin, Dactinoget, Dacmozen, Cosmegen

Daunorubicin Hydrochloride

Classification: Antibiotics, Antineoplastic

Chemical Name: (7S,9S)-9-acetyl-7-[(2R,4S,5S,6S)-4-amino-5-hydroxy-6-methyloxan-2-yl]oxy-6,9,11-trihydroxy-4-methoxy-8,10-dihydro-7H-tetracene-5,12-dione

Chemical Structure

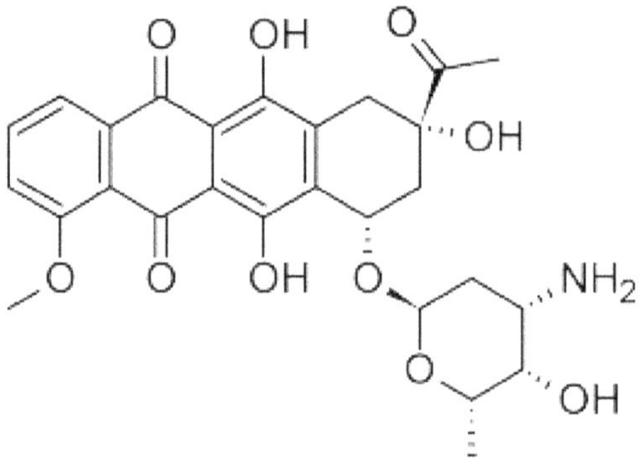

Uses
- For remission induction in acute nonlymphocytic leukemia (myelogenous, monocytic, erythroid) of adults and for remission induction in acute lymphocytic leukemia of children and adults.
- Daunorubicin is indicated in combination with cytarabine for the treatment of newly-diagnosed therapy-related acute myeloid leukemia (t-AML) or AML with myelodysplasia-related changes (AML-MRC) in adults and pediatric patients 1 year and older.

Stability
- Daunorubicin stored in polypropylene syringes at 4°C after diluting with water for injections was stable at least 43 days.
- Its degradation in aqueous solution was studied at 50°C and pH 0–14.
- The photodegradation of daunorubicin and stability of daunorubicin in infusion fluids have also been studied.

Storage Conditions
- Daunorubicin should be stored at 2 - 8°C, protected from light.

Different types of Formulations: Powder for solution, Injection powder for solution, Solution, Injection lipid complex, Suspension

Popular brand names: Daunotec, Dauneon, Daunoside

Doxorubicin Hydrochloride

Classification: Antibiotics, Antineoplastic

Chemical Name: (7*S*,9*S*)-7-[(2*R*,4*S*,5*S*,6*S*)-4-amino-5-hydroxy-6-methyloxan-2-yl]oxy-6,9,11-trihydroxy-9-(2-hydroxyacetyl)-4-methoxy-8,10-dihydro-7*H*-tetracene-5,12-dione

Chemical Structure

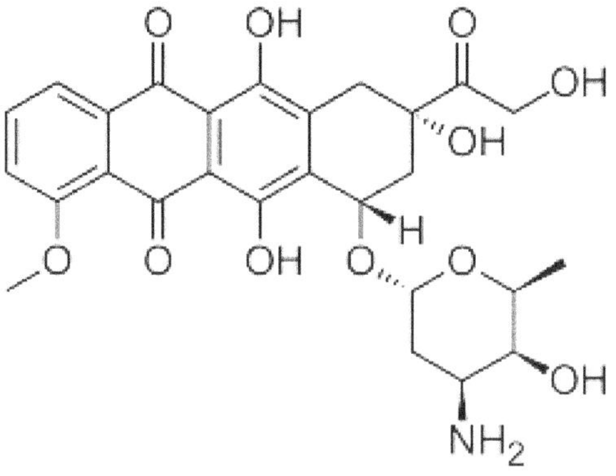

Uses

- Doxorubicin is used to produce regression in disseminated neoplastic conditions like acute lymphoblastic leukemia, acute myeloblastic leukemia, Wilms' tumor, neuroblastoma, soft tissue and bone sarcomas, breast carcinoma, ovarian carcinoma, transitional cell bladder carcinoma, thyroid carcinoma, gastric carcinoma, Hodgkin's disease, malignant lymphoma and bronchogenic carcinoma in which the small cell histologic type is the most responsive compared to other cell types.
- Doxorubicin is also indicated for use as a component of adjuvant therapy in women with evidence of axillary lymph node involvement following resection of primary breast cancer.

Stability

- Doxorubicin is stable (loss in potency of less than 10%) for 24 days.
- It is found extremely unstable to alkaline hydrolysis even at room temperature, unstable to acid hydrolysis at 80°C, and to oxidation at room temperature.

Storage Conditions

- Store in a refrigerator (2°C - 8°C).
- Keep the vial in the outer carton in order to protect from light.
- For storage conditions of the diluted medicinal product, in-use stability has been demonstrated in 0.9% sodium chloride injection and 5% dextrose injection for up to 28 days at 2 – 8°C and for up to 7 days at 25°C when prepared in glass containers protected from light.

Different types of Formulations: Solution, Powder for solution, Injection solution, Injection suspension, Injectable liposomal, Suspension

Popular brand names: Doxilyd, Adrim, Doxorex, Dobixin, Doxotero, Adrosal, Cadria, Doxox, Doxoform, Doxutec

Etoposide

Classification: - Antineoplastic Agents

Chemical Name: (5S,5aR,8aR,9R)-5-[[(2R,4aR,6R,7R,8R,8aS)-7,8-dihydroxy-2-methyl -4,4a,6,7,8,8a-hexahydropyrano[3,2-d][1,3]dioxin-6-yl]oxy]-9-(4-hydroxy-3,5-dimetho-xyphenyl)-5a,6,8a,9-tetrahydro-5H-[2]benzofuro[6,5-f][1,3]benzodioxol-8-one

Chemical Structure

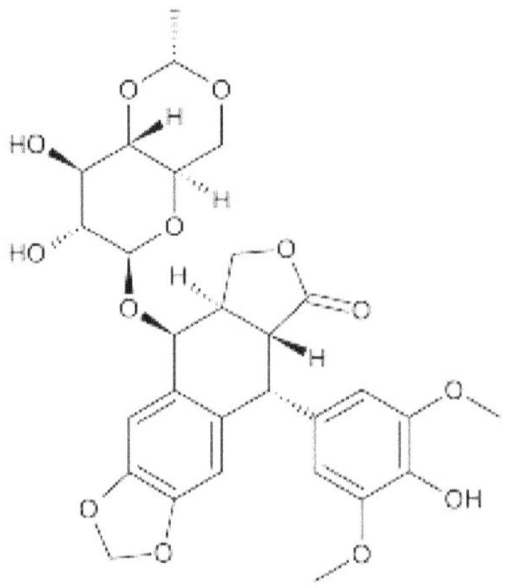

Uses

- For use in combination with other chemotherapeutic agents in the treatment of refractory testicular tumors and as first line treatment in patients with small cell lung cancer.
- Also used to treat other malignancies such as lymphoma, non-lymphocytic leukemia, and glioblastoma multiforme.

Stability

- Etoposide is supposed to be stable up to 96 h at 400 mg/L in a NaCl 0.9 % solution and in dextrose 5 % in water.

Storage Conditions

- Store solutions in DMSO at 4°C.
- For long term storage prepare aliquots and store at -20°C.
- Store the unopened vials under refrigeration 2° to 8°C
- Store lyophilized or in solution at -20°C, desiccated.

Different types of Formulations: Liquid, Injection powder, Injection solution, Injection lyophilized, Capsule, Solution

Popular brand names: Etoplast, Etosid, Etovel, Lastet, Posid, Etopa, Fytosid, Oncosid, Topok, Etoglan

Vinblastine Sulphate

Classification: Antineoplastic Agents

Chemical Name: methyl (1R,9R,10S,11R,12R,19R)-11-acetyloxy-12-ethyl-4-[(13S, 15R,17S)-17-ethyl-17-hydroxy-13-methoxycarbonyl-1,11-diazatetracyclo[13.3.1.0^{4,12}.0^{5,10}] nonadeca-4(12),5,7,9-tetraen-13-yl]-10-hydroxy-5-methoxy-8-methyl-8,16-diazapentacyclo[10.6.1.0^{1,9}.0^{2,7}.0^{16,19}]nonadeca-2,4,6,13-tetraene-10-carboxylate

Chemical Structure

Uses

- For treatment of breast cancer, testicular cancer, lymphomas, neuroblastoma, Hodgkin's and non-Hodgkin's lymphomas, mycosis fungoides, histiocytosis, and Kaposi's sarcoma.

Stability

- Vinblastine solutions in 0.9% sodium chloride solution for injection (1 mg/mL) in polypropylene syringes at 25°C protected from light are stable for up to one month.

Storage Conditions

- Store the intact vials at 2°C to 8°C (36°F to 46°F).
- Protect from light.

Different types of Formulations: Powder for solution, Liquid, Solution, Injection powder lyophilized for solution

Popular brand names: Cytoblastin, Vintest

Vincristine Sulphate

Classification: - Antineoplastic Agents

Chemical Name

methyl   (1*R*,9*R*,10*S*,11*R*,12*R*,19*R*)-11-acetyloxy-12-ethyl-4-[(13*S*,15*S*,17*S*)-17-ethyl-17-hydroxy-13-methoxycarbonyl-1,11-diazatetracyclo[13.3.1.0^{4,12}.0^{5,10}]nonadeca-4(12),5,7,9-tetraen-13-yl]-8-formyl-10-hydroxy-5-methoxy-8,16-diazapentacyclo[10.6.1.0^{1,9}.0^{2,7}.0^{16,19}]nonadeca-2,4,6,13-tetraene-10-carboxylate

Chemical Structure

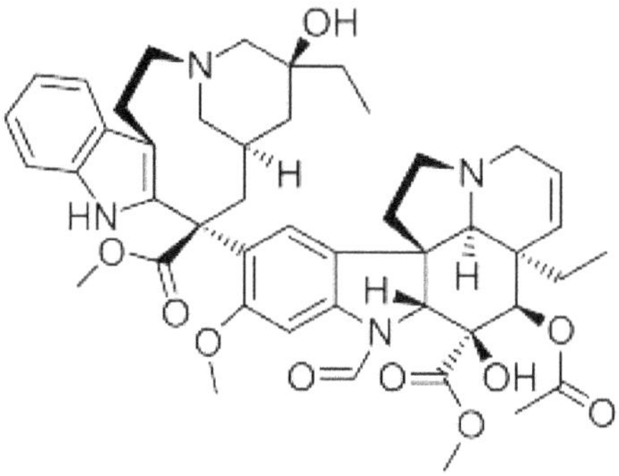

Uses

- Treatment of acute lymphocytic leukemia (ALL), Hodgkin lymphoma, non-Hodgkin lymphomas, Wilms' tumor, neuroblastoma, rhabdomyosarcoma.
- Liposomal vincristine is indicated for the treatment of relapsed Philadelphia chromosome-negative (Ph-) acute lymphoblastic leukemia (ALL).

Stability

- Vincristine Sulfate Injection, USP when diluted with 0.9% Sodium Chloride Injection in concentrations from 0.0015 mg/mL to 0.08 mg/mL is stable for up to 24 hours when protected from light or 8 hours under normal light at 25°C.

Storage Conditions

- Vials should be stored in refrigerator (2°C to 8°C) and protected from light.

Different types of Formulations: Liquid, Solution, Powder for solution, Kit, Injection solution

Popular brand names: Vinlon, Nucris, Onvinc, Kristina V, Vincryst, Vinrosa, Paracristine, Biocristin, Unicristin, Oncocristin

Cisplatin

Classification:

Chemical Name: azane; dichloroplatinum

Chemical Structure

Uses: For the treatment of metastatic testicular tumors, metastatic ovarian tumors and advanced bladder cancer.

Stability

- Cisplatin, both undiluted in glass containers and diluted with NaCl 0.9% in PE bags, remains stable (<10% degradation) for at least 30 days at room temperature when protected from light.

Storage Conditions

- Do not store above 25°C.
- Do not refrigerate or freeze.
- The diluted solution should be protected from light.
- Store injection vials at 15°C to 25°C (59°F to 77°F).
- Keep container in the outer carton in order to protect from light.

Different types of Formulations: Injection powder lyophilized for solution, Liquid, Solution, Injection solution

Popular brand names: Cistero, Celplat, Kemoplat, Cismax, Cistix, Ciswel, Cytoplatin, Platipar, Platikem, Duplant

Mitotane

Classification: Antineoplastic Agents

Chemical Name: 1-chloro-2-[2,2-dichloro-1-(4-chlorophenyl)ethyl]benzene

Chemical Structure

Uses

- For treatment of inoperable adrenocortical tumours; Cushing's syndrome.

Stability

- Significant degradation has been reported under basic, acidic stress, and UV light.

Storage Conditions
- Store bottles at 25°C (77°F); excursions permitted between 15°C and 30°C (59°F-86°F).

Different types of Formulations
- Tablet

Popular brand names: Lysodren

Dromostanolone Propionate

Classification: Androgenic anabolic steroid

Chemical Name: (2R,5S,8R,9S,10S,13S,14S,17S)-17-hydroxy-2,10,13-trimethyl-1,2,4,5,6,7,8,9,11,12,14,15,16,17-tetradecahydrocyclopenta[a]phenanthren-3-one

Chemical Structure

Uses
- Drostanolone is indicated in postmenopausal women with recurrent breast cancer, in a combined hormone therapy.

Stability
- Susceptible to thermal decomposition and Strong oxidizing agents. Formation of toxic gases is possible during heating or in case of fire.

Storage Conditions
- Vials for parenteral administration should be stored at room temperature (15 to 30°C).
- Keep away from heat, moisture and light.
- Keep all medicine out of the reach of children.

Different types of Formulations
- Injection

Popular brand names: Drolban, Masteril, Masteron, Drolban, Masteril

Multiple Choice Questions

1. Select the INCORRECT statement
   (a) The resistance towards 6-MP is due to alteration of HGPRT
   (b) Allopurinol increases the action of 6-MP
   (c) Azathioprine is prodrug of 6-MP
   (d) 6-MP is given with leucovorin

2. Select the INCORRECT statement
   (a) Leucovorin is given along with 5-FU to decrease megaloblastic anemia
   (b) Capecitabine is a prodrug of 5-FU converted by tumor specific thymidine phosphorylase
   (c) The dose of 5-FU should be reduced in dihydropyridine dehydrogenase deficient patients
   (d) Cytarabine inhibits DNA polymerase

3. The drug corresponding to letter 'O' in the R-CHOP regimen used for chemotherapy of lymphocytic leukemia is
   (a) Omalizumab   (b) OndanPageron
   (c) Vincristine   (d) Prednisone

4. The pathogenesis of cancer involves
   (a) Conversion of oncogenes to proto-oncogenes
   (b) Conversion of protooncogenes to oncogenes
   (c) Activation of tumor suppressor genes
   (d) Inactivation of anti-apoptic factors

5. Choose the WRONG statement
   (a) In the liver, cyclophosphamide splits in to phosphoramide mustard and acrolein
   (b) Phosphoramide mustard causes haemorrhagic cystitis
   (c) It is treated by N-Acetylcysteine
   (d) Cisplatin is a polar co-ordination complex

6. Rituximab is particularly used for
   (a) Breast cancer   (b) Prostate cancer
   (c) B-cell lymphomas   (d) Renal tumor

7. Which of the following anticancer agent produces crystalluria
   (a) Sulfamethoxazole   (b) Vincristine
   (c) 6-Mercaptopurine   (d) Methotrexate

8. The resistance to the majority of the anticancer agents is mainly due to
   (a) Increased metabolism
   (b) Alteration of enzymatic activity
   (c) Drug efflux from target tissues
   (d) Receptor down regulation

9. Choose the WRONG combination of drug and its main target
   (a) Irinotecan, topoisomerase I
   (b) Rituximab, HER2 antibody
   (c) Bevacizumab, vascular endothelium growth factor
   (d) Dactinomycin, DNA polymerase inhibitor

10. Choose the WRONG combination of drug and its main target
    (a) Imatinib, tyrosine kinase inhibitor
    (b) Gefitinib, Epidermal growth factor receptor
    (c) Trastuzumab, HER2 growth receptor
    (d) Etoposide, Topoisomerase I

Practicals

Experiment 01: Assay of Calcium Gluconate by Complexometry

AIM: To perform the assay of the given sample of Calcium Gluconate.

Requirements:

Apparatus required: Burette, Burette stand, pipette, conical flask, volumetric flask, funnel etc.

Chemicals required: Calcium gluconate, 0.05M EDTA solution, pH 10 buffer solution, calcium gluconate, ammonia, calcium chloride, ammonium chloride (NH4Cl), magnesium sulphate, hydrochloric acid, and solochrome black-T indicator or mordant black II.

Principle: The assay of calcium gluconate is based upon a replacement complexometric titration. Magnesium forms a complex with the mixture of indicator mordant black II which indicates the first colour. The magnesium-indicator complex is more stable compared to the calcium-indicator complex; hence calcium does not affect the magnesium-indicator complex. When titrated against disodium edetate, calcium and EDTA formed.When all of the calcium has been consumed, the drop of EDTA breaks the magnesium-indicator complex, allowing the free indicator to form a complex with the magnesium. The endpoint is determined by detecting the second colour at that time.

$$Mg^+ + In^- \longrightarrow Mg\text{-}In$$
$$Ca^+ + EDTA \longrightarrow Ca\text{-}EDTA$$
$$Mg\text{-}In + EDTA \longrightarrow Mg\text{-}EDTA + In^-$$

Preparation of 0.05M Magnesium Sulphate:
- Take 600 mg of anhydrous $MgSO_4$ and dissolve in 50 ml of distilled water in a volumetric flask, and properly mixing it.
- Once it has completely dissolved, make up the volume to 100 ml.

Preparation of Strong Ammonia- Ammonium Chloride Solution:

- Take 10 ml of water and 20 ml of strong ammonia solution in a beaker and saturate it with ammonium chloride.

Titration Procedure:

- All glassware should be cleaned and dried according to standard laboratory procedures.
- Before filling the burette for the titration, rinse it with distilled water and then pre-rinse it with a portion of the titrant solution. Pre-rinsing is required to make sure that all solution in the burette is the desired solution, not a contaminated or diluted solution.
- Take the unknown stock solution of titrant in a clean and dry beaker then fill the burette using the funnel.
- Remove air bubbles from the burette and adjust the reading to zero.
- Take 0.5 gm of calcium gluconate and pour it into a conical flask, and dissolve in 50 ml of warm water.
- Allow the solution to cool to ambient temperature, add 5 ml of 0.05 M magnesium sulphate solution
- Using a pipette, add 10.00 ml of strong ammonia-ammonium chloride solution.
- Then, as an indicator, add 2 drops of mordant black II mixture and properly mix it.
- Titrate the sample solution with standardized disodium edetate until the endpoint is reached. The actual endpoint is indicated by a change in the color of the solution.
- Properly record the readings of the burette.
- To get accurate results, repeat the titration three times.
- Take the precise reading of any two similar observations and calculate the percentage purity of calcium gluconate.
- For a blank reading (B), repeat the titration using the same procedure but without the calcium gluconate.

Observation Table:

Table 1 Titration of calcium gluconateVs disodium edetate

| S. No. | Content in conical flask | Burette reading | | Volume of titrant used (ml) (Precise reading) |
		Initial	Final	
1				
2				

Table 2 Titration of the Aspirin Sample

S. No.	Content in conical flask	Burette reading		Volume of titrant used (ml) (Precise reading)
		Initial	Final	
1				
2				

Calculation:

$$\%\text{purity} = \frac{V \times E \times AM \times 100}{W \times RM}$$

Where,

V is a volume of EDTA used

$$V = A - B$$

A is the volume of EDTA used in the titration with calcium gluconate

B is the volume of EDTA used in the titration without calcium gluconate

E is an equivalent factor

AM is an actual molarity

RM is a required molarity

W is the weight of the sample

For 0.1 ml of calcium gluconate, the equivalent factor of 0.05 M disodium edetate is 0.02242

Results: The percentage purity of calcium gluconate was found to be_____.

Precaution:

- Usually, an air bubble is present in the nozzle of the burette,it must be removed before taking the initial reading.
- There should not be any leakage from the burette during titration.
- Keep your eye in level with the liquid surface while taking the burette reading or while reading the pipette or measuring flask etc.
- Always read lower meniscus in case of colourless solution and upper meniscus in case of coloured solutions.
- Do not blow through the pipette to expel the last drop of solution from it,simply touch the inner surface of the titration flask with the nozzle of the pipette for this purpose.
- Shaking of the titration flask should be continuous during adding the solution from the burette.

- Use your index finger while pipetting the solution.
- Do not waste your time in bringing the burette reading to zero before each titration.

Experiment 02: Assay of Ferrous Sulphate by a Redox Titration

AIM: To perform the assay of the given sample of Ferrous Sulphate.

Requirements:

Apparatus required: Burette, Burette stand, pipette, conical flask, volumetric flask, funnel etc.

Chemicals required: Ferrous sulphate, 0.1N $KMnO_4$, 0.1N oxalic acid, dil. H_2SO_4.

Principle: Ferrous sulphate is an example of reducing agent and this is an example of redox titration. $KMnO_4$ is a powerful oxidant. In the presence of the dil.H_2SO_4 ferrous sulphate is oxidised to ferric sulphate. As soon as oxidation of ferrous sulphate is completed addition of drop of $KMnO_4$ to the resulting solution permanent pink colour is obtained which indicates the end point. No indicator is required as $KMnO_4$ is a self-indicator.

Theory: A redox titration is a titration in which the analyte and titrant react through an oxidation–reduction reaction. As in acid–base titrations, the endpoint of a redox titration is often detected using an indicator. Ferrous sulphate is an essential body mineral. It is used to treat and prevent iron deficiency anaemia as it is type of iron normally, we get from food. As iron helps body to make healthy red blood cells which carry oxygen around the body.

Procedure:

1. **Standardization of 0.1N Potassium permanganate solution:** Into a conical flask pipette out exactly 10 ml of 0.1 N oxalic acid.

   Add 10 ml dil H_2SO_4 and boil the contents of the flask at 60 to 70°C.

   Titrate the contents of the flask against 0.1 N $KMnO_4$ solution until a faint pink color is obtained.

   Repeat the titration to get concurrent values.

2. **For assay of ferrous sulphate:** Weigh accurately about 1 gm of $FeSO_4$ and dissolve in 20 ml of dilute H_2SO_4.

   Titrate against 0.1 N $KMnO_4$ solution till a permanent pink colour is obtained.

   Repeat the titration to get concurrent values.

   0.1 N oxalic acid = Weigh accurately 6.3 g $(COOH)_2.2H_2O$ and transfer it to a volumetric flask (1 litre), half-filled with distilled water. Shake well and make the volume up to the mark. Label it as N/10 oxalic acid solution.

   Note: If anhydrous oxalic acid (COOH) is available then dissolve 4.5 g of the acid in one litre of distilled water to get 0.1 N oxalic acid solution.

0.1 N KMnO4 = Dissolve 3.2 g $KMnO_4$ in one litre of distilled water. Boil it for 10-15 minutes and then allow to stand for few days and then filter it through glass wool.

Observation Table:

Table 1 Titration of 0.1 N oxalic acid Vs 0.1 N $KMnO_4$

Sr. No.	Content in conical flask	Burette reading		Volume of titrant used (ml) (Precise reading)
		Initial	Final	
1				
2				

Table 2 Titration of $FeSO_4$ solution Vs 0.1 N $KMnO_4$

Sr. No.	Content in conical flask	Burette reading		Volume of titrant used (ml) (Precise reading)
		Initial	Final	
1				
2				

Calculation:

$$\% \text{ Purity of } FeSO_4 = \frac{\text{Vol. of 0.1 N } KMnO_4 \times \text{I. P. Factor} \times 100 \times \text{N of } KMnO_4 \text{ (actual)}}{\text{Weight of } FeSO_4 \times \text{N of } KMnO_4 \text{ (exp)}}$$

IP Factor: Each ml of 0.1 N KMnO4 is equivalent to 0.0278 g of FeSO4.

Result: The percentage purity of the given sample of $FeSO_4$ is______.

Experiment 03: Assay of Sodium Chloride by Mohr's Method

AIM: To determine the percentage purity of given sample of sodium chloride using standard 0.1 N $AgNO_3$ (Mohr's Method).

Requirements:

Apparatus required: Burette, Burette stand, pipette, conical flask, volumetric flask, funnel etc.

Chemicals required: LR grade silver nitrate ($AgNO_3$), sodium chloride (NaCl), and potassium chromate (K_2CrO_4), etc.

Principle: Precipitation titrations are based upon reactions that yield ionic compounds of limited solubility. The most important precipitating reagent is silver nitrate. Titrimetric methods based upon silver nitrate are sometimes termed argentometric methods. Potassium chromate can serve as an end point indicator for the argentometric determination of chloride, bromide and cyanide ions by reacting with silver ions to form a brick-red silver chromate precipitate in the equivalence point region.

When silver nitrate is directly titrated against sodium chloride, it forms a white precipitate $AgNO_3$ with NaCl. When all of the NaCl has been consumed, it reacts with K_2CrO_4 and the endpoint is detected as a brick red colour due to the formation of silver chromate and potassium nitrate.

    A. Preparation and standardization of silver nitrate (0.1 M).

    B. To perform the assay of sodium chloride.

Preparation of 5% K_2CrO_4(indicator): 1.0 g of K CrO was dissolved in 20 mL of distilled water.

Standard Silver Nitrate (0.1M) Solution:
- Take 16.99 gm of silver nitrate using a pipette, dissolve in 500 ml of distilled water in a volumetric flask, and properly mixing it.
- Once it has completely dissolved, makc up thc volume to 1000 ml.

Standard Sodium Chloride (0.1M) Solution:
- Take 05.84 gm of previously dried sodium chloride and dissolve in 500 ml of distilled water in a volumetric flask, and properly mixing it.
- Once it has completely dissolved, make up the volume to 1000 ml.

Titration procedure:
- All glassware should be cleaned and dried according to standard laboratory procedures.

- Before filling the burette for the titration, rinse it with distilled water and then pre-rinse it with a portion of the titrant solution. Pre-rinsing is required to make sure that all solution in the burette is the desired solution, not a contaminated or diluted solution.
- Take the unknown stock solution of titrant in a clean and dry beaker then fill the burette using the funnel.
- Remove air bubbles from the burette and adjust the reading to zero.
- Take 10.00 ml of prepared sample solution of sodium chloride and pour it into a conical flask.
- Add 2-3 drops of potassium chromate solution as an indicator.
- Titrate the sample solution with silver nitrate solution until the endpoint is reached.
- The actual endpoint of the titration is indicated by a brick red color at the end of the reaction.
- To get accurate results, repeat the titration three times.
- Properly record the readings of the burette.
- Take their mean and calculate the molarity of the silver nitrate solution.

Observation Table:

Table 1 Standardization of $AgNO_3$

Sr. No.	Content in conical flask	Burette reading		Volume of titrant used (ml) (Precise reading)
		Initial	Final	
1				
2				

Table 2 Titration of Sodium Chloride Vs 0.1M Silver Nitrate

Sr. No.	Content in conical flask	Burette reading		Volume of titrant used (ml) (Precise reading)
		Initial	Final	
1				
2				

Calculation:

$$\% \text{ Sodium Chloride (NaCl)} = \frac{V \times E \times AM \times 100}{W \times RM}$$

Where,

V is a volume of silver nitrate used

E is an equivalent factor

AM is an actual molarity

RM is a required molarity

W is the weight of the sample

For 1 ml of 0.1 M silver nitrate, the equivalent factor of PHP is 0.005845

Results: The percentage purity of the sodium chloride (NaCl) sample was found to be_____.

Experiment 04: Assay of Ibuprofen by Alkalimetry

Aim: To perform the assay of Ibuprofen by alkalimetry.

Requirements:

Apparatus required: Burette, Burette stand, pipette, conical flask, volumetric flask, funnel etc.

Chemicals required: 20 tablets of ibuprofen, chloroform, sodium hydroxide.

Principle: The term alkalimetry refers to that part of volumetric chemical analysis which enables us to work out the concentration of an acid solution using an alkaline solution at a known concentration and a suitable indicator. Ibuprofen is NSAID mean non steroidal anti-inflammatory drug. Ibuprofen is used to reduce fever and treat pain or inflammation caused by many conditions such as headache, toothache, back pain, arthritis, menstrual cramps, or minor injury. It works by reducing hormones that cause inflammation and pain in the body.as for precaution do not use ibuprofen before or after heart surgery.

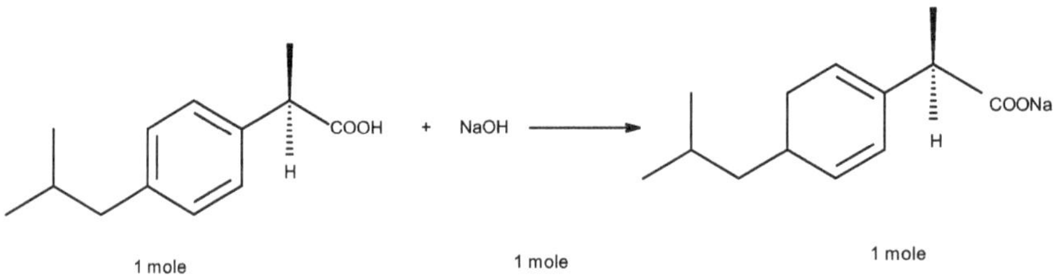

Procedure:

- 20 ibuprofen tablets which is previously selected at random is weighed and powdered.
- A quantity of powder containing 0.5 g ibuprofen with 20 ml chloroform is extracted for 15 minutes and filtered through a sintered glass crucible.
- The residue with 3 × 10 ml chloroform is washed and then combined. Filtrate is gently evaporated just to dryness in a current of air. Then the residue is dissolved in 100 ml with ethanol (96%) previously neutralized to phenolphthalein solution.
- The solution with 0.1M sodium hydroxide is titrated to end point with phenolphthalein solution as the indicator. The content of ibuprofen if each ml of 0.1M sodium hydroxide is equivalent to 0.02063 g of $C_{13}H_{18}O_2$ is calculated.

Observation Table:

Standardization of sodium hydroxide

Sr. No.	Content in conical flask	Burette reading		Volume of titrant used (ml) (Precise reading)
		Initial	Final	
1				
2				

Assay of ibuprofen

Sr. No.	Content in conical flask	Burette reading		Volume of titrant used (ml) (Precise reading)
		Initial	Final	
1.				
2.				
3.				

Blank titration

Sr. No.	Content in conical flask	Burette reading		Volume of titrant used (ml) (Precise reading)
		Initial	Final	
1.				
2.				
3.				

Calculation:

Equivalent factor

$$1 \text{ ml of } 0.1N \text{ NaOH} = 0.206 \text{ gm/mol of ibuprofen } (C_{13}H_{18}O_2)$$

For standardization

$$N1V1/ N2V2$$

Where,

N1 = Normality of NaOH given

V1 = Volume of primary standard

N2 = Calculated Normality (find out)

V2 = Burette reading

For Assay

$$\% \text{ Purity of } Ibuprofen = \frac{\text{Vol. of } 0.1 \text{ N NaOH} \times \text{I. P. Factor} \times 100 \times \text{N of NaOH (actual)}}{\text{Weight of Ibuprofen} \times \text{N of NaOH (exp)}}$$

Results: The percentage purity of the Ibuprofen was found to be______.

Experiment 05: Assay of Ascorbic Acid by Iodometry

Aim: To perform the ascorbic acid by iodometry.

Requirements:

Apparatus required: Burette, Burette stand, pipette, conical flask, volumetric flask, funnel etc.

Chemicals required: Vitamin-C tablets containing Ascorbic acid in the range of 100-500 mg, Potassium iodate, Ascorbic acid, sulphuric acid, sodium thiosulphate solution, starch as an indicator

Principle: Ascorbic acid otherwise known as Vitamin C is antiscorbutic. It is present in citrus fruits, gooseberry, bitter gourd etc. in high amount. Generally it is present in all fresh vegetables and fruits. It is water soluble and heat-labile vitamin. The method described below is easy, rapid and a large number of samples can be analyzed in a short time Ascorbic acid reduces the 2, 6-dichlorophenol indophenol dye to a colorless leuco-base. The ascorbic acid gets oxidized to dehydroascorbic acid. Though the dye is a blue coloured compound, the end point is the appearance of pink colour. The dye is pink colour in acidic medium. Oxalic acid is used as the titrating medium.

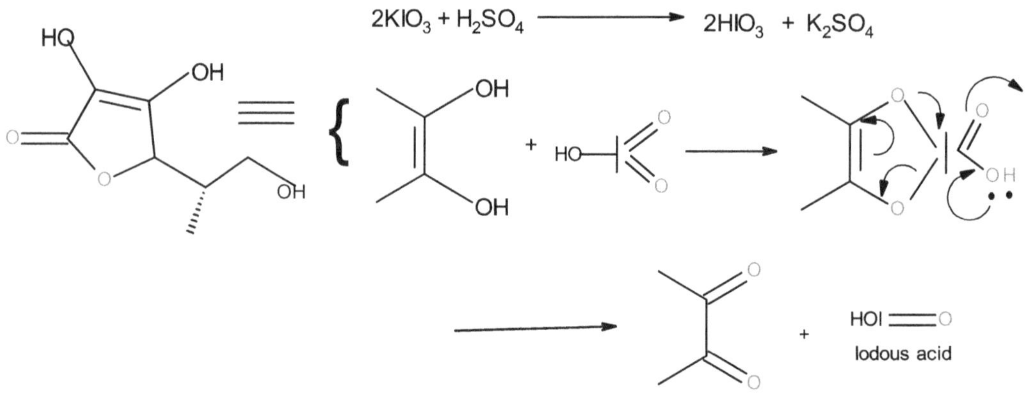

$$2KIO_3 + H_2SO_4 \longrightarrow 2HIO_3 + K_2SO_4$$

Procedure: In a typical experiment, a known excess of standard solution of potassium iodate is added to a known amount of ascorbic acid. After completion of the reaction, unreacted Potassium iodate is determined by iodometry. By carrying out a blank experiment simultaneously, the amount of potassium iodate consumed is determined. As the overall reaction requires one mole of CAT per molecule of ascorbic acid, which is equivalent to one mole of iodine, the molecular weight 'm' of the ascorbic acid is determined using the equation (1):

$$m = \frac{2000\ W}{V_1 - V_2}$$

where M-molarity of sodium thiosulphate, V_1 and V_2-volume of sodium thiosulphate consumed for experimental and blank titration. W-weight of ascorbic acid/tablet taken.

Determination of molecular weight of ascorbic acid

An accurately weighed (20-60 mg) sample of an ascorbic acid was dissolved in distill water (10 ml) in Erlenmeyer flask. To this, a solution 0.01 mol of potassium iodate (40 ml) was added. The reaction mixture was shaken well and kept aside at room temperature for about 30 min, after which 2N sulphuric acid (1 ml), 10% potassium iodide (1 ml) and water (2 ml) were added and liberated iodine was titrated against standard sodium thiosulphate solution (0.01 M) using starch as an indicator. In a similar way, a blank titration was conducted without adding ascorbic acid or ascorbic acid containing vitamin-C tablets. From the difference in the volume of sodium thiosulphate solution consumed, the molecular weight 'm' was calculated using equation (1)

Estimation of ascorbic acid in pharmaceutical vitamin tablets

A known amount of sample in the range of 10-60 mg of well-powdered vitamin tablets containing ascorbic acid in the range of 100-500 mg was dissolved in distilled water (10 ml) in an Erlenmeyer flask and then a solution of 0.01 mol of potassium iodate (40 ml) was added. The reaction mixture was shaken well and kept aside at room temperature for about 30 min followed by the addition of 2N sulfuric acid (1 ml), 10% potassium iodide (1 ml) and water (2 ml) and the liberated iodine was titrated against standard sodium phosphate solution (0.01M) using starch as an indicator. Similarly, a blank titration was conducted without adding ascorbic acid or ascorbic acid containing vitamin-C tablets.

Observation:

Assay of ascorbic acid

Sr. No.	Content in conical flask	Burette reading		Volume of titrant used (ml) (Precise reading)
		Initial	Final	
1				
2				

Blank titration

Sr. No.	Content in conical flask	Burette reading		Volume of titrant used (ml) (Precise reading)
		Initial	Final	
1				
2				

Calculation: From the difference in the volume of sodium thiosulphate solution consumed, the amount of ascorbic acid 'W' present in vitamin-C tablets was calculated using the following equation:

$$W = \frac{m(V_1 - V_2)M}{2000}$$

where M-molarity of sodium thiosulphate, V_1 and V_2 –volume of sodium thiosulphate consumed for experimental and blank titration, m-molecular weight of the ascorbic acid.

Results: The percentage purity of the ascorbic acid was found to be______

Experiment 06: Test for Purity of Pharmaceutical Aspirin

Aim: To identify and test for purity of pharmaceutical Aspirin

Requirements:

For identification test –
- Apparatus - Test tube, Hot plate, Pair of tongs
- Reagents - Water distilled, Ferric chloride TS

For test for purity/assay –
- Apparatus - Analytical Balance, Conical Flask, Burette, Water bath / Hot plate
- Reagents – Phenolphthalein TS, 0.5 N Sodium hydroxide, 0.5 N Sulfuric acid VS.

Theory

Aspirin, also known as acetylsalicylic acid, is a medication used to reduce pain, fever, or inflammation. Specific inflammatory conditions which aspirin is used to treat include Kawasaki disease, pericarditis, and rheumatic fever. Aspirin given shortly after a heart attack decreases the risk of death. It is a white crystal, which is commonly tabular or needle-like crystalline powder of white color. It is odorless or has a faint odor and stable in dry air; in moist air it gradually hydrolyzes to salicylic and acetic acids. It is freely soluble in alcohol; soluble in chloroform and ether; sparingly soluble in absolute ether; slightly soluble in water. Side effects of aspirin involve -conditions of excess stomach acid secretion, irritation of the stomach or intestines, nausea, vomiting, heartburn, stomach cramps.

Procedure for identification –
- Color test -
  - Take approximately about 0.5 g of sample into a test tube and add approximately about 10 ml of water. Heat the solution on a hot plate for about 3 minutes.
  - Cool it and add 1 or 2 drops of Ferric chloride TS.

Procedure for test for purity/assay –

Part I: Standardization of the NaOH solution

1. Obtain and prepare a burette for titration by washing and conditioning it with titrant solution (NaOH). Fill the burette, eliminate air bubbles, and have your instructor check for air bubble before starting your first titration. The burette is now ready for the rest of the lab (NOTE: You should not need more than 50 mL NaOH for all the titrations)

2. Record the initial burette reading to the correct number of decimal places. Don't forget to take the funnel out before all readings!

3. Locate a small vial of Potassium Hydrogen Phthalate (KHP) near the balance area. Tare a folded weigh-paper, and remove it from the balance pan. Use a

metal spatula to transfer a small amount of KHP to the paper, and then return the paper to the balance. Remove the paper to add KHP if necessary.

Never Return chemicals to the Stock Container! Record the mass, and transfer the Potassium hydrogen phthalate(KHP) to the flask, rinsing the paper with a gentle stream of DI water to ensure complete transfer. Place approximately 0.8 g of KHP (MW = 204.23 g/mol) in a clean 125 mL Erlenmeyer flask. Record the precise mass used. Dissolve the acid in 50 mL of distilled water and add 3 drops of phenolphthalein indicator.

4. Run slightly less (1-2 mL less) than this amount into the flask containing the acid, while swirling the flask. Use wash bottle to clean the walls of the flask of drops of base that may have splattered out the titration mixture add dropwise continue NaOH solution dropwise, swirling the flask constant type ensure full mixing. The volume estimated for complete reaction, add the NaOH more slowly, (one drop at a time) while continuing to swirl the flask and wash down the walls of the flask.

5. Stop the titration when the addition of a single drop of NaOH changes the color of the solution to a light pink, indicating that you have reached the endpoint. The endpoint should persist for 30 seconds without fading.

6. Record the final burette reading on you data table.

7. Repeat the titration. Your molarity should reflect the most significant figures you can obtain with the lab equipment, and the molarity obtained from two runs should agree within 5%. Foreach run:

Calculate the molarity of your NaOH solution. - Average the molarity of the first two runs, M - Compute the percent difference between the two runs: mL (approx. volume required)

$$\% \text{ Purity} = \frac{M_1 - M_2}{M} \times 100\% \text{difference}$$

- If run 1 and run 2 are within 5% agreement (of molarity), proceed to Part 2.
- If your runs are not in close agreement, run a third trial. Find the percent difference between the two closest runs, and report this in your Summary Table.
- If you omit a run explain why (i.e. over titrated sample; passed the endpoint).

Part II: Titration of the Aspirin Sample
- Obtain two tablets of commercially available aspirin, weigh them, and place them into a 250-mLflask. Record the brand name to identify your unknown.
- Obtain about 50 mL of 50% ethanol solution and add it to the flask.
- Allow the tablets to stand for a few minutes, and then tap the tablets using a glass stirring rod. They should disintegrate, and the solution will remain cloudy due to the insoluble starch binder. Swirl the mixture to dissolve the aspirin.

Aspirin itself does not dissolve well in water—an ethanol solution is used to dissolve the sample.

- Add several drops of phenolphthalein indicator. Slowly titrate the aspirin with the standardized NaOH solution. Record the initial and final burette readings to the correct number of significant figures. Calculate the percent purity of your sample.
- Repeat the titration. Calculate and report the percent purity of your aspirin sample. Do a third trial if percent difference in your percent purity is greater than 5% and time allows. Report the moles of acid found and percent difference in percent purity of the closest two trials.

Observation table:

Table 1 Standardization of NaOH

Sr. No.	Content in conical flask	Burette reading		Volume of titrant used (ml) (Precise reading)
		Initial	Final	
1				
2				

Table 2 Blank titration with content in conical flask Vs disodium edetate

Sr. No.	Content in conical flask	Burette reading		Volume of titrant used (ml) (Precise reading)
		Initial	Final	
1				
2				

Interpretation/ Calculation for test for purity/assay –

Calculate the assay of the Aspirin sample using the following formula –

$$\% \text{ Purity} = \frac{\text{Actual moles of Aspirin}}{\text{Theoretical moles of Aspirin}} \times 100$$

Results: The percentage purity of the aspirin was found to be______

Experiment 07: Identification and Test for Purity of Pharmaceuticals Paracetamol

Aim: To identify and test for purity of pharmaceuticals Paracetamol

Requirements –

For identification test-

- Reagents - conc. HCl, distilled water, potassium dichromate solution.

For test for purity/assay –

- Reagents – methanol, distilled water.

Theory: Paracetamol, also known as acetaminophen, is a medication used to treat fever and mild to moderate pain. Paracetamol is a commonly used medicine that can help treat pain and reduce a high temperature (fever). It's typically used to relieve mild or moderate pain, such as headaches, toothache or sprains, and reduce fevers caused by illnesses such as colds and flu. Paracetamol may relieve pain in acute mild migraine but only slightly in episodic tension headache. Some common side effects of paracetamol are nausea and abdominal pain. Chronic consumption of paracetamol may result in a drop in hemoglobin level, indicating possible gastrointestinal bleeding, and abnormal liver function tests. Acetaminophen is a p-aminophenol derivative with analgesic and antipyretic activities. Although the exact mechanism through which acetaminophen exert its effects has yet to be fully determined, acetaminophen may inhibit the nitric oxide (NO) pathway mediated by a variety of neurotransmitter receptors including N-methyl-D-aspartate (NMDA) and substance P, resulting in elevation of the pain threshold. The antipyretic activity may result from inhibition of prostaglandin synthesis and release in the central nervous system (CNS) and prostaglandin-mediated effects on the heat-regulating center in the anterior hypothalamus. It is freely soluble in water, alcohol; soluble in methanol, ethanol, dimethylformamide, ethylene dichloride, acetone, ethyl acetate; slightly soluble in ether; practically insoluble in petroleum ether, pentane, benzene.

Procedure for identification –

- Take 1 ml conc. Hydrochloric acid and add to the sample and stir well and add few drops of water and cool down the solution.
- Then add potassium dichromate solution to it.

Procedure for test for purity/assay:

- Dissolve accurately weighed 120mg of paracetamol in 10 ml methanol in a500 ml volumetric flask. Dilute with water up to volume and mix well.
- Transfer 5 ml of the solution to 100ml volumetric flask and dilute with water up to volume and mix well.

- Make a standard solution of paracetamol in the same medium of concentration 12µg/ml
- Absorbance is measured at 244 nm using water as blank.

Diagram:

Interpretation for identification – Violet color solution appears.

Calculation for test for purity/assay –

Calculate the quantity of paracetamol by the formula - 10C (Au/As)

    Where

    C = concentration in mg/ml of standard

    Au = absorbance of test sample

    As = absorbance of standard sample.

Results: The percentage purity of paracetamol was found to be_____

Experiment 08: Identification and Test for Purity of Pharmaceuticals Sulfanilamide

Aim: To identify and test for purity of pharmaceuticals Sulfanilamide

Requirements –

For identification test-

- Reagents –sodium hydroxide, copper sulfate.

For test for purity/assay –

- Reagents – HCl (0.2 and 0.5N), sodium hydroxide (0.1N), sodium nitrate, ammonium sulfamate, N-(1-napthyl)-ethylenediamidedyhidrochloride.

Theory - Sulfanilamide (also spelled sulphanilamide) is a sulfonamide antibacterial drug. Chemically, it is an organic compound consisting of an aniline derivatized with a sulfonamide group. Sulfanilamide is an organic sulfur compound structurally similar to p-aminobenzoic acid (PABA) with antibacterial property. Sulfanilamide competes with PABA for the bacterial enzyme dihydropteroate synthase, thereby preventing the incorporation of PABA into dihydrofolic acid, the immediate precursor of folic acid. This leads to an inhibition of bacterial folic acid synthesis and de novo synthesis of purines and pyrimidines, ultimately resulting in cell growth arrest and cell death. It is a white crystalline powder soluble in water, ethanol and insoluble in chloroform, ether, benzene.

Structure

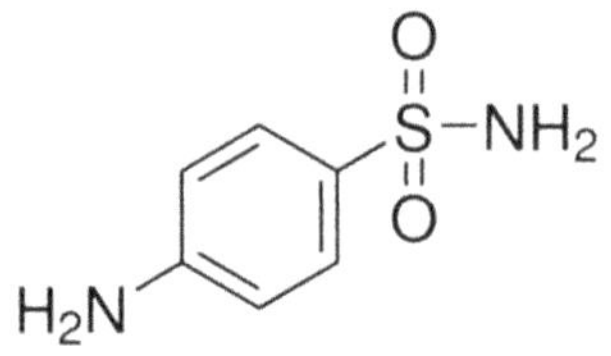

Procedure for identification –

- Take 1 ml of sample solution in a test tube and add few drops of sodium hydroxide 1N solution
- Add few drops of copper sulfate solution in the test tube.

Procedure for test for purity/assay –

- Firstly prepare 0.1N NaOH solution, 0.2N and 0.5N HCl solution, 0.1% $NaNO_2$ solution, 0.5% Ammonium sulfamate solution and 0.1% N-(1-napthyl)-ethylenediamidedyhidrochloride.
- For standard solution add 5 ml stock solution in 50 ml volumetric flask. To that add 3ml 0.2N and 5ml of 0.5N HCl solution. Lastly add 5ml $NaNO_2$ solution (0.1%).

- In blank solution add 5 ml of NaOH solution first in 50 ml volumetric flask. To that add 3ml 0.2N and 5ml of 0.5N HCl solution. Lastly add 5ml $NaNO_2$ solution (0.1%).
- In test solution add 5 ml of test sample in 50 ml volumetric flask then add 3ml 0.2N and 5ml of 0.5N HCl solution. Lastly add 5ml $NaNO_2$ solution (0.1%).
- Allow the solution to stand for 3 minutes in room temperature for diazotization.
- Then add 5ml of 0.5% Ammonium sulfamate solution and 5ml of 0.1% N-(1-napthyl)-ethylenediamidedyhidrochloride in all three solutions.
- Make up the volume upto 50ml using distilled water and read absorbance at 545 nm in a colorimeter within 15 minutes.

Interpretation for identification – greenish blue precipitate forms immediately, which if kept for 5 minutes forms blue sediment.

Interpretation/Calculation for test for purity/assay –

- Concentration of prepared standard solution = $C_1V_1 = C_2V_2$
- Concentration of the diluted test solution = $(A_2 + C_1)/A_1$
  - Concentration of standard solution = C_1
  - Volume of standard solution = V_1
  - Concentration of test solution = C_2
  - Volume of standard solution = V_2
  - Absorbance of standard solution = A_1
  - Absorbance of test solution = A_2
- Concentration of original test solution = $C_dV_d = C_tV_t$
  - C_d= calculated concentration of the diluted test solution
  - V_d = 50ml
  - C_t = concentration of original test solution
  - V_t = 5ml

Experiment 09: Identification Tests for Anions and Cations as per Indian Pharmacopoeia

Identification of ions means the detection of cations and anions present in a given sample of salt. The identification is made through the qualitative analysis of inorganic salts. In an inorganic salt, the part contributed by the acid is called anion, and the part contributed by the base is called a cation. In qualitative analysis, the reactions are carried out that is easily perceptible to our senses, such as sight and smell. Such reactions involve precipitate formation, colour change, the evolution of gas etc. The qualitative analysis of an inorganic salt involves the preliminary examination of solid salt and its solution, wet tests (reactions carried out in solution) and confirmatory tests for anions, wet tests and confirmatory tests for cations.

Aim: To identify the presence of different type of anion and cation in the sample.

Requirements: Test tube, burner, dropper, measuring cylinder, litmus paper, distilled water

Theory: Analytical chemistry's qualitative analysis approach is used to determine the elemental composition of inorganic salts. It is primarily focused with detecting ions in a salt aqueous solution.

The common procedure for testing any unknown sample is to make its solution and test this solution with various reagents for the ions present in it. Testing with various reagents gives characteristic reaction of certain ions, which may be a color change, a solid formation (Precipitation) or any other visible changes. Qualitative analysis of ions is verified through different identification tests

Cations are positively (+) charged ions. They are formed when a metal loses its electrons. They lose one or more electron and do not lose any proton. Hence carried net positive charge. Since cation have positive charge opposite to anion so they attracted towards anion.

Identification tests for Anions:

Aim: To identify the presence of different type of anion in a given sample such as acetate ion (CH_3COO^-), nitrate ion (NO_3^-), chloride ions (Cl^-) and sulphate ions (SO_4^-).

Requirement: Test tube, burner, dropper, measuring cylinder, litmus paper, distilled water

Theory: Anions are negatively (-) charged ions. These are formed when a metal gains the electrons. They can gain one or more electron. Therefor they carried negative charge and attract positive charge.

Procedure:

1. Procedure for identification of acetate ion (CH_3COO^-): -

(a) Test 1:
- 1gm of sample is taken in a test tube with 1ml of sulphuric acid.
- The test tube is heated gently then 3ml ethanol (95%) is added in it.
- Odour of ethyl acetate is evolved.

$$CH_3COOK + H_2SO_4 + C_2H_5OH \longrightarrow CH_3COOC_2H_5 + K_2SO_4 + H_2O$$

(b) Test 2:
- Sample containing acetate ion being examined is taken in a test tube.
- The test tube is heated with equal amount of oxalic acid.
- Acids vapours with a characteristic odour of acetic acid are liberated.

$$CH_3COONa + COOH\text{-}COOH \longrightarrow CH_3COOH + Na_2CO_3$$
$$\text{(Acetic acid)}$$

2. Procedure for identification of nitrate ion NO_3^- (Brown ring test):
- Sample in test tube containing nitrate ions ($NO3-$).
- Add dilute sulphuric acid in it and then add iron (II) sulphate solution and shake well to mix it.
- Sulphuric acid is carefully added to the side of test tube.
- Concentrated sulphuric acid react with the nitrate ion to form nitrogen monoxide molecule.
- And the nitrogen monoxide combines with iron (II) sulphate to form a brown complex which appear as a brown ring which confirm the presence of nitrate ion.

3. Procedure for the identification test for chloride ions (Cl^-): -
- 2 ml Sample is taken in a test tube and add dilute nitric acid in it.
- Addition of nitric acid prevent the precipitation of silver sulphate and silver carbonate in the test tube.
- Then add silver nitrate solution in it which help to form silver chloride (AgCl) and this silver chloride is insoluble salt and form white colour precipitate is seen.

4. Procedure for identification test for sulphate ions (SO_4^-):
- Sample is taken in a test tube and add dilute hydrochloride acid in it and shake gently.
- Barium chloride solution is added which form an insoluble white complex of barium sulphate which confirm the presence of sulphate ion in the given sample.
- Dilute hydrochloric acid is added to prevent the precipitation of barium carbonate.

5. Procedure for identification test for phosphate ion(PO_4^{2-}):

- Acidify sodium carbonate extract or the solution of the salt in water with conc. HNO_3 and add ammonium molybdate solution and heat to boiling.
- A canary yellow precipitate is formed.

6. Procedure for identification for Oxalate ions($C_2O_4^{2-}$):

- Take 1 mL of water extract or sodium carbonate extract acidified with acetic acid and add calcium chloride solution. A white precipitate insoluble in ammonium oxalate and oxalic acid solution but soluble in dil. HCl and dil. Nitric acid is formed.
- Take the precipitate from test and dissolve it in dilute H_2SO_4. Add very dilute solution $KMnO_4$ and warm. Color of $KMnO_4$ solution is discharged. Pass the gas coming out through lime water.
- The lime water turns milky.

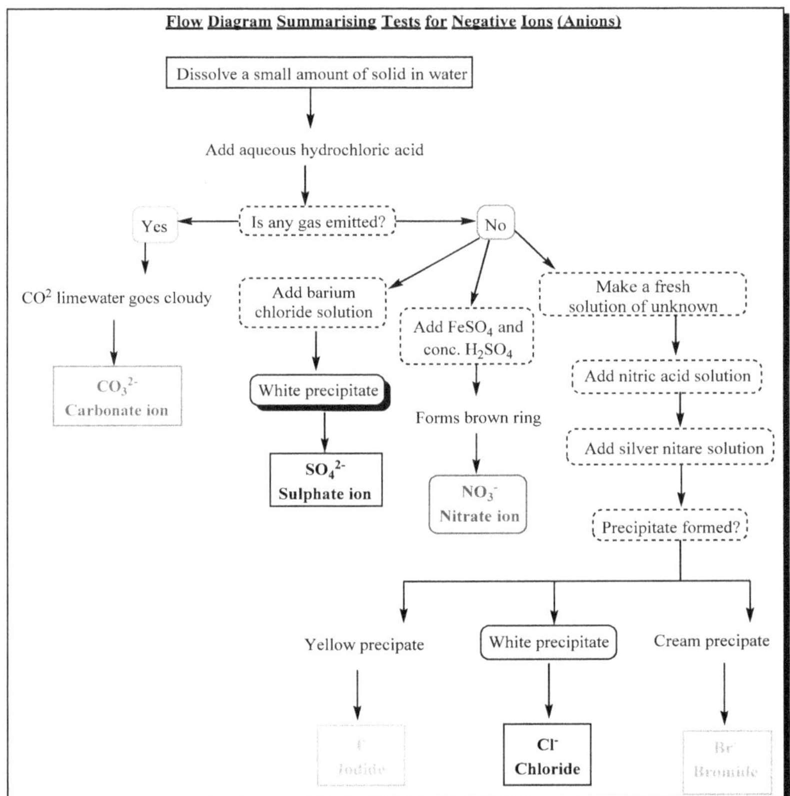

Fig. 1 Flow Diagram Summarising Tests for Negative Ions (anions).

Result: The given sample contains ....

Experiment 10: Identification Tests for Cations as Per Indian Pharmacopoeia

Aim: To identify the presence of different type of cations (NH_4^+, Fe_2^+, Al_3^+, Ca^{2+}, Pb^{2+}) in the given sample.

Requirements: Test tube, dropper, measuring cylinder, litmus paper

Theory: Cations are ions with a positive (+) charge and formed when metal loses its electrons. They lose one or more electrons while retaining all of their protons. As a result, it had a net positive charge. Because cations have a positive charge in the opposite direction of anion, they are attracted to it.

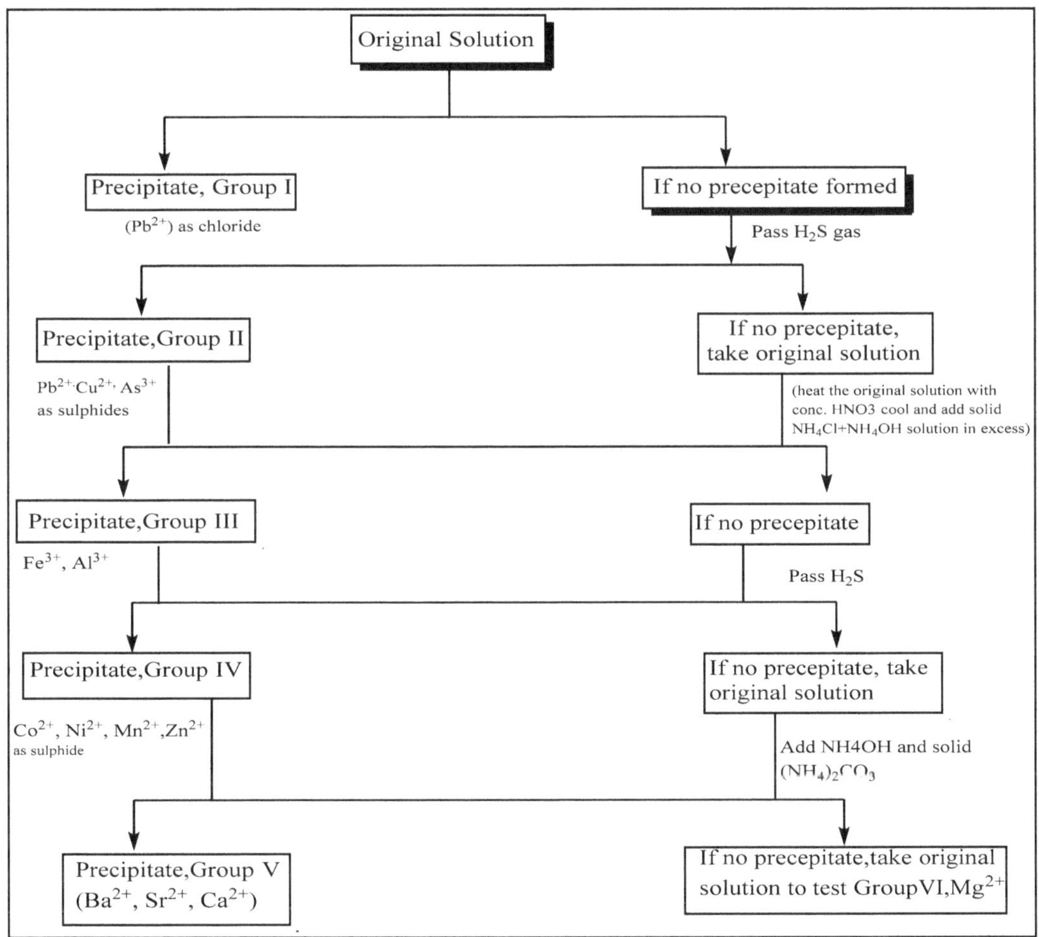

Fig. 2 Flow Diagram for the identification test of Cations

Procedure:

1. To identify the presence of **Ammonium ion (NH$_4^+$)**
   - About 2 mL of ammonium chloride solution is poured into a test tube.
   - About 4 mL of dilute sodium hydroxide solution is added to the test tube and the mixture is shaken well.
   - The mixture is carefully heated and the gas liberated is tested with a piece of moist red litmus paper.

   Observation: The colorless gas evolved **turns red litmus paper blue**.

   Explanation: Heating an ammonium salt with an alkali produces ammonia gas. $NH_4^+(aq) + OH^-(aq) \rightarrow NH_3(g) + H_2O(l)$. The alkaline ammonia gas turns red litmus paper blue which indicate the presence of ammonium ions.

2. Identification test of **Iron(II) ion (Fe^{2+})**
   - About 2 mL of iron(II) sulphate solution is poured into a test tube.
   - A dropper is used to add **potassium hexacyanoferrate (III), K$_3$Fe(CN)$_6$ solution**, drop by drop into the test tube.
   - Any change that occurs is recorded.

   Observation: A **dark blue** precipitate is obtained.

   Explanation: The iron(II) ion combines with a complex ion in the reagent to produce a dark blue precipitate.

   $$Fe^{2+}(aq) + Fe(CN)_6^{3-}(aq) \rightarrow \text{dark blue precipitate}$$

3. **Identification test of Aluminium (III) ion (Al^{3+}):**

   (a) Lake test: Aluminium hydroxide formed in the group analysis dissolves in dil. HCl to form soluble aluminium chloride. The aluminium chloride thus formed reacts with ammonium hydroxide to reform aluminium hydroxide. Blue colour of litmus solution is adsorbed on this precipitate.

   $$Al(OH)_3 + 3HCl \longrightarrow AlCl_3 + 3H_2O$$
   $$AlCl_3 + 3NH_4OH \longrightarrow 3NH_4Cl + Al(OH)_3$$

   Aluminium hydroxide

   (Blue color adsorbed on this precipitate)

   (b) **Charcoal cavity/Cobalt nitrate test:** In this test, aluminium oxide is produced in the charcoal cavity test reacts with CoO in cobalt nitrate test to produces a blue mass due to the formation of Al$_2$O$_3$.CoO.

   $$Al_2O_3 + CoO \longrightarrow Al_2O_3.CoO \text{ (Blue color mass)}$$

4. **Identification test of Calcium ion (Ca^{2+}):** The white precipitate of calcium carbonate formed in the group analysis dissolves in hot dil. acetic acid due to the formation of soluble calcium acetate.

$$CaCO_3 + 2CH_3COOH \longrightarrow (CH_3COO)_2Ca \text{ (Calcium acetate)} + CO_2 + H_2O$$

(a) **Ammonium oxalate test:** Calcium acetate (formed by dissolving calcium carbonate in dil. acetic acid) reacts with ammonium oxalate to form a white precipitate of calcium oxalate.

$$(CH_3COO)_2Ca + (NH_4)_2C_2O_4 \longrightarrow 2 CH_3COONH_4 + CaC_2O_4$$

(White precipitate of Calcium oxalate)

(b) **Flame test:** Calcium imparts brick red color to the flame.

5. Identification test of Magnesium ion (Mg^{2+})

(a) **Ammonium Phosphate test:** Mg^{2+} ions react with ammonium phosphate in presence of NH_4Cl and NH_4OH to form white precipitate of magnesium ammonium phosphate.

$$MgCl_2 + NH_4OH + (NH_4)2HPO_4 \longrightarrow Mg(NH_4)PO_4 + 2NH_4Cl + H_2O$$

Magnesium ammonium phosphate

(White precipitate)

(b) **Charcoal cavity/Cobalt nitrate test:** In this test, magnesium oxide produced in the charcoal cavity test reacts with CoO in cobalt nitrate test to produces a pink mass due to the formation of MgO.CoO.

$$MgO + CoO \longrightarrow MgO.CoO \text{ (Pink mass)}$$

6. Identification test of lead (II) ion (Pb^{2+})

Procedure:

- About 2 mL of lead (II) nitrate solution is poured into a test tube.
- A dropper is used to add about 1 mL of potassium iodide solution into the test tube.
- About 3 mL of distilled water is added and the mixture is boiled.
- The mixture is then cooled using running water from the tap.
- Any change that occurs is recorded.

Observation: A yellow precipitate formed which dissolves in hot water and on cooling, golden yellow crystals are formed.

Explanation: Iodide ion from potassium iodide combines with lead (II) ion to form a yellow precipitate of lead (II) iodide.

$$Pb^{2+}(aq) + 2I^-(aq) \longrightarrow PbI_2(s)$$

The precipitate is insoluble in cold water but soluble in hot water.

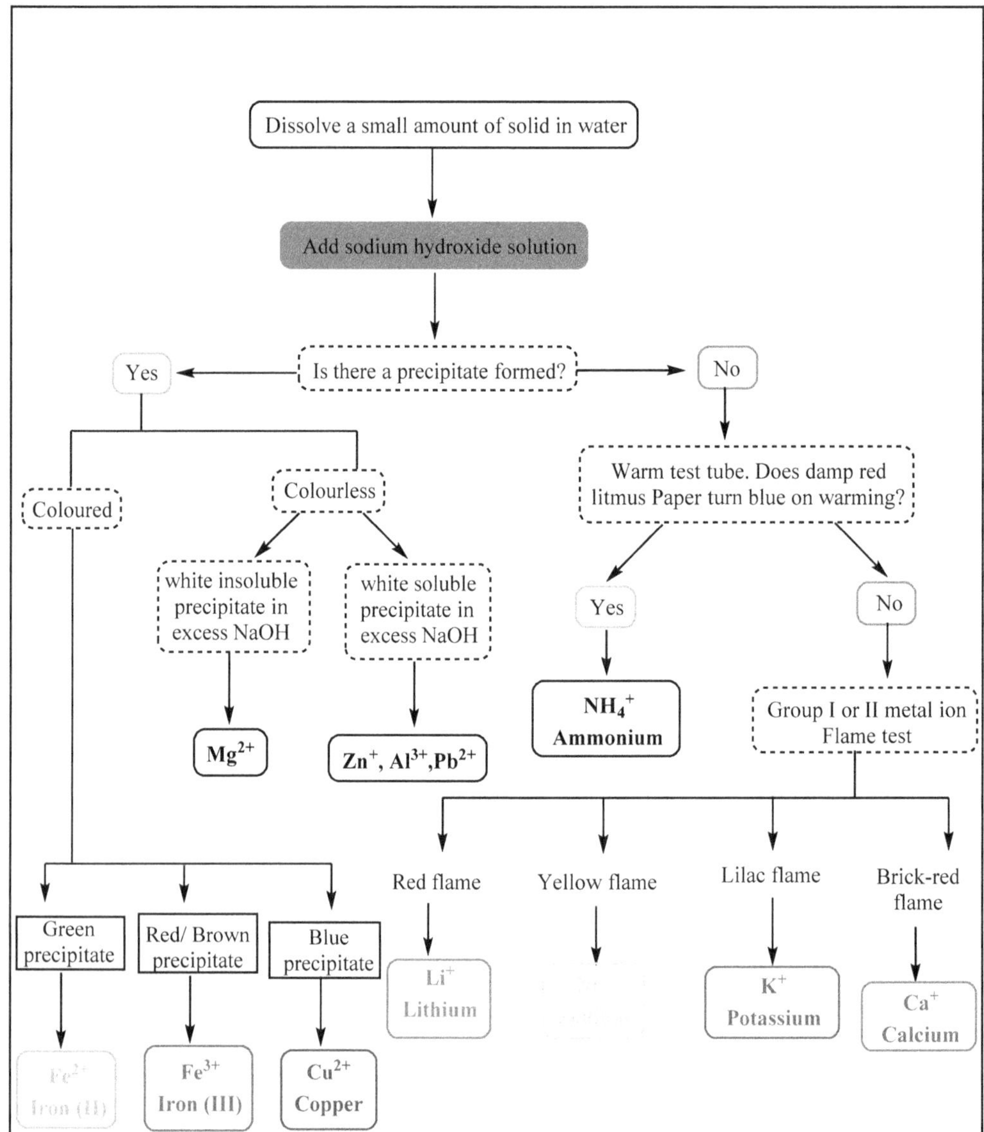

Fig. 3 Flow Diagram for the identification test of Cations

Result: The given sample contains …………………….

Experiment 11: Limit Test of Chlorides

Aim: Limit test of chlorides

Requirements:

Apparatus Required: Nessler cylinders, Glass rod, Stand

Chemicals Required: Dilute nitric acid (10%), Silver nitrate (5%), Sodium chloride

Theory: Limit Test for Chloride is based upon the chemical reaction between silver nitrate and soluble chloride in the presence of dilute nitric acid to give opalescence of silver chloride. The opalescence produced is compared with the standard solution. If the opalescence in the sample is less than the standard, it passes the test. If it is more than the standard, it fails the test.

Chemical Reaction:

$$NaCl + AgNO_3 \xrightarrow{HNO_3} AgCl + NaNO_3$$

Procedure: Take two 50 ml Nessler cylinders. Label one as "Test" and the other as "Standard"

Standard	Test
1. Place 1 ml of 0.05845% w/v solution of NaCl in a Nessler cylinder.	1. Dissolve the specified quantity of the substance in distilled water and transfer it to the Nessler cylinder.
2. Add 10 ml of dilute. HNO_3.	2. Add 10 ml of dilute. HNO_3.
3. Dilute to 50 ml with water and add 1 ml of silver nitrate solution.	3. Dilute to 50 ml with water and add 1 ml of silver nitrate solution.
4. Stir immediately with a glass rod and allow to stand for 5 minutes.	4. Stir immediately with a glass rod and allow to stand for 5 minutes.
5. Observe the opalescence developed and compare it with that of the sample.	5. Observe the opalescence developed and compare it with that of the standard.

Observation: The opalescence produce in sample solution should not be greater than standard solution. If opalescence produces in sample solution is less than the standard solution, the sample will pass the limit test of chloride and visa versa.

Reasons:

- Nitric acid is added in the limit test of chloride to make solution acidic and helps silver chloride precipitate to make solution turbid at the end of process.

Result: The opalescence produces in sample solution was ....

Experiment 12: Limit Test of Heavy Metals

Aim: Limit test of heavy metals.

Apparatus Required
- Nessler cylinders
- Glass rod
- Stand

Chemicals Required for the Limit Test for Heavy Metals
- Dilute CH_3COOH (10% v/v)
- Dilute ammonia (10% v/v)
- Hydrogen sulphide solution (saturated solution of H_2S) (or sodium sulphide solution)
- Standard lead solution (10 ml of the lead nitrate stock solution diluted to 100 ml with water). (20 ppm of lead).
- Lead nitrate stock solution: Dissolve 0.1598 gm of lead nitrate in 100 ml of water, add 1 ml of concentrated. HNO_3 and dilute to 1000 ml with water.

Theory: Limit test of heavy metals is based on the reaction of metallic impurities with hydrogen sulfide in acidic medium to form brownish colour solution. Metals that response to this test are lead, mercury, bismuth, arsenic, antimony, tin, cadmium, silver, copper, and molybdenum. The metallic impurities in substances are expressed as parts of lead per million parts of the substance. The usual limit as per Indian Pharmacopoeia is 20 ppm.

Chemical Reaction:

$$Pb(NO_3)_2(Pb^+) + H_2S \longrightarrow PbS \downarrow + 2HNO_3$$

$$PbCl_2 + Na_2S \longrightarrow PbS \downarrow + 2NaCl$$

Procedure: The Indian Pharmacopoeia has adopted three methods for the limit test of heavy metals.

Method I: Use for the substance which gives clear colorless solution under the specific condition.

Test sample	Standard compound
1. Solution is prepared as per the monograph and 25 ml is transferred in Nessler's cylinder	1. Take 2 ml of standard lead solution and dilute to 25 ml with water
2. Adjust the pH between 3 to 4 by adding dilute acetic acid 'Sp' or dilute ammonia solution 'Sp'	2. Adjust the pH between 3 to 4 by adding dilute acetic acid 'Sp' or dilute ammonia solution 'Sp'
3. Dilute with water to 35 ml	3. Dilute with water to 35 ml
4. Add freshly prepared 10 ml of hydrogen sulphide solution	4. Add freshly prepared 10 ml of hydrogen sulphide solution

Contd...

Test sample	Standard compound
5. Dilute with water to 50 ml	5. Dilute with water to 50 ml
6. Allow to stand for five minutes	6. Allow to stand for five minutes
7. View downwards over a white surface	7. View downwards over a white surface

Observation: The color produce in sample solution should not be greater than standard solution. If color produces in sample solution is less than the standard solution, the sample will pass the limit test of heavy metals and vice versa.

Method II: Use for the substance which do not give clear colorless solution under the specific condition.

Test sample	Standard compound

1. Weigh specific quantity of test substance, moisten with sulphuric acid and ignite on a low flame till completely charred
  • Add few drops of nitric acid and heat to 500 °C
  • Allow to cool and add 4 ml of hydrochloric acid and evaporate to dryness
  • Moisten the residue with 10 ml of hydrochloric acid and digest for two minutes
Neutralize with ammonia solution and make just acid with acetic acid
	1. Take 2 ml of standard lead solution and dilute to 25 ml with water

2. Adjust the pH between 3 to 4 and filter if necessary	2. Adjust the pH between 3 to 4 by adding dilute acetic acid 'Sp' or dilute ammonia solution 'Sp'
3. Dilute with water to 35 ml	3. Dilute with water to 35 ml
4. Add freshly prepared 10 ml of hydrogen sulphide solution	4. Add freshly prepared 10 ml of hydrogen sulphide solution
5. Dilute with water to 50 ml	5. Dilute with water to 50 ml
6. Allow to stand for five minutes	6. Allow to stand for five minutes
7. View downwards over a white surface	7. View downwards over a white surface

Observation: The color produce in sample solution should not be greater than standard solution. If color produces in sample solution is less than the standard solution, the sample will pass the limit test of heavy metals and vice versa.

Method III: Use for the substance which gives clear colorless solution in sodium hydroxide solution.

Test sample	Standard compound
1. Solution is prepared as per the monograph and 25 ml is transferred in Nessler's cylinder or weigh specific amount of substance and dissolve in 20 ml of water and add 5 ml of dilute sodium hydroxide solution	1. Take 2 ml of standard lead solution
2. Make up the volume to 50 ml with water	2. Add 5 ml of dilute sodium hydroxide solution and make up the volume to 50 ml with water
3. Add 5 drops of sodium sulphide solution	3. Add 5 drops of sodium sulphide solution
4. Mix and set aside for 5 min	4. Mix and set aside for 5 min
5. View downwards over a white surface	5. View downwards over a white surface

Observation: The color produce in sample solution should not be greater than standard solution. If color produces in sample solution is less than the standard solution, the sample will pass the limit test of heavy metals and vice versa.

Result: The color produce in sample solution was ……………………………..

Experiment 13: Limit Test for Sulphate

Aim: Limit test for Sulphate

Apparatus Required: Nessler cylinders, Glass rod, Stand

Chemicals Required:
- Dilute hydrochloric acid
- 0.5 M Barium chloride: 122.1 g of Barium chloride dissolved in distilled water.
- Barium sulphate reagent containing 0.5 M barium chloride in 1000 ml of water. (This is prepared as follows: Mix 15 ml of 0.5 M BaCl2, 55 ml of water and 20 ml of sulphate free alcohol. Add 5 ml of 0.0181% w/v potassium sulphate. Dilute to 10 ml with water and mix.)

Theory: Limit Test for Sulphate is based upon the chemical reaction between barium chloride and soluble sulphate in the presence of dilute hydrochloric acid. The turbidity produced is compared with the standard solution. Barium chloride reagent contains barium chloride, sulphate-free alcohol and a small quantity of potassium sulphate. The inclusion of a small quantity of potassium sulphate in the reagent increases the sensitivity of the test. Alcohol prevents supersaturation and more uniform turbidity develops. If the turbidity produced in the test is more intense than the standard turbidity, then the drug fails the test, otherwise, it passes the test.

Reaction:

$$SO_4^{2-} \; + \; BaCl_2 \; \xrightarrow{\text{dil } H_2SO_4} \; BaSO_4 \downarrow \; + \; 2Cl^-$$

Procedure: Take two 50 ml Nessler cylinders. Label one as "Test" and the other as "Standard"

Standard	Test
1. Place 1 ml of 0.1089% w/v solution of K₂SO₄ in a Nessler cylinder.	1. Dissolve the specified quantity of the substance in distilled water and transfer it to the Nessler cylinder.
2. Add 2 ml of dilute. HCI.	2. Add 2 ml of dilute. HCI.
3. Dilute to 45 ml with water and add 5 ml of barium sulphate reagent.	3. Dilute to 45 ml with water and add 5 ml of barium sulphate reagent.
4. Stir immediately with a glass rod and allow to stand for 5 minutes.	4. Stir immediately with a glass rod and allow to stand for 5 minutes.
5. Observe the turbidity developed and compare it with that of the sample.	5. Observe the turbidity developed and compare it with that of the standard.

Observation: The turbidity produce in sample solution should not be greater than standard solution. If turbidity produces in sample solution is less than the standard solution, the sample will pass the limit test of sulphate and vice versa.

Reasons

- Hydrochloric acid helps to make solution acidic
- Potassium sulphate is used to increase the sensitivity of the test by giving ionic concentration in the reagent.
- Alcohol helps to prevent super saturation.

Result: The turbidity produce in sample solution was………………..

Experiment 14: Limit test for Iron

Aim: Limit test for Iron.

Apparatus Required: Nessler cylinders, Glass rod, Stand

Chemicals Required:
- Standard Iron solution Ferric ammonium sulphate (1.726 g) dissolved in 10 ml of 0.1 N H_2SO_4 and sufficient water to produce 1000 ml.
- Sulphuric acid (0. 1 N): 10.0 ml.
- Iron-free citric acid solution (20% w/v): 2.0 ml.
- Thioglycolic acid: 0.1 ml.
- Iron-free ammonia solution: 20 ml.

Theory: Limit Test for Iron depends upon the reaction between ferrous iron and thioglycolic acid in the presence of ammonia. A pale pink to deep reddish-purple colour is produced. Ferric iron is reduced to ferrous iron by the thioglycolic acid and the compound produced is ferrous thioglycollate. Citric acid forms a soluble complex with iron and prevents its precipitation by ammonia as ferrous hydroxide. Ferrous thioglycollate is colourless in neutral or acid solution. The colour develops only in the presence of alkali. It is stable in the absence of air but fades when exposed to air due to oxidation to the ferric compound. Therefore, the colours should be compared immediately after the time allowed for the full development of colour is over.

Reaction:

$$Fe^{2+} + \underset{\underset{\text{Thioglycollic acid}}{COOH}}{\overset{CH_2SH}{|}} \longrightarrow \underset{\text{Ferrous thioglycollate}}{\overset{CH_2SH \qquad OOC}{\underset{COOH \qquad HSH_2C}{>Fe<}}} + 2H^+$$

Procedure: Take two 50 ml Nessler cylinders. Label one as "Test" and the other as "Standard".

Standard	Test
1. Dilute 2 ml of standard iron solution with 20 ml of water in a Nessler cylinder.	1. Dissolve the specified quantity of the substance in distilled water and transfer it to the Nessler cylinder.
2. Add 2 ml of 20% w/v solution of iron-free citric acid and 0.1 ml of thioglycolic acid and mix.	2. Add 2 ml of 20% w/v solution of iron-free citric acid and 0.1 ml of thioglycolic acid and mix.
3. Make alkaline with iron-free ammonia solution.	3. Make alkaline with iron-free ammonia solution.
4. Dilute to 50 ml with water.	4. Dilute to 50 ml with water.
5. Observe the intensity of the purple colour developed by viewing vertically and compare it with that of the sample.	5. Observe the intensity of the purple colour developed by viewing vertically and compare it with that of the standard.

Earlier ammonium thiocyanate reagent was used for the limit test of iron. Since thioglycolic acid is more sensitive reagent, it has replaced ammonium thiocyanate in the test.

Observation: The purple color produce in sample solution should not be greater than standard solution. If purple color produces in sample solution is less than the standard solution, the sample will pass the limit test of iron and vice versa.

Reasons:

- Citric acid helps precipitation of iron by ammonia by forming a complex with it.
- Thioglycolic acid helps to oxidize iron (II) to iron (III).
- Ammonia to make solution alkaline

Result: The color produce in sample solution was…………………………..

Answers

Chapter-1

1. D	2. C	3. A	4. B	5. C
6. C	7. A	8. A	9. D	10. B
11. D	12. B	13. A	14. B	15. C
16. C	17. A	18. A	19. C	20. A

Chapter-2

1.	2. D	3. D	4. D	5. D
6. C	7. C	8. B	9. C	10. B
11. A	12. B	13. B	14. C	15. D
16. C	17. C	18. B	19. C	20. D

Chapter-3

1. A	2. A	3. C	4. C	5. C
6. C	7. A	8. B	9. B	10. A

Chapter-4

1. A	2. C	3. C	4. B	5. B
6. D	7. B	8. C	9. B	10. A
11. B	12. D	13. B	14. B	15. A
16. D	17. C	18. C	19. A	20. B

Chapter-5

1. A	2. C	3. B	4. D	5. B
6. B	7. E	8. B	9. A	10. B

Chapter-6

1. B	2. B	3. A	4. B	5. A
6. B	7. C	8. B	9. B	10. C

Chapter-7

1. D	2. C	3. C	4. D	5. C
6. E	7. D	8. A	9. A	10. A

Chapter-8

1. C	2. A	3. C	4. A	5. B
6. D	7. A	8. B	9. A	10. B

Chapter-9

1. D	2. B	3. A	4. B	5. D
6. D	7. C	8. B	9. D	10. B

Chapter-10

1. D	2. C	3. D	4. E	5. B
6. B	7. B	8. D	9. B	10. A

Chapter-11

1. A	2. D	3. C	4. D	5. B
6. A	7. D	8. A	9. C	10. D
11. B&C	12. C	13. A	14. A	15. B
16. C	17. A	18. A	19. C	20. A

Chapter-12

1. D	2. D	3. C	4. A	5. A
6. C	7. D	8. B	9. C	10. A

Chapter-13

1. D	2. A	3. C	4. B	5. B
6. C	7. D	8. C	9. B	10. D